# Health Visiting

# Health Visiting

## SPECIALIST COMMUNITY PUBLIC HEALTH NURSING

*Third Edition*

**Edited by**

PATRICIA BURROWS,
MSc, PGDIP, BSc (Hons), RGN, RM, HV, FiHV
*Senior Lecturer Public Health, Programme Director*
*Public Health Nursing (District Nursing, Health visiting & School Nursing),*
*School of Health Sciences, City, University of London, London, United Kingdom*

JEAN COWIE
PhD, MSc, BA, Dip Nursing (London),
Dip HV, PGCE - Tertiary Level Teaching,
RHV, RM, RGN
*Principal Educator, Women, Children, Young People and Families Programme,*
*Nursing, Midwifery and Allied Health Professionals Directorate,*
*NHS Education for Scotland, Edinburgh, United Kingdom*

ELSEVIER

First edition © Harcourt Publishers Limited 2001
Second edition © 2005, Elsevier Limited. All rights reserved.

---

**Notices**

Practitioners and researchers must always rely on their own experience and knowledge in evaluating and using any information, methods, compounds or experiments described herein. Because of rapid advances in the medical sciences, in particular, independent verification of diagnoses and drug dosages should be made. To the fullest extent of the law, no responsibility is assumed by Elsevier, authors, editors or contributors for any injury and/or damage to persons or property as a matter of products liability, negligence or otherwise, or from any use or operation of any methods, products, instructions, or ideas contained in the material herein.

---

ISBN: 978-0-7020-8007-4

*Content Strategist*: Poppy Garraway
*Content Project Manager*: Shubham Dixit
*Design*: Bridget Hoette
*Illustration Coordinator*: Anitha Rajarathnam
*Marketing Manager*: Austin O'Saben

Printed in Great Britain

Last digit is the print number: 9 8 7 6 5 4 3 2 1

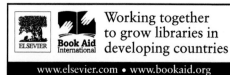

Working together
to grow libraries in
developing countries

www.elsevier.com • www.bookaid.org

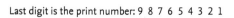

# CONTENTS

## PART 1

### Foundations of Public Health and Health Visiting

1 FOUNDATIONS OF PUBLIC HEALTH AND HEALTH VISITING ......................3
MARIA HORNE ▪ PATRICIA OWEN

2 THE HISTORY OF HEALTH VISITING ......23
MICHELLE MOSELEY ▪ KATE PHILLIPS

3 PROFESSIONAL PRACTICE AND PRACTITIONER WELL-BEING .................45
RACHEL STEPHEN ▪ ROBERT NETTLETON

4 SOCIAL POLICY, CONTEXT OF PUBLIC HEALTH AND THE ORGANISATION OF HEALTH VISITING SERVICE PROVISION ...............71
ALISON HACKETT ▪ KATHLEEN CLARKE ▪ JOYCE WILKINSON

## PART 2

### Fundamentals of Health Visiting Practice

5 HOME VISITING AND THERAPEUTIC RELATIONSHIP-BUILDING TO SUPPORT THE TRANSITION TO PARENTHOOD ....89
LIZ STURLEY ▪ LYNETTE SHOTTON ▪ BRIDGET HALNAN

6 ASSESSMENT ........................111
FELICITY JONES

7 EVIDENCE-BASED PRACTICE AND EARLY INTERVENTION TO SUPPORT CHILDREN AND FAMILIES........................131
CLARE MCGUIRE ▪ CLAIR GRAHAM ▪ DIANE ALLCOCK ▪ JANINE STEWART

8 LEADERSHIP SKILLS FOR LEADING HEALTH VISITING PRACTICE................153
KAREN STANSFIELD ▪ VICKY GILROY

9 TECHNOLOGY AND HEALTH VISITING PRACTICE ............................173
RITA NEWLAND

10 FACILITATING HEALTHY BEHAVIOUR – AN EMPOWERMENT APPROACH ..............191
KAREN ADAMS ▪ MICHELLE CLARK

## PART 3

### Health Visitor Practice-Focused Interventions

11 CHILDHOOD ADVERSITY AND TRAUMA ...............................211
BERNADETTE BRADLEY ▪ JAMES MCTAGGART

12 BUILDING EFFECTIVE SAFEGUARDING SKILLS: A SHIFT FROM THE 'WHAT' TO THE 'HOW' IN PRACTICE ....................231
JANE HATT ▪ ALISON J. HACKETT

13 PERINATAL MENTAL HEALTH .............251
PATRICIA BURROWS ▪ MARY MALONE ▪ SHARIN BALDWIN

14  EMOTIONAL AND MENTAL HEALTH
    WELL-BEING AND DEVELOPMENT OF
    INFANTS AND CHILDREN ....................279
    KIRSTEN COULL ▪ AMANDA HOLLAND

15  COMMUNICATION AND LANGUAGE
    DEVELOPMENT...................................301
    JOANNE GIBSON ▪ JEAN COWIE ▪ MICHELLE SCOTT

16  MANAGEMENT OF COMMON
    CHILDHOOD AILMENTS AND ACCIDENT
    PREVENTION .......................................323
    VAL THURTLE

17  TRANSITION TO SCHOOL ...................343
    JAMES McTAGGART ▪ RUTH ASTBURY

INDEX .........................................................355

# CONTRIBUTORS

KAREN ADAMS, DEd, MA, PgDip HPE, RN, RM, RHV, RNT, FHEA, QN, FiHV, CMgr MCMI
Head of Post Registration Business and Enterprise, Department of Nursing and Midwifery, School of Human and Health Sciences, University of Huddersfield, Queensgate, United Kingdom

DIANE ALLCOCK, MSc PRIMARY CARE, PG DIP HV, SPQ PRACTICE NURSING, RN, RM
Practice Development Nurse and Health Visitor, NHS Greater Glasgow and Clyde, Glasgow, United Kingdom; Panel Chair, Children's Hearing Scotland, Edinburgh, United Kingdom

RUTH ASTBURY, DNurs, MSc (NURSING), RGN, RSN, RHV, PGCert (ED)
Programme Leader for the PgD, SCPHN School Nursing Programme, University of the West of Scotland, Glasgow, United Kingdom; External Examiner, SCPHN School Nursing Programme, Liverpool John Moores University, Liverpool, United Kingdom

SHARIN BALDWIN, RN, RHV, BSc (HONS), PG DIP, MSc, PhD, QN, FiHV
Clinical Doctoral Fellow (NIHR DSE Award), University of Warwick, Coventry, United Kingdom

BERNADETTE BRADLEY, MSc, PgD HEALTHCARE IN HIGHER EDUCATION, RNT, HV, RGN, FHEA
Programme Leader Health Visiting, Glasgow Caledonian University, Glasgow, United Kingdom

MICHELLE CLARK, BSc (HONS), MSc, DPSYCH HEALTH, C PSYCHOL
Clinical Health Psychologist, Specialist Research and Training Lead/Principal Educator - Health Improvement Workstream; Psychology Directorate, NHS Education for Scotland, Bexley, United Kingdom

KATHLEEN M. CLARKE, NURS. D, MSc, BA, PGCE, RGN, RMN, RHV, RNT, FHEA
Lecturer, Faculty of Health Sciences and Sport, University of Stirling, Stirling, UK

KIRSTEN COULL, DCLINPSYCH, MSc, BSc (HONS), HPCP REGISTERED CLINICAL PSYCHOLOGIST
Clinical psychologist, NHS Lothian & NHS Education for Scotland, HCPC & BPS, Edinburgh, United Kingdom

JOANNE GIBSON, MSc, PGCE, BSc SPEECH AND LANGUAGE THERAPY, HPCP REGISTERED SPEECH AND LANGUAGE THERAPIST
Speech and Lanaguage Therapist, NHS Lanarkshire; Senior Educator, AHP Practice Education Coordinator, NHS Education for Scotland, Glasgow, United Kingdom

VICTORIA JANE GILROY, RGN, RSCN, RHV, PGCE, MSc, FiHV
Head of Projects & Evaluation, Institute of Health Visiting, London, United Kingdom

CLAIR GRAHAM, PROF DR, MPC, PG CERT TLHE, BSC, DIP COMMUNITY HEALTH, CERT FP, SFHEA, HV, RM, RN
Senior Lecturer Specialist Nursing, School of Health and Life Sciences, University of The West of Scotland, Glasgow, United Kingdom

ALISON J. HACKETT, MSC, BA, BSC, PGCE, RN-ADULT, SCPHN-HV, RNT, FHEA
Lecturer Early Years, Programme Director MSc Early Years Practice (Health Visiting), University of Stirling, Stirling, United Kingdom

BRIDGET HALNAN, MScM RHV, RGN, FHEA, FIHV
Senior Lecturer, Anglia Ruskin University, Cambridge, United Kingdom

JANE HATT, RGN, RHV, BA (HONS), MA, PGCAP
Senior Teaching Fellow, King's College London, London, United Kingdom

AMANDA HOLLAND, MSc SCPHN, PGCE, BN HONS (ADULT), RHV, RN
Lecturer and Programme Manager of the Specialist Community Public Health Nursing Programme, Cardiff University, Cardiff; CPHVA Chair for Wales, United Kingdom

MARIA HORNE, PHD, MA (HEALTH RESEARCH), BA (HONS), DIP COMMUNITY HEALTH STUDIES, SCPHN (HV), SCM, RGN, SENIOR FELLOW IHV AND QUEENS NURSE
Associate Professor, London South Bank University, London, United Kingdom

FELICITY JONES, BSc (HONS), PGCERT, RN-ADULT, SCPHN HV
Teaching Fellow in Integrated Care (Population Health), Director of Studies for Specialist Practice and Pathway Lead for Health Visiting, University of Surrey, Surrey, United Kingdom

MARY MALONE, PHD, MSc, PGDIP (EDUCATION), PGDIP HEALTH VISITING, BA (HONS) HISTORY, RN, RM
Vice Dean (Education) and Professor of Nursing, Florence Nightingale Faculty of Nursing, Midwifery and Palliative Care, King's College London, London; Previous role: Director of the Oxford School of Nursing and Midwifery, Oxford Brookes University, United Kingdom

CLARE MCGUIRE, MSc, BSc (HONS), DIPHE, RN, SCPHN-HV, TEACHER
Head of Programme: Women, Children, Young People & Families, NHS Education for Scotland, Glasgow, United Kingdom

JAMES MCTAGGART, MA (OXON), DIPPSYCH, MSc, CPSYCHOL
Early Years Educational Psychologist, The Highland Council, Inverness, United Kingdom

SCOTT MICHELLE, DIPHE-RGN, BSc NURSING, BSc (HONS), SQCPHN, PG DIP CHILD PROTECTION, MSc HEALTH STUDIES
Practice Educator, NHS Education for Scotland, Glasgow, United Kingdom

MICHELLE E. MOSELEY, BSc (COMMUNITY HEALTH STUDIES), MSc (ADVANCED NURSING PRACTICE), PGCE (HP) RGN, RSCN, RHV, SFHEA, IHV MEMBER, CPHVA, RCN, AOCPP (ASSOCIATION CHILD PROTECTION PROFESSIONALS)
Education and Lifelong learning adviser, RCN Wales, Cardiff, United Kingdom

ROBERT NETTLETON, DED, MSc (NURS), PGDIPED, BNURS, RN, RSCPHN-HEALTH VISITING, NDNCERT, FHEA, FIHV
Education Lead, Institute of Health Visiting, London, United Kingdom

Rita Newland, MSc, PGDIP, BSc (Hons), RN, RM, RHV, DN, SFHEA, Registered Prescriber, Registered Teacher, Senior Fellow iHV and Queens Nurse
Associate Professor, London South Bank University, London, United Kingdom

Patricia Owen, PhD, MPH, BSc, Cert Ed (FE), RN, SCPHN (HV), MIHPE
Emerita Professor, Keele University, Newcastle, United Kingdom

Kate Phillips, MSc SCPHN, BN (Hons), PGCertEd for Healthcare Professionals, RN (Adult & Child), RHV SFHEA, CPHVA
Lecturer Child Nursing, University of Leeds, Leeds, United Kingdom

Lynette H. Shotton, EdD, MSc, BSc (Hons), PgCert PCET, RGN, SCPHN/HV, Senior Fellow Advance HE
Director of Access and Participation, Head of Subject Education and Community Well-being, Department of Social Work, Northumbria University, Newcastle, United Kingdom

Karen Jane Stansfield, DBA, MMedSci, BSc (Hons), RGN, RHV, fellow iHV
Professor and Dean, Faculty of Health Studies, University of Bradford, Bradford, West Yorkshire, United Kingdom

Rachel Stephen, MSc, BSc (Hons), RGN, DN, HV
Professional Development Officer – Emotional Wellbeing at Work, Institute of Health Visiting, London, United Kingdom

Janine Stewart, RGN, HV, Community Nurse Prescriber, Teacher, MSc (Health and Social Care Education), BA (Community Health), PG Cert (Sexual and Reproductive Health), FHEA
Senior Educator, NHS Education for Scotland, Glasgow, United Kingdom

Liz Sturley, Dip HE Adult Nursing, BSc (Hons) Public Health Practice (Health Visiting), PG Cert Learning, FHEA
Open University Professional Lead for Nursing in Scotland, Edinburgh, United Kingdom

Val Thurtle, Doc HC, MA, BSc (Hons), RN, SCPHN(HV), FIHV
School of Health Sciences, City, University of London, London, United Kingdom

Joyce Wilkinson, PhD, BA, PGCE, RSCN, RGN, RHV, RNT, FHEA
Lecturer, University of Stirling, Stirling, United Kingdom

# FOREWORD

It is a pleasure to write a foreword for a text-book specifically about health visiting, especially at this time. December 2021 marked the 20-year anniversary of the Nursing and Midwifery Order 2001, which removed the title 'health visiting' from the UK statute books. At the time, it was said "It's up to us now, to ensure the title remains in use. If it continues to have currency in practice, it will continue." This has happened and fierce debates of that time, about whether or not health visitors should stop using their professional title, have largely ceased. Parents and families have, consistently, made clear that they understand and value health visitors, but are not accustomed to the statutory title of 'specialist community public health nurse (SCPHN),' which has gained familiarity with neither public nor professionals. The NMC have published new draft standards for SCPHN training[1], which propose distinct pathways for each of the three occupations (health visitors, school nurses, occupational nurses) represented on that part of their register. If approved, their implementation will begin the process of re-establishing legal recognition for the health visiting qualification and profession, in the same year that this book is published.

It is a tough time for health visitors at present, not only because of the many constraints and pressures caused by the Covid-19 pandemic, but also because the size of their workforce has been significantly reduced in England. Government cuts to the public health grant that funds them have led to there being only 6279 whole time equivalent (WTE) health visitors employed by the NHS in September 2021[2]. Even allowing for the fact that between 1000 and 1500 more are employed in local authorities or by private sector providers, that means there are fewer health visitors overall than at any time in the last 50 years. The Royal Commission on the NHS[3] recorded 6,403 WTE health visitors in the whole of Great Britain in 1967, rising to 10,248 ten years later – with 8477 in England alone in 1977[4]. Whilst birth rates have fallen during the intervening years, the population has risen markedly, and health needs continue.

Indeed, this book will stand as a marker of the enduring need for health visitors, which is described so eloquently in chapters outlining the faltering growth in life expectancy, increase in child poverty, rising inequalities in infant and public health, along with many other worsening statistics. More positively, it explains the increasing clarity of evidence about how health visitors can, and do, help to improve the lot of new parents and their pre-school children. Whilst services are struggling in too many places in England, those in other UK home nations are responding to the mounting evidence about the importance of the first 1000 days of life. Full information is given about the enhanced health visiting pathway, now embedded in Scotland, with early signs of benefits[5] and a wider evaluation underway[6]. Flying Start Wales, likewise, has clarity, purpose and the staff to implement effective health visiting services for those of their youngest citizens living in deprived areas, as part of a wider programme. An evaluation of linked routine data suggests better outcomes for children at school entry, although the extent of engagement between health visitors and the families they visit has yet to be fully examined[7]. Whilst those are national examples of excellence, there are many local examples from Northern Ireland and England as well. Overall, the way that government decisions affect service provision is well explained through these and other comparative examples in the text, along with the part that health visitors need to play in influencing policies at local and national levels, to counter some of the disparities that arise between different parts of the country.

The second half of the book shows the very practical nature of health visiting, in providing both an explanation and an evidence base for working with some of the most important groups and issues that practitioners will face on a daily basis. Here, the skills they need and the increase in evidence that health visitors have to draw upon shines through. Advances in neurological science and epigenetics illustrate the connection between the social and physical dimensions of life[8]. Exposure to nurturing care at key moments of human development, particularly the first 2000 days of life (that is, from conception until age five)[9], shows the importance of that age-range as a focus for health visitors. Supportive parenting and early experiences can both protect children from risks and expose them to positive opportunities. In turn, these shape a child's capacity to form future relationships, benefit from future learning (development of language/communication and executive function) and manage responses to life stressors.

We know, now, how to support early attachment, how to prevent, identify and treat postnatal depression and other early mental health problems affecting parents or children, and so much more. Physical health, child growth and development, unintentional injuries and safeguarding have been important features of the health visitors' day since the service began – and will continue as staple fare. I predict the chapter on 'Management of common childhood ailments and accident prevention' will be the most thumbed and frequently referred to in practice, by student and novice health visitors, if not by their more experienced peers checking out new approaches and evidence! And different forms of service organisation are at least being critiqued now, even if there is far too little evidence about how the different formats affect practice.

This book is being published 160 years after the Salford Ladies' Missionary Association (described in the 'history of health visiting' chapter) first decided to raise money, to employ local women to visit the homes of families living in difficult circumstances, offering practical help, support and advice 'where accepted'[10]. The decision was a radical departure from the many extant schemes (in 1862) for delivering 'improving' religious tracts, or providing nursing care for the sick, or of middle-class women visiting homes themselves. Instead, the Ladies hoped that sending someone who would understand the issues faced by mothers (in those gender-divided days, it was only mothers!) and their families, would make their 'health-bringing mission' more acceptable. Since that time, the health visiting profession has grown and developed, changing and developing, whilst retaining its original commitment to enhancing health and life chances for people facing disadvantage. It continues to offer a deeply satisfying career, as well as contributing greatly to the wellbeing of the population. Health visitors are needed now more than ever, so this text will serve the needs of many future students, as well as being suitable for updating their qualified and experienced colleagues.

Dame Sarah Cowley
December 2021

## REFERENCES

1. Nursing and Midwifery Council. (2021). Standards of proficiency for specialist community public health nursing – draft 11th January 2021. https://www.nmc.org.uk/globalassets/sitedocuments/post-registration/final-documents/standards-of-proficiency-for-specialist-community-public-health-nursing-.pdf. Accessed 22nd December 2021.
2. NHS Digital. NHS Workforce Statistics September 2021, Provisional statistics. https://digital.nhs.uk/data-and-information/publications/statistical/nhs-workforce-statistics/august-2021. Accessed 22nd December 2021.
3. Royal Commission on the NHS. (1979). Chapter 7 https://www.sochealth.co.uk/national-health-service/royal-commission-on-the-national-health-service-contents/royal-commission-on-the-nhs-chapter-7/. Accessed 22nd December 2021.
4. Royal Commission on the NHS. (1979). Chapter 13 https://www.sochealth.co.uk/national-health-service/royal-commission-on-the-national-health-service-contents/royal-commission-on-the-nhs-chapter-13/. Accessed 22nd December 2021.
5. Doi, L., Jepson, R., & Hardie S (2017). Realist evaluation of an enhanced health visiting programme. *PLoS ONE, 12*(7), e0180569. https://doi.org/10.1371/journal.pone.0180569. Accessed 22nd December 2021.
6. Doi, L., Morrison, K., Astbury, R., et al. (2020). Study protocol: - a mixed-methods realist evaluation of the Universal Health Visiting Pathway in Scotland. *BMJ Open, 10*, e042305. doi: 10.1136/bmjopen-2020-042305. https://bmjopen.bmj.com/content/bmjopen/10/12/e042305.full.pdf. Accessed 22nd December 2021.
7. Welsh Government (2021). Analysis of Flying Start outcomes using linked data: childcare and Foundation Phase baseline assessments https://gov.wales/analysis-flying-start-outcomes-using-linked-data-childcare-and-foundation-phase-baseline-assessments-html. Accessed 22nd December 2021.
8. Center on the Developing Child at Harvard University. (2010). The Foundations of Lifelong Health Are Built in Early Childhood. https://developingchild.harvard.edu/resources/the-foundations-of-lifelong-health-are-built-in-early-childhood/. Accessed 23rd December 2021.
9. World Health Organization, United Nations Children's Fund, World Bank Group. Nurturing care for early childhood development: A framework for helping children survive and thrive to transform health and human potential. Licence: CC BY-NC-SA 3.0 IGO. Geneva: World Health Organization, 2018. https://apps.who.int/iris/bitstream/handle/10665/272603/9789241514064-eng.pdf.
10. Dingwall, R. (1977). Collectivism, regionalism and feminism. Health visiting and British social policy 1850-1975. *Journal of Social Policy, 6*, 291–315.

# ACKNOWLEDGEMENTS

The editors wish to acknowledge, with grateful thanks, all the authors and contributors for their time and commitment to the third edition. A very special thanks to Sarah Cowley for her valuable contribution in the foreword.

# INTRODUCTION TO THE THIRD EDITION

The first edition of this book, published in 2005, became established as a core text in public health nursing education programmes. This third edition has been revised substantially to incorporate many changes to the policy context of health visiting.

After a long period of poor acknowledgement of the role of health visiting in promoting the health and well-being of the population, the value and worth of health visiting was recognised by reinvestment in health visiting (DH 2011) with the Call to Health Visiting in England, and similarly in Scotland with the refocusing of the health visiting service and commitment by the Scottish Government (2015) to increase the number of health visitors in Scotland.

On publication of the previous edition (2005) the Nursing and Midwifery Council (NMC) introduced the new Specialist Community Public Health Nursing part of the NMC Register (NMC 2004),[1] and as this book is being produced the Nursing and Midwifery Council are once again reviewing these Standards of proficiency for specialist community public health nurses (SCPHNs),[2] as well as other post-registration standards. As this book goes into publication, the role of the health visitor has never been more needed. The World Health Organization (WHO) declared the coronavirus, Covid-19, pandemic in January 2020 and in March 2021 the whole of the UK went into lockdown. Schools, colleges, universities, workplaces, places of worship, shops and hospitality all closed. People were told to stay at home, to work from home if possible and only to venture out if it was essential. The NHS was overwhelmed by the impact of Covid-19. Many staff, including health visitors, were redeployed, and over the course of the pandemic the impact of the redeployment of health visitors became apparent with increasing evidence indicating a rise in violence in the home, putting women and children at great physical and mental health risk. Evidence also highlights an increase in emotional and mental health concerns in families including women and children.[3-6] Some health visitors continued working in their role as health visitor during the pandemic or returned to their health visiting role after a period of redeployment. Many used their professional judgement and, while abiding by the government's pandemic restrictions, risked their own health to visit and support vulnerable families at home. Others learned to use new technologies to contact and support families remotely, as discussed in Chapter 9 of this textbook. True to the spirit of health visiting, and as if history were repeating itself, health visitors have shown their versatility and flexibility by adapting to the crisis at hand and embracing new ways of working and new technologies to support women and families.

This is the first pandemic to affect the UK in our generation and, although devastating, it has also led to some positive changes in ways of working and will continue to do so for some time yet. Health visitors have already proven that they are adaptable and responsive to change; however, the full impact of the pandemic on the physical, emotional and mental health well-being of families is not yet fully realised. In producing this book, we are grateful to all the authors for reviewing and, where relevant, revising their chapters to include the emerging evidence of new knowledge and practice evolving from the Covid-19 pandemic.

The devastation caused by the pandemic will live with us for a long time yet and will present new challenges for health visitors. Like those before them, we are confident that the health visitors of the future will adapt and meet these challenges and changes.

The aim, as in previous editions, has been to provide a comprehensive textbook that takes into consideration the breadth of health visiting and the current context in which it is practised. The book contains 17 chapters divided into three sections:

**Part 1: Foundations of Public Health and Health Visiting Practice** encompasses chapters on Public Health, the History of Health Visiting, Professional Practice and Practitioner Well-being, the Social policy context of public Health and the organisation of health visiting service provision.

**Part 2: Fundamentals of Health Visiting Practice** encompasses chapters on Home Visiting and therapeutic relationship building to support the transition to parenthood, Assessment, Evidence-based practice and early intervention to support children and families, Leadership skills for leading health visiting practice, Technology and Health Visiting practice and facilitating heathy behaviour and lifestyle change.

**Part 3: Health Visitor Practice-focused Interventions** encompasses chapters on Childhood adversity and trauma, Safeguarding, Perinatal Mental Health, Emotional & Mental Health well-being and development of infants and children, Communication and language development, Management of common childhood ailments and accident prevention, and Transition to school.

The chapters contain thinking spaces and the opportunity for you to reflect on key aspects of learning. We encourage you to work at these individually and in groups. The chapter content is as follows:

**Chapter 1** outlines the nature and complexity of public health set within health visiting practice and discusses the underlying principles, history and contemporary perspectives of public health. The concepts of public, health, public health and health promotion are considered with an examination of the role of health promotion within contemporary public health.

**Chapter 2** discusses the history and context of health visiting with its relevance in public health and health promotion delivery. The complex role of the health visitor is highlighted within the varied service provision across the United Kingdom and it is recognised that the philosophy of the service has remained the same with a clear goal to promote health, prevent disease and safeguard the health and well-being of children and families.

**Chapter 3** recognises the importance of practitioner well-being for effective professional health visiting practice. The challenge of adapting and transitioning from student to health visitor, and the value of preceptorship and clinical or restorative supervision for new and experienced health visitors. Strategies to strengthen resilience and create more joy at work are considered.

**Chapter 4** aims to develop understanding of social policy, public health policy and the welfare state, as well as the similarities and differences in health visiting provision between the devolved nations of the UK. Whilst differences in health visiting service provision do exist, commonality across the four nations includes a focus on the early years, early intervention and prevention, human rights and the reduction of health inequalities.

**Chapter 5** highlights the importance of home visiting and establishing an effective therapeutic health visiting relationship with parents and families. Strategies to help health visitors develop and build effective relationships with parents are discussed within this chapter. Consideration is also given to the needs of fathers and diverse families as well as the impact and experience of trauma on parents themselves and parenting behaviours.

**Chapter 6** recognises that assessment is core to the role of the health visitor requiring professional knowledge, intuition, knowledge of assessment tools and support of organisational guidelines. The most used assessment tools in health visiting practice are discussed with a focus on partnership working with families using a strength-based approach.

**Chapter 7** provides a meaningful overview of research, evidence-based practice and quality improvement and measures, and their value in underpinning health visiting practice. The chapter focuses on the early years and aims to enhance the health visitor's knowledge and skills in using the available evidence to support, inform and develop their own professional practice as well as health visiting services.

**Chapter 8** discusses leadership and leadership styles and aims to develop understanding of the importance of effective leadership in health visiting practice. A leadership development model for health visiting is presented and described which challenges health visitors to reflect on their own leadership skills and leadership identity.

**Chapter 9** considers technological advancements and the increasing use of technology within health visiting practice. Whilst the use of technology to support record keeping has become commonplace for some health visitors, the impact of the recent Covid-19 pandemic has seen enormous technological developments, with technology increasingly being used to communicate with, and to support families.

**Chapter 10** considers the art and science of behaviour change in relation to health visiting practice and the role of the health visitor in working with individuals, families and communities. It summarises the historical and contemporary approaches to promoting health and facilitating healthy behaviour. An empowerment approach is proposed as most appropriate to the work of health visitors with families and communities. The role of health visitors in the evaluation of interventions they design and deliver to improve outcomes for the communities they support is considered.

**Chapter 11** provides an overview of psychological trauma and childhood adversity, and the impact this has on children's development and outcomes. The importance of understanding the evidence base and careful and respectful assessment and analysis with families is emphasised. The role of the health visitor is discussed in working with parents and carers to support the provision of the physical environment, resources, attachment relationships, experience of moderate and resolved stress and developmentally appropriate stimulation required by children. The chapter concludes by discussing the effects of working with trauma and adversity on the health visitor and the importance of health visitors looking after their own well-being.

**Chapter 12** aims to provide an understanding of the complex dynamics in child safeguarding. The aspects of family engagement and challenge within practice are critically discussed, acknowledging the importance of being equipped with the skills to build strong relationships with children and their families. The significance of dangerous dynamics, intuitive and intercultural competency and self-reflection in achieving unconscious competence are explored. The relevance of safeguarding supervision in supporting competent and accountable practice is also explored.

**Chapter 13** discusses the complex issue of perinatal mental health disorders. Consideration is given to maternal mental health in the antenatal and postnatal periods as well as the mental health well-being of adoptive parents and fathers. The impact of Covid-19 on maternal and paternal mental health is also highlighted. Interventions and strategies to support women experiencing perinatal mental health disorders and their families are also included.

**Chapter 14** provides an overview of infant mental health and its impact on the developing child. The significance of the health visitor in being key to early identification of risk factors that can impact on infant/child mental health and well-being is discussed. The range of evidence-based therapeutic interventions which can facilitate family attachment, parental sensitivity and positive mental health development are examined.

**Chapter 15** discusses the importance of speech, language and communication development in the healthy development of children. The chapter aims to develop an understanding of the health visitor's role in the assessment and identification of factors that may lead to an increased risk of speech language and communication need in children. Consideration is given to the role of the health visitor executing early interventions and strategies to promote speech, language and communication development, and minimise speech, language and communication need in young children.

**Chapter 16** provides an overview of accident prevention and common minor ailments in the preschool child. Consideration is given to the role of the health visitor in supporting families to care for a child with a common minor ailment; readers are signposted to recognised national health service websites for further information and advice.

**Chapter 17** aims to develop understanding of the complex process of the transition of children to school. This chapter considers this transition through the lens of the child, as well as the parent, and challenges health visitors to reflect on their role in preparing and supporting children and their parent for going to school.

We would like to thank our publisher and authors for their support and dedication in writing new chapters for this edition. All the hard work and expertise are greatly appreciated.

## REFERENCES

1. NMC (2021). Building on ambitions for community and public health nursing - The Nursing and Midwifery Council. https://www.nmc.org.uk/about-us/consultations/past-consultations/2021-consultations/future-community-nurse/.
2. NMC (2004). Standards for Specialist Community Public Health Nurses. https://www.nmc.org.uk/standards/standards-for-post-registration/standards-of-proficiency-for-specialist-community-public-health-nurses/
3. Deoni, S. C., Beauchemin, J., Volpe, A., Dâ Sa, V.; RESONANCE Consortium. (2021). Impact of the COVID-19 Pandemic on Early Child Cognitive Development: Initial Findings in a Longitudinal Observational Study of Child Health. medRxiv [Preprint]. doi: 10.1101/2021.08.10.21261846. PMID: 34401887; PMCID: PMC8366807. https://pubmed.ncbi.nlm.nih.gov/34401887/
4. Sunders, B., Hogg, S. (2020). Babies in Lockdown: Listening to parents to build back better. https://parentinfantfoundation.org.uk/our-work/campaigning/babies-in-lockdown/
5. Coronavirus: Domestic violence 'increases globally during lockdown'. https://www.bbc.co.uk/news/av/world-53014211
6. Kourti, A., Stavridou, A., Panagouli, E., Psaltopoulou, T., Spiliopoulou, C., Tsolia, M., Sergentanis, T. N., Tsitsika, A. (2021). Domestic Violence During the COVID-19 Pandemic: A Systematic Review. Trauma Violence Abuse. doi: 10.1177/15248380211038690. Epub ahead of print. PMID: 34402325. https://pubmed.ncbi.nlm.nih.gov/34402325/

# PART 1

# Foundations of Public Health and Health Visiting

PART OUTLINE

1 FOUNDATIONS OF PUBLIC HEALTH AND HEALTH VISITING

2 THE HISTORY OF HEALTH VISITING

3 PROFESSIONAL PRACTICE AND PRACTITIONER WELL-BEING

4 SOCIAL POLICY, CONTEXT OF PUBLIC HEALTH AND THE ORGANISATION OF HEALTH VISITING SERVICE PROVISION

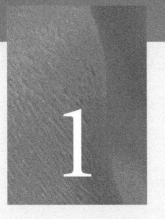

# 1

# FOUNDATIONS OF PUBLIC HEALTH AND HEALTH VISITING

MARIA HORNE ■ PATRICIA OWEN

## CHAPTER CONTENTS

INTRODUCTION

OVERVIEW OF PUBLIC HEALTH

UNDERPINNING THE PHILOSOPHY AND PERSPECTIVES OF PUBLIC HEALTH

THE HISTORY OF PUBLIC HEALTH: DOES IT MATTER?

HEALTH PROMOTION: PROMOTING THE PUBLIC'S HEALTH

HEALTH VISITING AND PUBLIC HEALTH

CHANGES TO THE DELIVERY OF HEALTH VISITING

CHANGES IN TIMES OF CRISIS

CONCLUSION

## LEARNING OUTCOMES

*To:*

■ explore the concepts of public, health, public health and health promotion

■ explore the history and context of public health

■ examine the role of health promotion within contemporary public health

■ examine and understand the context and practice of contemporary public health work

■ explore alternative ways of working

## INTRODUCTION

As Health Visitors are Specialist Community Public Health Nurses registered on the third part of the Nursing and Midwifery Council Register, this chapter focuses on the public health aspect of the role. It aims to outline the nature and complexity of public health set within health visiting practice and discuss the underlying principles, history and contemporary perspectives of public health. It also situates health promotion within public health practice and society.

## OVERVIEW OF PUBLIC HEALTH

Public health remains a complex area of activity that has seen several phases of development associated with changes in the nature of society, political and societal value judgements, and the emergence of various threats to population health.[1] Although the origins of health visiting are traditionally rooted in public health, the concepts and frameworks commonly used to describe public health remain[2,3] a widely contested area.[4–6]

To understand the nature and complexity of public health, and how these are translated into practice, it is necessary to define some commonly used terms and concepts – epidemiology, health, public and public health. Epidemiology, the study of disease in populations, is the underpinning science of public health, providing data about the factors associated with different health problems.[7,8] Contemporary public health also acknowledges the importance of the behavioural and social sciences as equally important in public health practice and improving public health – these being psychology, sociology and anthropology.[9] The terms 'health promotion' and 'public health' are often used interchangeably, although health promotion is generally seen as a means of achieving public health goals.[10]

Health is a broad concept that has been interpreted in several ways depending on the perspective of the practitioner. The biomedical interpretation of health is seen as a negative, narrow, physical or biophysical view of health as it conceptualises health as merely the absence of disease. Broader interpretations of health conceptualise it as well-being in its widest, positive sense: for example, the World Health Organisation (WHO) definition of health as '...*a state of complete physical, mental and social well-being and not merely the absence of disease or infirmity*'.[11] Health has also been defined as a resource for life, which sees health as embedded in the processes and actions of everyday life, enabling people to lead individually, socially and economically productive lives. For example, the WHO's[12] definition of health as 'a *resource for everyday life, not the object of living. It is a positive concept emphasising social and personal resources as well as physical capabilities*'. The latter interpretations of health as a positive concept emphasise its social, environmental and psychological aspects,[13] which involve, not only the individual's physical health, but also their environment, place in the social environment, and mental health. Well-being is connected to these positive approaches to health in describing the meaning of health as more than just the 'absence of disease'.[14]

The term 'public health' means different things to different people. Unquestionably, it is about the health of the public, but how we define 'public' remains open to interpretation.

Interpretations of the 'public' in 'public health' have been considered by Verweij and Dawson,[15] who propose two interpretations: (i) as an aggregate of the health experiences of the individuals that make up a population, and (ii) collective and organised action either by the state or groups of people.

## Interpretation and definitions of public health

Interpretations and definitions of public health mirror the aforementioned deliberations about the meaning of health and well-being. How we interpret public health influences its practice. It has been classified into narrow and broad perspectives.[15] Narrow perspectives of public health focus on how long people can remain free from disease, whilst broader perspectives view public health in terms of protecting the health of the population, health promotion, and disease prevention.[15] These perspectives reflect societal priorities for improving the health of the public and are driven by the prevailing political climate.[16] They have also developed from our understanding of health, which now recognises that it is not just the absence of disease, but overall physical, mental and social well-being. In practice, defining public health in narrow terms is going to focus on specific diseases and problems, but a possible consequence may be an emphasis on treatment and care provision without considering the wider influences on health. By contrast, broader approaches to public health, which include and consider wider influences on health, may be too ambiguous and, as such, difficult to translate into practice.

Many definitions of public health have been proposed, but these are largely based on the multifaceted notion of health discussed above. For example, public health has been defined as:

*The science and art of preventing disease, prolonging life and promoting health through the organised efforts of society.*[16]

*The science and art of preventing disease, prolonging life and promoting health through the organised effects and informed choices of society, organisations, public and private, communities and individuals.[17]*

*The science and art of preventing disease, prolonging life and promoting health through the organized efforts and informed choices of society, organizations, public and private, communities and individuals.[18]*

*Collective action for sustained population-wide health improvement.[19]*

There is some diversity among these definitions: some are broad in their nature and scope, while one has a narrower scope, mirroring the definitions of health outlined earlier. However, there are commonalities. First, they define health in its broadest sense, not merely as the absence of disease. Second, they are concerned with the improvement of population health, recognising the influence of the wider determinants of health.[20,21] Third, they acknowledge the need for collective action, shared responsibility and partnerships with organisations outside the health sector and the population being served to improve and promote health, prevent disease and prolong life.[22] These definitions convey the 'public', 'societal' elements of improving health, whether it is through interventions or policies.[8] The role of the state in public health is implicit and linked to a concern for the underlying socio-economic determinants of health and the need to address its inequalities, defined as differences in the health status between different population sub-groups.

Based on these definitions, one can see that public health uses collective or population approaches to provide conditions under which people can maintain health, improve their health and well-being, or prevent the deterioration of their health, whilst clinical interventions are targeted at individuals to improve the health of individuals. As the population consists of individuals, the two approaches are unsurprisingly interrelated. Collective interventions (e.g. policies) affect individuals and require individual participation, whilst interventions for individuals can also directly affect the population, for example in the control of communicable diseases. Contemporary public health is based on a social model, which recognises that the health and well-being of individuals, communities and the public are determined by a wide range of social, economic and lifestyle factors, in addition to heredity and health care – many of these factors are modifiable and form the basis of public health interventions to improve health and well-being. We discuss this further in the **Health promotion: promoting the public health** section below.

Public health also focuses on a life course approach to preventing ill health and promoting health and well-being. Therefore, public health action aims, not only to eradicate specific diseases, but also to provide personal services to individuals, such as vaccinations, behavioural counselling or health advice. This includes legislation to promote behavioural change by changing social norms: for example, the introduction of non-smoking in public places. The vehicle used to encourage public health is health promotion. In the UK, the terms public health and health promotion are used interchangeably. The latter is often seen as a means to achieving the health of the public.[23]

Public health raises political and ethical issues linked to the relationship between individuals and society. These are based on various philosophies and perspectives, which seek to justify how interventions are delivered to promote and protect the public's health.

THINKING SPACE

Which interpretation aligns with your own perspective of public health practice and why?

# UNDERPINNING THE PHILOSOPHY AND PERSPECTIVES OF PUBLIC HEALTH

This section aims to provide a general overview of the main underpinning philosophies and perspectives that influence the practice of public health.

## Paternalism and utilitarianism

*Paternalism* is a philosophy of intervention based on an inequality of power, authority and status. It involves the external assessment of individual needs by a higher authority[24] and has been defined as *'the interference of a state or an individual with another person, against their will, and justified by a claim that a person interfered with will be better off or protected from harm'*.[25]

This philosophy of public health is generally associated with inhibiting an individual's freedom and liberty of action to protect or promote their welfare.[6,25] However, there are occasions where external assessment of individual, community and population needs by a higher authority is required to protect population groups that would be considered: (i) vulnerable: for example, child protection, as children are not in a position to make rational decisions for themselves[26] and (ii) where adults may not act rationally to protect their health and well-being: for example, smoking, excessive alcohol consumption and narcotic use.[6] A recent example of this approach is the European and UK governments' call for lockdown during the Coronavirus-19 (COVID-19) pandemic. External assessment of individual, community and population needs by governments deemed it necessary to protect the population, particularly older adults and those with comorbidities, through lockdown and restriction of movement.

*Utilitarianism* provides a philosophical basis for interventions in public health and welfare that overrides individual choices and freedoms.[6]

Public health interventions often justify policies and actions on utilitarian grounds, based on the interest of the majority.[27,28] These principles are closely aligned with collectivist and socialist perspectives and founded on social justice. An example of utilitarianism is the European and UK governments' call for lockdown during the COVID-19 pandemic. Lockdown and restrictions of movement overrode individual choice of movement outside the home and was seen as a necessary public health intervention to prevent the spread of the virus in the interests of the majority.

## Collectivism and socialism

As a public health philosophy, *collectivism and socialism* emphasise the beneficial role of the state and other collective arrangements, for example cooperatives.[6] From this perspective, public health is founded on social justice (deriving from theories of justice and fairness), understanding people in their social context, rather than as individuals. Therefore, individual liberties are balanced with promoting a social good that is embedded within a broader commitment to securing a sufficient level of health for all and to narrow inequity and inequalities.[29] This approach adopts a broader definition of public, privileging action on the social determinants of health[30] and enabling people to do things through collective action, a principle of *'empowerment'*.

## Liberal-individualistic perspectives

Liberal-individualistic ideological perspectives on public health are focused on individual liberty and non-domination as a primary moral and political value. Therefore, this perspective seeks to safeguard negative liberty, whereby individuals are free to pursue activities without interference from the state with the proviso that others are not harmed in the process.[6] Individuals must take responsibility for their own health, make informed choices rather than being dictated to by the *'nanny state'*.[6]

This ideological perspective privileges consensus reform.[30] However, there are difficulties in applying liberal-individualist ideological perspectives to public health as public health is predominantly focused on populations and population-level perspectives. In addition, it shapes how we understand what makes something a 'public' versus a private matter, as well as the concept of health.[31]

### Environmental and green perspectives

The links between the natural environment and indirect and direct health outcomes are now well recognised.[32] *Environmental and green perspectives* emphasise the role of individuals and small, local groups in promoting the local environment,[6] acknowledge the environmental determinants of public health and the need for social equity. Public health approaches adopt an ecological model of health, emphasising environmental influences on health and well-being and the dynamic interplay between the individual and the environment. Therefore, individual behaviour is placed within an environmental context, with the individual's interaction with the natural environment seen as the crucial factor in maintaining health.[6] Thus, more holistic solutions are needed to improve the population's health: for example, sustainable development, balancing economic, social and environmental considerations, in addition to 'precautionary' principles, such as early intervention to prevent damage to the environment and health.[6] These perspectives are closer to *collectivist and socialist* perspectives in relation to social justice and the belief in collective action.[6]

### Summary

- Paternalism and Utilitarianism are philosophies which underpin theories of public health practice and are concerned with inequity of power and the balance of individual choice versus the welfare of the population.
- The concepts of social justice, empowerment and cooperation are important aspects of public health theory and practice.
- Liberal-individualistic philosophies can pose challenges to public health practice.
- Sustainability and the impact on health of the natural world are important facets of public health action.
- These perspectives have been played out in the recent discussions around how to manage the 2020 Coronavirus pandemic.

## THE HISTORY OF PUBLIC HEALTH: DOES IT MATTER?

As well as understanding the underlying principles of public health it is important to understand the history of public health in the UK specifically because, in order to understand the future, it is important to consider the past. So, if we view public health as integral to health visiting practice then it is important to consider its historical development. As with any story over time, there are some aspects to bring forward.

Firstly, the history and development of public health practice cannot be considered in isolation from the **context of the people and the society** of the day. The health problems people face and have faced in the past, and which have required the solutions of public health interventions to ameliorate them, are dependent on the social, economic, environmental and political influences affecting society and health at that point in history. Each era, therefore, has endured particular threats to population health due to factors arising from society's effect on health at that time. One of the health challenges of today is obesity, with population levels increasing since the late 1990s.[33] This is due to a rise in unhealthy food consumption by the population of the UK for an extensive range of reasons related to modern living, including social and economic deprivation, as outlined in the original Marmot Review.[34] One of the challenges of a different era (the 1800s) was high mortality from communicable disease during the industrial revolution. This was arguably due to the unprecedented number of people moving to live in cities, which resulted in some negative **health consequences** for the population. So, the factors affecting the health of people in different periods of history are dependent on the economic and social conditions of that society at that time. The health of the public cannot be divorced from the society within which it resides.

Secondly, it is possible to identify, across the timeframe we are considering, people who at different times have had a large impact on enhancing population health. They may have been instrumental in developing social policy or in the discovery of causes and treatments of disease. These people we would consider as **public health leaders**.

The development of public health has not always progressed in an even and systematic manner across the decades. To articulate this, there have been different definitions of the way public health history is described. Jones and Douglas[33] refer to the 'phases' of public health development over time, identifying each phase's main focus: for example, 'sanitary reform' in the early 1800s or 'the New Public Health' in the 1980s. Armstrong[35] refers to 'regimes' of public health: for example, the regime of quarantine, inclusion or exclusion and its dominance up until the middle of the 19th century. He relates each regime to methods of social control. Hanlon et al[36] suggest **'waves' of public health** improvement. The wave metaphor is useful. We can visualise how a wave rises and falls as it comes onto a shore and this metaphor is used to demonstrate that each 'wave' of public health practice rises out of its forerunner and peaks but then declines. There follows a 'trough of activity' of the wave, which remains despite not having the same impact as when at its peak.[36] This analogy is used to explain that public health development has been '...*cumulative and interactive, if not entirely smooth. Overall health and social progress has been maintained by a new wave starting, while an established wave is*

*still rising*'.[36] The waves of public health in the UK since the 19th century and the possible **lessons to learn** are discussed below.

Although there are well-documented examples of public health practice across the world and throughout history dating back to ancient Greek times – for example, when an unidentified fatal epidemic swept through Athens in 430 BC[37] – it is usually accepted that modern public health and the practice of enhancing the health of the population, dates back to the early part of the 19th century in the UK. Hanlon et al[36] identify four 'waves' of public health, starting with the first in the 19th century. They also moot a fifth.

(i) **The first wave (1830–1900): implications of the industrial revolution**

**The societal context:** Prior to the industrial revolution, many people worked in agriculture or in craft jobs. As a mainly agrarian economy, people in the UK often lived in the countryside. With the advancement of industry, the opening of factories and mills, the rapid increase in the use of machines to mass-produce, and the ensuing requirements for an increase in labour, there was a movement of people into cities to support the enlargement of an industrial and manufacturing society. This led to overcrowding in the cities, which had not been built to withstand such a swift enlargement of population. Overcrowding led to a range of health issues which affected, not just those working in the manufacturing industry at the time, but the whole of society.

**The health consequences:** The first medical officers identified the consequences of overcrowding and poverty. With the increase of people living with poor sanitation, unclean water and homelessness came a rise in communicable disease, notably cholera and tuberculosis. Cholera is a disease which results in severe diarrhoea, vomiting and dehydration, causing death at rates of 50%[38] in the squalor of the 19th century and the ignorance of its cause and treatment. Cholera can be treated today by hydration and antibiotics.

Global cholera pandemics hit the UK between about 1830 and 1851, resulting in high mortality. Dorling,[39] for example, identifies that cholera arrived in the UK around 1831; by 1832 30,000 people had died from it. The large-scale effects of the cholera pandemics provided an impetus for early leaders to identify causes and implement strategies to improve health.

**Public Health Leaders:** The early leaders in public health during that time laid the foundations of epidemiology and population strategies for preventing disease that we are familiar with today. Indeed, the early forerunners to health visitors came about at this time in response to the poor health of the working people. We know that health visiting was not a branch of nursing but developed independently from the Ladies Branch of the Manchester and Salford Sanitary Society (The Ladies Health Society) in the 1860s in order to support working-class families in education and practice around hygiene, nutrition and to improve infant mortality.

The tragedy of the cholera epidemic brought about a need for an explanation: medics began to map and plot the outbreaks in order to try and monitor the disease. The most famous case of mapping was the work undertaken by Dr John Snow, who is considered to be the founding father of modern epidemiology. The story of the Broad Street cholera outbreak in 1854 and Dr Snow's plotted map of the area is well documented, but other figures were instrumental in mapping the spread of the disease and producing explanations of its causation: for example, Dr Henry Gaulter in Manchester (1833) and Dr William Budd in Bristol (1842). The realisation that poor sanitation was connected to the ill health of the population was recognised over time and supported by the publication of Chadwick's seminal report.[40]

**Learning and criticality:** During this 'wave', the importance of systematic recording and reviewing of information in order to understand disease formation and progression is apparent. It demonstrated how this new understanding could be used to organise sections of society to improve health. The self-interest of the ruling classes also played a part in the improvement of sanitation and drinking water due to the ability of cholera to affect all strata of society.

(ii) **Second wave (1890–1950): implications of war**

**The societal context:** The Boer War was fought between Britain and Dutch settlers in South Africa between 1899 and 1902 and the First World War occurred between 1914 and 1918. Winter (1980) identified that between 40% and 60% of potential military recruits around this time were turned down due to being deemed unfit for service. This was an alarming statistic for the country and was due to the malnourishment and poor health of the mainly working-class recruits that were turned away from a military career. During the

First World War the extent and types of military injury were on a scale not previously seen, as war became increasingly mechanised. This mechanisation of arms continued throughout the next decade and was seen extensively in the Second World War (1939–1945), culminating in the devastation of the atomic bomb.

**The health consequences:** As a consequence of the poor health of military recruits for the Boer War, The Committee on Physical Deterioration was set up by the government in 1903. Recommendations included: medical inspections for school children, free school meals for the poor, and education for working-class mothers. Although legislation came about to bring these recommendations into statute, it was not soon enough to improve the health of the working man rapidly, or for the First World War. Therefore, the Ministry of Health was set up following the war, becoming responsible for the organisation of hospitals and medical training. Mortality was not only due to the injuries caused by the new weaponry and ways of warfare, but also to the infections which came about due to the poor conditions soldiers had to endure, and which became a major cause of mortality during these conflicts. In addition to the policy implementation which improved public health at this time (e.g. the 1907 Education Act, which introduced medicals for school children), major public health initiatives were based on the acceptance of germ theory during the late 1860s. This enabled microbiology, immunology, radiology and medical science to become prevalent; as a consequence, antibiotics, immunisa-

tions and radiography became key public health interventions.

**Public health leaders:** Scientists were the key figures to emerge during this wave, led by Koch, Pasteur, Fleming and Curie. Other pioneers of particular medical interventions include: McIndoe, who developed burns treatment in London; Harken, who pioneered the removal of shrapnel and bullets from open hearts, which led to work underpinning heart surgery; and Gillies, who developed plastic surgery, especially for facial wounds.

**Learning and criticality:** The response to the trauma, disfigurements and disablements of war led to the creation of a range of policy and medical interventions which we now take for granted. Arguably, the most effective public health intervention – vaccination – was developed at this time. However, we can also see the rise of the 'expert' and, because of the growth of this scientific specialist, paternalistic ways of working in health became evident, as outlined above.

(iii) **Third wave (1940–1980): implications of Beveridge's 'five giant evils'**

**The societal context:** 'Want, Ignorance, Disease, Squalor and Idleness' were the five giant challenges to society in the post-Second World War era, as identified by William Beveridge in his report of 1942. Initially set up to review national insurance schemes, the report went far wider and drew on the challenges people were facing in post-war Britain. Society was framed by severe housing shortages due to the Second World War destruction of towns and cities; people having no income if they were ill and having not paid into local insurance schemes; and, much of the population living in poverty and being malnourished with no support for the disabled or chronically ill. These were some of the factors underpinning the recommendations made by Beveridge. Following the war and the election of the Labour Government of 1945, universal health care and a social welfare system were implemented to care for people from 'the cradle to the grave'. This ensured that not only health care, but education, social financial security and housing – all factors which affect the public's health – were centrally organised and managed, influenced by the philosophies of Marx and Engels, for example, in the pre- and post-war eras.

**The health consequences:** The National Health Service (NHS) was the main health consequence for people in the post-war era. As well as hospital services if one was ill and required in- or out-patient care, a system of primary care (including dentists and opticians) was developed alongside the NHS to provide comprehensive health care to everyone, free at the point of delivery. This included health visitors, at this time managed by local authorities, not the NHS.

**Public health leaders:** According to Hanlon et al,[36] the public health leaders of the time were not scientists but politicians. Clement Attlee's post-war government, which brought in not only the NHS, but social affordable housing on a large scale, welfare benefits for the marginalised, and universal education, had great impact on the health of the population.

**Learning and criticality:** Population health is determined by multiple factors

and the connections between each wave as history progresses is clear to see. The science of the second wave of public health was continuing to be played out in the third wave, as exemplified post-war by the rise in state scientific research and the rise of biomedicine.[41]

(iv) **Fourth wave (1960–2000): implications of a post-industrial society**

**The societal context:** During this wave society changed fundamentally and rapidly. Traditional institutions, industry, work and the roles of men and women were affected. This rapid change affected North America, Asia and Europe particularly, as service and knowledge economies replaced traditional manufacturing. People had more choice about how they led their lives, attitudes to marriage, divorce and children born outside marriage changed. Birth control enabled women to have more work choices outside the home and the new economies had less use for the physical strength of men. Societal inequalities were increasingly acknowledged.

**The health consequences:** With an increasingly complex society came increasing complexity in health and lifestyle behaviours. Risk-taking became more prevalent around diet, exercise, smoking and drug and alcohol abuse. Mental ill health also became more widely diagnosed due to people's changing attitudes towards mental illness and the impact of a changing society on mental and emotional health. With an increasing focus on inequality in society came the recognition of a large gap in the health status of the 'haves' and the 'have-nots'.

**Public health leaders:** Health researchers and academics became influential in this timeframe; Hanlon et al[36] cite, for example, the work of Sir Richard Doll, whose work on cigarette smoking and lung cancer became seminal, and Sir Michael Marmot, who continues to research and publish on inequalities in health.[42]

**Learning and criticality:** Hanlon et al[36] show that, as new challenges arise, a new 'wave of public health' rises to meet them. They go on to identify new challenges which the fourth wave may not be able to meet – for example, obesity and sustainability.

**Fifth wave: implications of a post-modern society**

Since 2000, society has become increasingly digitalised and technical. There has been tension and debate around the effect of humankind on the planet and an exponential growth in many areas of global society. Hanlon et al[36] argue that a fifth wave is beginning to rise up to meet these new challenges. New ways will be identified to meet new health challenges and new leaders emerge. Davies et al[43] suggest that these new challenges will be met by different groups contributing in different ways to predecessors, especially around climate change, agricultural policies, transport and food standards. They identify, for example, that in Croydon, London, the local authority is considering the use of planning powers to limit the density of fast food outlets, and consequently reduce obesity levels in the area. The global COVID-19 pandemic is another example of the globalisation of public health approaches and the integration of technology in public health activity. Worldwide there has been implementation of contract tracing of people using technology, often via mobile phone apps, which have met with different levels of success and which have sometimes challenged the privacy of the individual.

***Summary***

- Hanlon et al (2011) suggest there have been 'waves' of public health intervention over time which may have had a cumulative but not fluent effect.
- The '5 Waves' commenced in the 1830s through to the present day, with each having a distinct focus.

## THINKING SPACE

Reflect on your own health visiting practice and consider which aspects of the five waves apply and why.

## HEALTH PROMOTION: PROMOTING THE PUBLIC'S HEALTH

In addition to the definitions of public health described earlier in the chapter, Beaglehole and Bonita[22:147] identified the essential elements of public health theory and practice. These are:

- 'it's emphasis on collective responsibility for health and the prime role of the state in protecting and promoting the public's health;
- a focus on whole populations;
- an emphasis on prevention, especially the populations strategy for primary prevention;
- a concern for the underlying socioeconomic determinants of health and disease, as well as the more proximal risk factors;
- a multi-disciplinary basis which incorporates quantitative and qualitative methods as appropriate; and
- partnership with populations served'.

It is possible to determine these themes throughout the history of public health discussed above. Arguably, these themes are also the basis of health visiting theory and practice and can be identified in the principles of health visiting.[2,44]

Promoting the public's health, therefore, is central to public health and health visiting practice.

Today's health promotion approaches have their roots in the practice of 'health education', in which different methods of delivering healthy messages were dispensed with the expectation that people would take appropriate action upon receiving the relevant education. It is recognised now that changing people's and group's behaviours is much more complicated than giving them information. The Lalonde Report[45] is seen as a seminal document as it provides different ways to consider and promote health than the medically focussed practices which prevailed after World War War 2. The report outlines for the first time a conceptual framework consisting of four elements, and called the 'Health Field' concept. The four elements are Human Biology, Environment, Lifestyle and Healthcare Organisation. The report states that 'these four elements were identified through an examination of the causes and underlying factors of sickness and death'.[46:31] This view, that the attainment of health is dependent on a range of factors, not just medical intervention, was developed further by the World Health Organisation in 1977, with the declaration at Alma Ata of 'Health for All' at the 30th World Health Assembly.[46] There was, for the first time, a focus on primary care as a setting for promoting health.

However, it was in January 1984 that the WHO defined health promotion as 'the process of enabling people to increase control over and to improve their health',[47] which was encapsulated two years later in the Ottawa Charter at the first International Conference on Health Promotion.[12] Subsequent International Conferences on Health Promotion considered a range of issues, including healthy public policy making and building capacity to promote health. The last conference, in Shanghai, China in 2016, located health promotion within the Sustainable Development Goals.[48]

The WHO has identified 17 Sustainable Development Goals (SDGs),[49] one of which, SDG no 3, is focussed on health promotion. It is broad in scope, stating 'enable healthy lives and promote well-being for all at all ages' and consists of 13 particular targets; targets in the other goals are also linked to SDG 3. Throughout the SDGs is the acknowledgement of the impact of social determinants on health. As identified in the history of public health above, and outlined in the Lalonde Report, society and the context in which people live impact on population health. Dahlgren and Whitehead[20] demonstrated the interrelationship of social, economic and cultural conditions, which affects health in their model of the main determinants of health. Figure 1.1 identifies those factors which are an individual's constitutional factors – for example, age or sex – and demonstrates how these are interrelated with individual lifestyle factors, social and community networks and, at the macro level, the general socio-economic, cultural and environmental conditions that affect the person. The determinants of health may have negative or positive effects on the health of individuals and groups. For example, if housing is in poor condition or damp it may exacerbate respiratory problems in children, providing a negative health effect; on the other hand, well-planned housing provides green space for exercise or activity, resulting in a positive health effect.

In 2015, the UK government published 'All our Health', a framework to support the promotion of health for individuals, communities and whole populations. The framework has developed into a range of resources which support preventative work, supporting individuals and communities to make healthy choices and 'Making Every Contact Count' (MECC), an approach to maximise brief opportunistic interventions by all health professionals. The development of public health policy – that is, the state's role in intervention as compared with the autonomy of the individual – has been debated widely and outlined above. Beattie's model (Fig. 1.2) of health promotion[50] can enable analysis of different

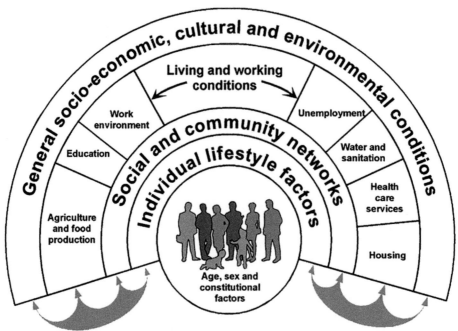

**Figure 1.1** ■ The determinants of health (Based on Dahlgren and Whitehead, 1991. Policies and strategies to promote social equity in health. Stockholm. Institute of Future Studies).

approaches to enhancing the health of the population. It[50] identifies four quadrants, split by two axes: 'focus of intervention' and 'mode of intervention'. The 'focus of intervention' runs along a continuum between the individual and the collective. The 'mode of intervention' is another continuum between negotiated and authoritative. In each quadrant, split by the two axes, are four different approaches to health promotion, and arguably policy. So, the authoritative and individualistic approach of 'health persuasion' is seen in the upper left quadrant: the state paternalistically persuading the individual to enhance their health. At the other end of the continuum, the negotiated and collective, the approach of 'community development' is seen, in which the community is empowered to play a part in negotiating how their health may be enhanced. The other two approaches in this model, 'legislative action' and 'personal counselling', are also

at either end of the continuum, in terms of the extent to which the approach is focussed on the collective or the individual, and the extent to which the approach is empowering or authoritative. During the 2020 COVID-19 pandemic the initial approaches to protecting the health of the public was focussed very much on the authoritative end of the continuum. This included persuading the population, through mass media and government messaging, to comply with measures, and also legislative action, to reduce the geographical movement of people in an attempt to reduce the spread of the disease.

Another tool for analysing health-promoting public health policy in terms of approaches to intervention is the Nuffield Bioethics Intervention Ladder.[51] This iterative 'ladder' of explanations of intervention starts at the very bottom with no intervention at all, where nothing is done about a situation and so the individual or

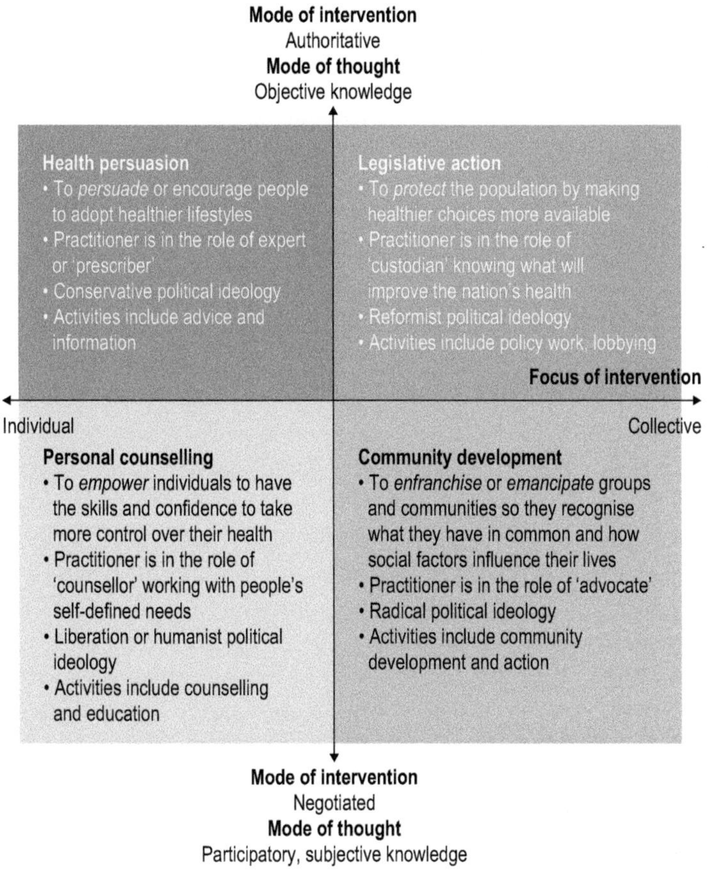

**Mode of intervention**
Authoritative
**Mode of thought**
Objective knowledge

Health persuasion
- To *persuade* or encourage people to adopt healthier lifestyles
- Practitioner is in the role of expert or 'prescriber'
- Conservative political ideology
- Activities include advice and information

Legislative action
- To *protect* the population by making healthier choices more available
- Practitioner is in the role of 'custodian' knowing what will improve the nation's health
- Reformist political ideology
- Activities include policy work, lobbying

**Focus of intervention**

Individual ◄─────────────────────────────► Collective

Personal counselling
- To *empower* individuals to have the skills and confidence to take more control over their health
- Practitioner is in the role of 'counsellor' working with people's self-defined needs
- Liberation or humanist political ideology
- Activities include counselling and education

Community development
- To *enfranchise* or *emancipate* groups and communities so they recognise what they have in common and how social factors influence their lives
- Practitioner is in the role of 'advocate'
- Radical political ideology
- Activities include community development and action

**Mode of intervention**
Negotiated
**Mode of thought**
Participatory, subjective knowledge

Figure 1.2 ◼ Beattie's model of health promotion (Naidoo, J., & Wills, J. (2009). Foundations for health promotion. Elsevier.)

community continues without intervention. At the top of the intervention ladder is where choice is eliminated and legislation, for example, occurs so that the individual or community has no choice at all in the matter. MECC, for example, could be seen in this model as being '*providing information*'. On this 'rung' the intervention enables the health professional to signpost and educate the individual in the brief intervention.

## HEALTH VISITING AND PUBLIC HEALTH

The essence of health visiting, throughout its history, has been the enhancement of the health of the public. In the early years of the profession,

the focus was on the enhancement of maternal and family health, which has been a key focus of health visiting over the last 150 years or so. Dingwall identifies that, at its inception, health visiting was a '*radical women's occupation, run largely by women for women*'.[52:315] In considering Beaglehole and Bonita's definition of public health above, it is clear that the role of health visiting is synonymous with the principles of public health they outline. For example, an emphasis on primary prevention and a concern for the underlying socio-economic determinants of the health of the population, as well as a multi-disciplinary approach. However, there has also been a tension within health visiting, between a public health population approach to health improvement and an approach which focuses on the welfare of the individual and/or family. Brookes and Rafferty identify a dichotomy in the role between '*an agent for reform and surveillance*', on the one hand, and the '*mother's friend*', on the other.[53:143] At different times throughout its history, the health visitor's role has changed from one purely focussed on population health to an approach focussed on the health of the individual, providing a universal integrated package of immunisation, screening, surveillance, health promotion and parenting support for families and children from birth to about five years of age.[54] Such activities that are directly undertaken to meet the health needs of individuals and families are considered to be public health interventions: they contribute to the health of the whole population.[55]

The underpinning principles of health visiting,[2,44] which are interconnected, have clear parallels with the principles of public health practice outlined by Beaglehole and Bonita.[22:9] As such, these principles form the basis of preventative work and health improvement (health promotion), inform practice with individuals, families and communities and focus work on individuals, families and communities identified as being in need, thereby reducing inequalities in health.

The four principles of health visiting are as follows:

(i) **the search for health needs** – seen as a fundamental aspect of health visiting practice and the starting point for health improvement and addressing health inequalities. This often involves undertaking a health needs assessment, but the focus of the search for health needs is on *health and well-being*, rather than disease or illness. Hence, when addressing needs, the focus is on maximising health, as opposed to what health concern(s) there may be. This focus takes a preventative approach to public health practice that acknowledges the wider determinants of health and is based on a social model of health which recognises that the health and well-being of individuals, families and communities is determined by a wide range of social, economic and lifestyle factors in addition to heredity and health care.

(ii) **the stimulation of an awareness of health needs** – information collected through the search for health needs feeds directly into raising awareness of health needs to determine a suitable public health response. This encompasses public health action at three levels: (a) enabling individuals, families and communities to maximise opportunities for improving health and well-being through strength-based approaches; (b) enabling commissioners and service providers to organise services that promote the health and well-being of individuals, families and communities, and reduce inequalities in health, and (c) politicians and policymakers to raise awareness of policies that affect the health and well-being of individuals, families and communities.[2]

(iii) **the influence on policies affecting health** – although recognised as a challenging principle,[2] the political nature of public health, which is dependent on influencing and developing policies to improve health and well-being, challenges practitioners to advocate on behalf of individuals, families and communities to ensure that policies positively impact health and well-being. This approach draws on, and aims to strengthen, the community's capacity to take collective action, and subsequently leads to changes in health or the social determinants of health. This approach can also be undertaken through engaging professional organisations to take action.

(iv) *the facilitation of health-enhancing activities* – focuses on the socio-environmental factors and how these may influence activities undertaken by individuals, families and communities to enhance their health and well-being.[2] This public health approach to practice directly acknowledges the wider determinants of health. It is based on a social model of health which acknowledges the need to facilitate changes in the socioeconomic environment to enable active participation of individuals, families and communities in promoting health and well-being through multidisciplinary approaches.

The underpinning principles of health visiting form the foundation of the Standards of Proficiency for Specialist Community Public Health Nurses[56] and are reflected in the Public Health Skills and Knowledge framework.[57] The framework, updated in response to the introduction of the Health and Social Care Act[58] and the consequent redistribution of public health workers across England, reflects ongoing changes to public health policy, practice and workforce planning in health and social care across the UK.

## CHANGES TO THE DELIVERY OF HEALTH VISITING

The New Labour government of 1997, led by Tony Blair, revitalised the public health agenda in the UK. Wide-ranging initiatives included the appointment of a Minister for Public Health and a series of White Papers and reports on public health. Health visitors and school nurses were the most frequent practitioners identified in these reports to be 'specifically identified' with public health work.[59:141] However, there was confusion as to the meaning of public health within health visiting and the extent to which students were educated about its implementation in health

visiting.[60] Debate continued as to the focus of the role. Lowenhoff,[61] for example, advocated investing in intensive infant and mother support programmes to promote early attachment rather than a general population approach to health improvement. When the coalition government of 2010 came into power, the focus was to recruit 4200 health visitors in a nationwide recruitment drive with the Health Visitor Implementation Plan.[62] Although that plan was realised in 2015, and came to an end shortly afterwards, due to the new Conservative government's budget cuts health visitor numbers began to fall. This occurred at the same time as health visitors were transferred into local authorities rather than being employed by the NHS, the first time that health visitors were not a part of the NHS since 1974. Under local authority control, and with local authority public health budgets reduced between 2015–2016 and 2019–2020,[63] health visitor numbers across the UK also reduced; different ways of delivering the Healthy Child Programme are currently (2021) in operation across the UK.

The integrated 4–5–6 model for health visitors (and school nurses), along with six High Impact Areas for early years (health visiting), as well as six High Impact Areas for school-aged years (school nursing), came into force in 2016 to focus the role of health visitors in their work with families and communities by improving access, experience, outcomes and reducing health inequalities, and by helping children and families to achieve their potential in these areas (PHE 2016) – see Box 1.1. High impact areas support delivery of the Healthy Child Programme – pregnancy and the first five years of life – and form the basis of the Public Health England routine monitoring of the health and well-being outcome indicators relating to the nought to five years population. The integrated 4–5–6 model also supports the effective commissioning of health visitor and school nurse services across the whole nought to 19 age range, which is the responsibility of the local authority.[57]

**BOX 1.1**

**4–5–6 MODEL FOR HEALTH VISITORS (AND SCHOOL NURSES)[57]**

Four levels of service:
- Your community
- Universal
- Universal plus
- Universal partnership plus

Five universal health reviews (mandated for 18 months):
- Antenatal
- New baby
- Six to eight weeks
- One year
- Two to 2½ years

Six high impact areas:
- Transition to parenthood
- Maternal mental health
- Breastfeeding
- Healthy weight
- Managing minor illness and accident prevention
- Healthy 2-year-olds & school readiness

It must be recognised that, since the introduction of the Health and Social Care Act in 2012,[58] whereby health visiting services were moved from NHS to local authority responsibility, different service models in the delivery of health visiting services have developed, based on how Local Authority's prioritise and structure their local services. Local authorities now commission health services, which NHS Trusts and independent and private provider organisations deliver.

## CHANGES IN TIMES OF CRISIS

In a changing and uncertain world – and certainly during the 2020 COVID-19 pandemic – the public health issues facing the population and affecting health visiting practice can take a different focus. For example, there were reports of an increase in domestic violence during the lockdown period in the UK,[64] with corresponding implications for health and social work professionals, as well as the police and the judiciary. The uncertainty of how the course of the pandemic would progress may have led to social isolation and mental health issues. With communities experiencing a reduction in salaries, job losses and other financial restrictions, further deprivation can impact on communities and groups which are already adversely affected by socio-economic disadvantage.

The use of technology to deliver public health messages, and manage aspects of public health intervention, is clearly a part of the post-modern world. Mobile phone apps to support contact tracing, information (and dis-information) being shared on social media, communication via websites and digital interventions are a new arm in public health activity to protect the public and prevent further ill health. Health visitors prioritise workload in their usual working week, but during times of crisis this results in different working practices. For example, during the COVID-19 pandemic in 2020, some health visitors were reallocated to acute care provision in NHS Trusts, while others undertook new birth visits via telephone or online consultation. It may be too soon to identify future lessons for public health practice as a consequence of the Coronavirus pandemic, but those will be detected following review and enquiry.

## CONCLUSION

It is clear that there are four basic factors underlying public health practice: (i) decision-making that is evidence-based; (ii) a focus on populations rather than individuals; (iii) the goal of social justice and equity; and, (iv) an emphasis on prevention rather than curative care.[65] The development of these factors over time can be seen in the history of public health outlined above, as well as the inherent principles of health visiting.[2,44] Public health and health visiting have a shared history and a shared future. The next chapter will discuss further the development of health visiting in the light of public health and contemporary health visiting practice.

## KEY LEARNING POINTS

- Examination and understanding of the contested concepts of public, health, public health and health promotion.
- Acknowledgement of the waves of public health and their location in a socio-political context over time.
- Examination of health promotion within contemporary public health.
- Examination and understanding of health visiting and public health.
- Acknowledging alternative ways of working.

## FURTHER RESOURCES

Public Health England. https://www.gov.uk/government/organisations/public-health-england.

The King's Fund, Public Health. https://www.kingsfund.org.uk/topics/public-health.

The Best Start in Life. https://www.england.nhs.uk/ltphimenu/children-and-young-people/best-start-in-life/.

What is Public Health? https://www.healthcareers.nhs.uk/working-health/working-public health/what-public-health.

Centre for the History of Public Health. https://www.lshtm.ac.uk/research/centres/centre-history-public-health.

## REFERENCES

1. Lyon, A. (2003). *The fifth wave.* Edinburgh: Scottish Council Foundation.
2. Cowley, S., & Frost, M. (2006). *The principles of health visiting: Opening the door to public health practice in the 21st century.* London: Community Practitioners and Health Visitors' Association.
3. Cowley, S., Whittaker, K., Grigulis, A., Malone, M., Donetto, S., Wood, H., et al. (2013). Why health visiting? A review of the literature about key health visitor interventions, processes and outcomes for children and families. London: National Nursing Research Unit, King's College.
4. Orme, J., Powell, J., Taylor, P., & Grey, M. (Eds.), (2007). Mapping public health. In Public health for the 21st century: New perspectives on policy, participation and practice (2nd ed.). Maidenhead: Open University Press.
5. Verweij, M., & Dawson, A. (2009). The meaning of 'public' in 'public health'. In A. Dawson, & M. Verweij (Eds.), *Ethics, prevention, and public health.* Oxford: Oxford University Press.
6. Baggott, R. (2011). *Public health policy & politics* (2nd ed.). Houndmills, Basingstoke: Palgrave MacMillan.
7. Adetunji, H. A. (2009). Chapter 7: Principles of epidemiology. In Wilson, F., & Mabhala, M. (Eds), *Key concepts in public health.* http://dx.doi.org/10.4135/9781446216736.n8.
8. Middleton, J. (2017). Public health in England in 2016 – the health of the public and the public health system: A review. *British Medical Bulletin, 121*(1), 31–46.
9. Public Health England. (2018). *Improving people's health: Applying behavioural and social sciences to improve population health and well-being in England.* PHE Publications.
10. Naidoo, J., & Wills, J. (2016). *Foundations for health promotion* (4th ed). China: Elsevier.
11. WHO, (1946). Definition of health. Preamble to the Constitution of the World Health Organisation as adopted by the International Health Conference. Geneva: WHO.
12. World Health Organisation. (1986). *Ottawa Charter for Health Promotion, First International Conference on Health Promotion, Ottawa 17–21 November:* Copenhagen: WHO Regional Office for Europe.
13. Aggleton, P. (1990). *Health.* London: Routledge.
14. Naidoo, J., & Wills, J. (2011). *Foundations for health promotion* (4th ed.). Edinburgh: Bailliere Tindall/Elsevier.
15. Verweij, M., & Dawson, A. (2009). The meaning of 'public' in 'public health'. In A. Dawson, & M. Verweij (Eds.), *Ethics, prevention, and public health.* Oxford: Oxford University Press.
16. Acheson, D. (1988). *Public health in England.* London: Department of Health.
17. Wanless, D. (2002). *Securing our future health: Taking a long-term view. Final report.* London: HM Treasury.
18. Winslow, C. E. A. (1920). The untilled fields of public health. *Science, 51,* 23.
19. Beaglehole, R., & Bonita, R. (2004). *Public health at the crossroads: Achievements and prospects* (2nd ed.). Cambridge: Cambridge University Press.
20. Dahlgren, G. & Whitehead, M. (1991). *Policies and strategies to promote social equity in health* (1st ed.). Stockholm: Institute of Future Studies.

21. Morgan, A., & Cragg, L. (2013). Chapter 7: The determinants of health. In L. Cragg, M. Davis, & W. Macdowall (Eds.), *Health promotion theory (understanding public health)* (2nd ed.). Maidenhead: Open University Press.

22. Beaglehole, R., & Bonita, R. (Eds), (1997). *Public health at the crossroads*. Cambridge: Cambridge University Press.

23. Naidoo J., & Wills J. (2016). *Foundations for health promotion* (4th ed.), Edinburgh: Bailliere Tindall.

24. Dworkin, G. (1972). Paternalism. *The Monist, 56*, 64–84.

25. Dworkin, G. (2002). Paternalism. https://plato.stanford.edu/entries/paternalism/. Accessed 2 April 2020.

26. Gostin, L. O. (2007). Meeting the survival needs of the world's least healthy people: A proposed model for global health governance. *The Journal of the American Medical Association, 298*(2), 225–228.

27. Goodin, R. (1995). *Utilitarianism as a public health philosophy*. Cambridge: Cambridge University Press.

28. Scarre, G. (1996). *Utilitarianism*. London: Routledge.

29. Powers, M., & Faden, R. (2006). *Social justice*. New York: Oxford University Press.

30. Wills, J. (2012). Understanding and using theories and models. In L. Jones, & J. Douglas (Eds.), *Public health: Building innovative practice*. London: Sage/Open University Press.

31. Viens, A. M. (2016). Public health and political theory: The importance of taming individualism. *Public Health Ethics, 9*(2), 136–138.

32. Hartig, T., Mitchell, R., de Vries, S., & Frumkin, H. (2014). Nature and health. *Annual Review of Public Health, 35*(1), 207–228.

33. Jones, L., & Douglas, J. (2012). *Public health: Building innovative practice*. London: Sage Publications in association with the Open University.

34. Marmot, M. (2010). Fair society, healthy lives: Strategic review of health inequalities in England. http://www.instituteofhealthequity.org/resources-reports/fair-society-healthy-lives-the-marmot-review/fair-society-healthy-lives-full-report-pdf.pdf. Accessed 28 February 2020.

35. Armstrong, D. (1993). Public health spaces and the fragmentation of identity. *Sociology, 27*(3), 393–410.

36. Hanlon, P., Carlisle, S., Hannah, M., Reilly, D., & Lyon, A. (2011). Making the case for a 'fifth wave' in public health. *Public Health, 125*, 30–36.

37. Detels, R., McEwen, J., Beaglehole, R., & Tanaka, H. (2004). *Oxford textbook of public health* (4th ed.). Oxford: Oxford University Press.

38. Berridge, V., Gorsky, M., & Mold, A. (2011). *Public health in history: Public health, policy and practice*. Maidenhead: Open University Press.

39. Dorling, D. (2013). *Unequal health: The scandal of our times*. Bristol: The Policies Press.

40. Chadwick, E. (1842). *Report on the sanitary conditions of the labouring population of Great Britain*. London: W. Clowes and Sons.

41. Quirke, V., & Gaudilliere, J. (2008). The era of biomedicine: Science, medicine and public health in Britain and France after the Second World War. *Medical History, 52*, 441–452.

42. Marmot, M. (2020). *Health equity in England: The marmot review 10 years on*. http://www.instituteofhealthequity.org/resources-reports/marmot-review-10-years-on. Accessed 28 February 2020.

43. Davies, S., Winpenny, E., Ball, S., Fowler, T., Rubin, J., & Nolte, E. (2014). For debate: A new wave in public health improvement. *The Lancet, 384*, 1889–1895.

44. Council for the Education and Training of Health Visitors (CETHV). (1977). *An investigation into the principles of health visiting*. London: CETHV.

45. Lalonde, M. (1974). *A new perspective on the health of canadians. Ottawa:* Ministry of National Health and Welfare. https://www.phac-aspc.gc.ca/ph-sp/pdf/perspect-eng.pdf. Accessed 28 February 2020.

46. World Health Organisation. (1978). Declaration of Alma Ata. International Conference on Primary Health Care. 6–12 September, Alma Ata, Geneva: WHO.

47. World Health Organisation. (1984). *Health promotion, a discussion document on the concepts and principles*. Copenhagen: WHO.

48. World Health Organisation. (2020). *WHO global health promotion conferences*. https://www.who.int/health-promotion/conferences/en/. Accessed 28 February 2020.

49. World Health Organisation. (2015). *Health in 2015: From MDGs, Millennium Development Goals to SDGs, Sustainable Development Goals*. https://www.who.int/gho/publications/mdgs-sdgs/en/. Accessed 28 February 2020.

50. Beattie, A. (1991). Knowledge and control in health promotion: A test case for social theory. In J. Gabe, M. Calnan, & M. Bury (Eds.), *The sociology of the health service*. London: Routledge; 162–201.

51. Nuffield Council on Bioethics. (2007). Public health ethical issues. https://www.nuffieldbioethics.org/publications/public-health. Accessed 6 March 2020.

52. Dingwall, R. (1977). Collectivism, regionalism and feminism. Health visiting and British social policy 1850–1975. *Journal of Social Policy, 6*, 291–315.

53. Brookes, J., & Rafferty, A. M. (2010). Education and role conflict in the health visitor profession 1918–1939. *Nursing Inquiry, 17*(2), 142–150.

54. Cowley, S., Whittaker, K., Malone, M., Donetto, S., Grigulis, A., & Maben, J. (2015). Why health visiting?

Examining the potential public health benefits from health visiting practice within a universal service: A narrative review of the literature. *International Journal of Nursing Studies, 52*, 465–480. https://doi.org/10.1016/j.ijnurstu.2014.07.013.

55. Keller, L. O., Strohschein, S., Lia-Hoagberg, B., & Schaffer, M. A. (2004). Population-based public health interventions: Practice-based and evidence-supported. Part I. *Public Health Nursing, 21*(5), 453–468.

56. Nursing and Midwifery Council (NMC). (2004). Standards for specialist community public health nurses (updated 2018). https://www.nmc.org.uk/standards/standards-for-post-registration/standards-of-proficiency-for-specialist-community-public-health-nurses/. Accessed 2 April 2020.

57. Public Health England. (2016). *Public health skills and knowledge framework 2016*. PHE Publications.

58. Health and Social Care Act. (2012). London: Stationery Office. http://www.legislation.gov.uk/ukpga/2012/7/contents/enacted. Accessed 2 April 2020.

59. Plews, C., Billingham, K., & Rowe, A. (2000). Public health nursing: Barriers and opportunities. *Health and Social Care in the Community, 8*(2), 138–146.

60. Carr, S. M. (2005). Refocusing health visiting—sharpening the vision and facilitating the process. *Journal of Nursing Management, 13*, 249–256.

61. Lowenhoff, C. (2004). Have talents: Need liberating! *Community Practitioner, 77*(1), 23–25.

62. Department of Health. (2011). *The Health Visitor Implementation Plan 2011–2015*. https://www.gov.uk/government/publications/health-visitor-implementation-plan-2011-to-2015. Accessed 15 March 2020.

63. Local Government Association. (2019) The reduction in the number of health visitors in England briefing paper. https://www.local.gov.uk/sites/default/files/documents/LGA%20briefing%20-%20Reduction%20in%20the%20number%20of%20health%20visitors%20in%20England%20WEB.pdf. Accessed 15 March 2020.

64. Nicola, M., Alsafi, Z., Sohrabi, C., Kerwan, A., Al-Jabir, A., Isoifidis, C., et al. (2020). The socio-economic implications of the Coronavirus pandemic (Covid-19): A review. *International Journal of Surgery, 78*, 185–193.

65. Koplan, J. P., Bond, T. C., Merson, M. H., Reddy, K. S., Rodriguez, M. H., Sewankambo, N. K., et al. (2009). Towards a common definition of global health. *Lancet, 373*, 1993–1995.

# 2

# THE HISTORY OF HEALTH VISITING

MICHELLE MOSELEY ■ KATE PHILLIPS

## CHAPTER CONTENTS

INTRODUCTION

HEALTH VISITING – A GLOBAL
PERSPECTIVE

THE HISTORY OF HEALTH VISITING
WITHIN THE UNITED KINGDOM

THE NEED FOR A HEALTH VISITING
SERVICE

UK HEALTH VISITING IN THE 21ST CENTURY

PROPORTIONATE UNIVERSALISM

EARLY INTERVENTION

PUBLIC HEALTH PRIORITIES

INTEGRATED SERVICES

CONCLUSION

## LEARNING OUTCOMES

*To:*

- explore the history of health visiting and how its evolved since its conception
- develop an understanding of contemporary health visiting practice from a UK-wide perspective, underpinned by the principles of health visiting
- re-visit the principles of health visiting
- compare and contrast health visitor provision across the UK

## INTRODUCTION

This chapter will explore and discuss the history of health visiting, incorporating its relevance in public health and health promotion delivery. Global comparisons of the service will be referred to, leading into its history from conception within the UK to current-day practice. The definition of the principles of health visiting will be key and how they are relevant from an early intervention and prevention perspective. We recognise how the role has evolved over the last 150 years, with a focus on searching for health needs and the relevance of the early intervention and prevention agenda. The role is complex and ever-changing, and its delivery is varied across the UK, as well as 'general' health visiting, specialist health visitor roles also exist.

## HEALTH VISITING – A GLOBAL PERSPECTIVE

Health visiting has been in place for societies since the late 1800s within the United Kingdom (UK), although the term 'health visiting' is specific to the UK, Norway, Finland and Denmark, the role exists in various formats across the world. Sweden uses the term 'Public Health Nurse', Belgium uses the term 'Social Nurse', with Pakistan using the terminology 'Lady Heath Visitor' and 'Lady Health Worker'. In New Zealand, the role is named a 'Plunket nurse'.[1] The New Zealand ethos is making a difference within the first 1000 days of a child's life, to positively impact future generations, giving children the most favourable start in life to enhance their future potential within society. The Plunket nurse role has been in place for over 100 years. Within the United States of America (USA), public health nurses are named 'Maternal Child Nurses': they work within the remit of family–nurse partnerships. The role has been in place for over four decades with the aim to support new mothers with an overarching remit of developing trusting relationships to achieve 'extraordinary outcomes'.[2] The partnership targets new mothers rather than utilising a universal approach to their service. Australia uses the term 'Child Health Nurse', and Russia uses 'District Paediatric Nurse'.[3] Their input/service delivery varies but has a public health focus for children and their families.

In the UK, health visitors are qualified nurses or midwives who have undertaken further training at post-graduate diploma or Masters level to attain the qualification of 'Specialist Community Public Health Nurses (SCPHNs)'. The term SCPHN refers to health visitors, school nurses and occupational health nurses.[4] The level of training varies throughout the UK amongst education providers which are Accredited Educational Institutions (AEIs)/Universities. The qualification can be attained at Level 6 or 7 (Post-graduate Diploma or Masters level). Their remit is to work with children aged 0 to 5 years and their families. The practitioner focus of this chapter is on the role of the health visitor. The term health visitor and SCPHN will be interchanged based on more evolving, contemporary, literature, policy and guidance specific to the role.

## THE HISTORY OF HEALTH VISITING WITHIN THE UNITED KINGDOM

The earliest health visitors were members of the Ladies Sanitary Reform Association and evolved within Manchester and Salford. This association was established in 1852 with records of district nurses and health visitor-type roles being established in 1862. The Association was originally formed to address 'temperance', which relates to moderating certain indulgences (alcohol, appetite), general 'health laws' and 'personal and domestic cleanliness'.[5] The Ladies Sanitary Reform Association was a separate committee within the main association and is recorded as an example of one of the first health visiting services.[6] These early health visitors visited families who had poor living conditions and poor sanitation in a time when infant mortality was significantly high. The first health visiting training programme is recorded as being established in 1892, by Florence Nightingale, who was responsible for the role being developed and used more widely. She recognised the role health visitors could play in supporting the population from a public health perspective and recommended the need for formal training for nurses to develop as health visitors.[7] This was particularly forward-thinking for the time, with Florence Nightingale seeing the benefit of home visiting and the public health role these nurses could undertake. The reputation of Florence Nightingale is well known, deemed as the 'lady of the lamp', she was a nursing visionary of her time and instrumental in caring for the wounded in the Crimea War, and improving sanitation within the field hospital. In 1860, she established the first school of nursing in St Thomas's Hospital, London.[8] The now Royal Society for Public Health (previously the Royal Sanitary Institute), established the first recognised education programmes for health visitors in 1916. The first statutory qualification is dated from 1919 and was awarded from the Ministry of Health. The programme was equally divided between theory and practice.[6]

The 1919 programme included:

*'elementary physiology, methods of artisan cookery and household management, hygiene, infectious and communicable diseases, maternity and infant child welfare and elementary economics and social problems'.*[7,6:3].

It seems health visiting in the early 1900s had a grasp on the health needs of the populations they served, and they responded to those needs as they changed. The Notification of Birth Acts of 1907[9] and 1915[10] and the Maternity and Child Welfare Act of 1918[11] promoted the development of maternal and child services, and this led to the development of the first health visiting education programme. The content of that 1919 health-visiting programme reflected the health needs of the time: poor sanitation and reducing the rise of deaths from infectious diseases. From 1945, health visitors were expected to have a midwifery and/or nursing qualification prior to commencing their training. This was governed by the then Ministry of Health.[6] Health visitor caseloads from 1918 are recorded as one health visitor to 400 births; this was later reduced in the 1930s to one health visitor per 250 births.[12]

The National Health Service (NHS) was established in 1948, and the health-visiting role was recognised as essential in relation to working with parents, especially focussing on the health and well-being of mothers and their children. The role of the health visitor began to broaden and expand, though there was some confusion as to where it sat – with general practitioners in primary care settings, or with medical officers within the hospital setting.[13] The Jameson Report referred to the working party who trained and recruited *'visitors'* and the Younghusband Report[14] defined social work practice. To provide further clarity, Jameson[15] defined health visitors as *'generalist case finders'* due to how they accessed families within their

homes. Social workers were defined as *'case workers'*, as the families they dealt with had particular problems. It could be argued that the roles overlap from a social well-being perspective. Today, health visitors, social workers and social care teams work in partnership with each other, especially from a safeguarding perspective, but also within the remit of early intervention and prevention.

As the health visiting role became more established, health visiting became a statutory body with the first principles of health visiting being established in 1977 (Council for the Education of health visitors (CETHV)).[16] The role continues to evolve (Table 2.1). By the 1970s, it was defined as a professional practice which:

*consists of planned activities aimed at the promoting of health and prevention of ill health. It therefore contributes substantially to individual and social well-being, by focussing attention at various times on either an individual, a social group or a community*[16:7]

The role of the health visitor has evolved over the past century, as has the definition. Cowley and Frost[17] define health visiting as consisting of 'planned activities', which relate to improving the health and well-being of the population. These activities encompass the individual's physical, mental, emotional and social well-being with an aim of preventing disease and reducing health inequalities, the main aim of health visiting being to empower families in improving their health and well-being status. They do this by identifying health needs and working within the remit of their four principles,[17:1] which are:

- The search for health needs.
- The stimulation of an awareness of the health needs.
- The influence of policies affecting health.
- The facilitation of an awareness of health needs.

### TABLE 2.1

| Year | Key developments within health visiting 1970–2020 |
|------|--------------------------------------------------|
| 1970 | Council for the Education and Training of health visitors (CETHV) established |
| 1975 | CETHV and Council for the Education and Training of Social Workers separated. All nursing bodies reviewed. |
| 1977 | Principles of health visiting defined by CETHV |
| 1979 | Nurses, Midwives and Health Visitor Act |
| 1983 | CETHV abolished. United Kingdom Central Council for Nursing, Midwifery and Health Visiting (UKCC) developed. |
| 1984 | English and Welsh National Nursing Boards established |
| 2001 | Nursing and Midwifery Council (NMC) removed health visiting as a distinct profession in statute |
| 2004 | Health visiting register closed. The new register included health visitors as Specialist Community Public Health Nurses (SCPHNs). |
| 2004 | SCPHN, NMC proficiency standards published |
| 2006 | Principles of health visiting reviewed by Cowley and Frost |
| 2009 | Healthy Child Programme launched[18] |
| 2010 | UK government review of health visiting – commitment to increase health visiting numbers by 4200 in England[19] |
| 2010 | A Framework for the Child Health Promotion Programme in Northern Ireland[20] |
| 2012 | 150 years of health visiting celebrations |
| 2012 | 'A Vision for Health Visiting' (Welsh government 2012) launched in Wales[21] |
| 2015 | Universal Health Visiting Pathway – Scotland[22] |
| 2016 | Launch of the Healthy Child (Wales) Programme[23] |
| 2019 | A review of health visiting in England undertaken by the Institute of Health Visiting (iHV)[24] |

These four principles continue to be as relevant today as they were in the 1970s, when they were developed. They underpin health visitor practice within the UK. They are also relatable to the earlier health visiting practice of the late 19th century, where there was a clear search for health needs, with appropriate interventions being delivered to families within their local areas. Health visitors work collaboratively with families and the community with an aim to improve and enhance children's health, well-being and development. They advise, educate and empower individuals and families, as well as the wider agencies they work with. The principles are fundamental daily health visiting practice.

### THINKING SPACE

*If you are a health visitor*, reflect on how you apply the principles of health visiting to your daily practice. Are you supported by resources which allow health needs to be met? If not, how can you influence that? Think about how you use the principles proactively to enhance service delivery.

*If you are student*, think about how health visitors apply the principles of health visiting in practice to improve the health and well-being of individuals and their families. Here are some example scenarios:

A young family with their first baby is having difficulty maintaining breastfeeding.

A family states that they want to wean their 16-week infant onto solid food.

You receive two Accident and Emergency Department notifications relating to two children in the same family, aged 2 and 4. The injuries include: the 2-year-old sustained a scald from tea. The 4-year-old attended with a bruised forehead after falling off a trampoline.

A father discloses that his mental health has deteriorated since the birth of his daughter 6 weeks ago.

The health needs of populations are evolving constantly, and health professionals respond to these as governed by policy, legislation and recommendations from public health bodies, such as: the World Health Organisation (WHO), departments of health and country-specific public health departments. Pertinent public health, health promotion and safeguarding policy from a macro (global), meso (national, UK) and micro level (home nation or local) perspective, underpin health visitor practice along with the most up-to-date evidence-based research. Health visitors are a skilled workforce undergoing further training from their nursing and/or midwifery qualifications to gain the Specialist Community Public Health Nursing–Health Visitor qualification.

The health visiting curriculum from the early 1900s is somewhat replicated in today's SCPHN programmes across the UK in line with the SCPHN, NMC standards.[4] The academic programme is still divided between 50% theory and 50% practice, as it was in the early 1900s. Although the content of the programme has changed drastically, there are some elements of similarity with a focus of promoting the general health and well-being of families. Today's health visiting curriculum varies across higher education institutions (HEIs). All programmes are validated by the NMC and, in general, broadly consist of: research skills in health and social care improvement, contemporary approaches to health visiting practice, health promotion and public health, leadership in health visiting and safeguarding children and young people.

The health needs of the 21st century reflect global and national drivers to reduce the impact of obesity, non-communicable disease, poor dental health and poor mental health. Caseload sizes currently vary across the UK and service delivery is very different within the home nations (Wales, Scotland, England and Northern Ireland). The Community Practitioner and Health Visitor Association (CPHVA) continue to recommend a ratio of one health visitor per 250 births, but this is exceeded in many areas, according to anecdotal evidence. Some areas within the UK report caseloads of 800–1000 children. The Department of Health[25] recommends one health visitor per child under the age of 5. The iHV[24] continues to support the recommendation of 250 children per caseload, which should be reduced if the caseload is categorised as high need or deprived.

The health-visiting role has never been more significant within the 21st century with an emphasis on the delivery of necessary, early intervention and prevention. The recent Marmot Review[26] depicts a static life expectancy in England and gross health inequality continues; this is not dissimilar to the health inequality in the other home nations of the UK. In 2010, within Marmot's Fair Society, Healthy Lives, six areas of policy change were recommended.[27] This was published after the health visitor implementation plan – A Call to Action.[19] The six key areas identified were:

- Providing children with the best start in life.
- Enabling society – children, young people and adults – to reach their potential within their lives.
- The creation of 'fair' employment and 'good work for all'.
- Exposure to a 'healthy standard of living'.
- The creation of healthy and 'sustainable' communities.[26:3]

The key areas identified by Marmot in 2010 are particularly applicable to health visiting practice and underpinned the drive for more health visitors in England at that time. All of the above policy objectives are crucial to improve the health and well-being of our future generations and health visitors, by delivering the principles of health visiting, and can play a key role in early intervention to improve general health and well-being and influence policies that affect health.

## THINKING SPACE

What are the caseload numbers in your area? Do they sit above 250?

Identify any inequalities in your area of practice?

Think about how/if the resources available support the families in your caseloads, and how you influence their general health and well-being.

## THE NEED FOR A HEALTH VISITING SERVICE

Cowley et al[28] set out to explore the benefits of a universal health visiting service and rationalise its positive impact on wider health improvement measures and in the reduction of health inequalities. Their aim was to determine what health visitors do, and the extent in which their role and purpose is reflected in England's Call for Action Health Visitor (HV) Implementation Plan.[19] Their results – following a systematic, narrative analysis – showed that health visiting practice is 'characterized by a particular orientation to practice' (p465). This characterisation refers to health visitors' values, skills and attitudes, which enables them to carry out a universal service. This universal service relates to a 'core' service provided by health visitors. The core health visiting service varies across the UK, but the common thread is that the health visitor remit covers working with children and their families, from birth to 5 years. The universal service within the Cowley et al[28] paper refers to the importance of the first 1000 days. This is the time from pregnancy up to the child's second birthday.[29] It's a time when intervention from a health visitor can positively influence parenting, attachment, feeding decisions (breast or formula), as well as form a therapeutic relationship whilst searching for health needs.

Cowley et al[28] refer to salutogenesis, a concept explored by Aaron Antovosky.[30] It has a central role within public health and health promotion. Promoting health and working within public health agendas are two key practice roles undertaken by health visitors on a daily basis. Cowley et al,[28:465] define salutogenesis as 'health creating'. Salutogenesis is thought to be essential in addressing issues and raising the key public health agenda through promoting health. Antovosky's focus was prioritising the needs of people by working within their strengths and capacity and within the resources available – to promote

health.[31] Therefore, as a concept, salutogenesis fits with, and is demonstrated to be within, HV practice. It is also shown to be within the four principles of health visiting. These refer to searching for health needs, stimulating an awareness of health needs, the facilitation of health enhancing activities and the influence on polices that affect health.[17] Health visitors build therapeutic relationships with clients, assessing their needs, their capacity, and how they can address specific health needs locally with the resources available to them. The aim is to promote positive health and wellbeing – hence, creating health and demonstrating a salutogenic approach to their practice.

The Cowley et al[28] narrative review captures how health visiting could look in an ideal world. It has a thought-provoking title of 'Why health visiting?', which prompts discussion around problematising health visiting and its role in healthcare, and subsequently, British society. Health visiting practice is underpinned by the principles as identified above, as well as observing and monitoring child development, prevention, detection and supporting in safeguarding children and young people, leadership and research applicable to its field.[17,32] The first 3 years of a child's life are critical in building foundations for their future, and this is well documented.[33] The first 1000 days are a time where attachments to close family members and carers are built; the child starts an explorative journey, learning and communicating at a fast rate. This includes brain development, where building blocks are set in place for future health and wellbeing.[33] Epigenetics also needs to be taken into consideration. This is a new concept within scientific research that purports that gene structure can be altered based on early childhood experiences.[34] This supports research undertaken by Bellis et al[35] in relation to the impact of adverse childhood experiences in adult life. Therefore, the need for a service which accesses pregnant women and their families, as well as within early childhood, is essential. These therapeutic relationships have the potential to offer support and enhance or 'generate positive epigenetic structures that activate genetic potential'.[34] The health visitor is well placed, therefore, to support families with their pre-school children.

Cowley et al[28] reflect on what is known about the early years and the role health visitors play. During these early years of child development, parents/carers require support in various formats. This could be one-to-one support, group support or signposting for specific support. For example, from a voluntary agency, such as Women's Aid or Barnardo's. Both of these agencies offer specific support based on the service user's need. The support health visitors offer is vast. As already mentioned, it could relate to feeding problems (breast or formula), and assessment of attachment. It can also include support sleep issues, weaning (commencement of solid food), parental mental health, parental substance misuse, post-natal depression or psychoses, housing difficulties, child development concerns, responses to hospital admissions or accidents and domestic abuse or child protection concerns. A home visiting service utilising the health visitor role has been deemed an effective and essential one in offering such support,[28] and use of a targeted approach is based on the health needs of the family. A targeted approach is used throughout the UK in varying formats. The purpose of this targeted, universal approach is to offer all children and their families support and advice, and to offer a 'progressive' universal approach, which allows them to be supported. For those with the greatest needs, this support will be enhanced.[36] The targeted approach throughout the UK is addressed later on within this chapter as the number of contacts health professionals have with families varies across all UK home nations. The aim of these contacts from the antenatal period is to offer a best start in life allowing individuals to meet their full potential emotionally and physically. The health visitor has contact within the child's first 5 years, when the aforementioned relationships can be established, and when they can make 'every contact count' in relation to delivering health promotion messages and promoting behaviour change with the aim of mitigating non-communicable disease in later years.[37] This is supported by research relating to early identification of adverse childhood experiences by health visitors[38] and emphasises a need for an increased awareness of epigenetics.

Cowley et al[28] relate the role of the health visitor to the seminal work of theorists, namely, Antonovsky,[39] Rogers[40] and Brofenbrenner.[41] This offers further evidence to demonstrate the validity of the health visitor role and its place in nursing and society, particularly from an early intervention and prevention perspective, linking once again to the potential enhancement of life chances influenced by behaviour change. Antonovsky's work in relation to salutogenesis[39] is linked to the pro-activeness health visitors demonstrate in identifying need and their solution-focussed approach. By applying the principles of health visiting, client needs are established and acted upon. Health visitors recognise that any intervention is 'needs led' by the client (the parent/carer within health visiting practice). Bradshaw[42] defines this as 'felt need'. Health visitors value the person; they offer a person-/client-centred approach to any intervention. Hence, the link to Rogers.[40]

Rogers'[40] work is extremely relevant to the underpinning ethos of health visiting practice, which seeks to empower individuals and help them realise their full potential. This refers to children here as well as parents/carers. Rogers' theory[40] considers the personal growth of individuals: every person can grow, but they need a certain environment to do this, a positive environment, where they can express themselves, be open and honest and feel accepted. Once goals or wishes are achieved, self-actualisation takes place. This self-belief offers a way forward for individuals, especially if a behaviour change is involved or change in lifestyle, parenting style and feeling empowered to leave an abusive relationship. The feeling of self-worth (self-efficacy) is powerful in motivating change. Health visitors are key professionals in delivering such interventions in their work with families based on building therapeutic relationships of respect and mutual trust.

The UK home nations offer the health visiting service in different ways, and it appears the priorities of governments vary. The priorities here relate to health visitor provision throughout the UK. Devolution has evolved in the last century, with all four home nations taking further responsibility away from central Parliament. Each home nation has its own public health department, which is also instrumental in the delivery of health services. The latter half of this chapter will explore how health visiting is delivered in each of the UK home nations.

### THINKING SPACE

What is salutogenesis?

How do you apply a salutogenic approach within your health visiting practice, with the resources available to you?

Are you an influencer within your own caseload, local area or an influencer of policy?

Think about the importance of influencing policy affecting health.

## UK HEALTH VISITING IN THE 21ST CENTURY

Throughout history, the underpinning philosophy of the health visiting service has not changed and remains committed to improve the health and well-being of children, families and communities, ensuring they are not disadvantaged by their social and environmental circumstances. Health visitors in the 21st century continue to provide a public health universal service to families with children aged 0 to 5 years in local communities

by assessing health needs and providing support and practical advice that promotes good health and well-being. Contemporary health visiting practice continues to evolve and develop in response to new emerging evidence, political direction and the changing needs of society. Political strategic direction across the four nations of the United Kingdom is driven to prioritise the importance of early intervention and laying firm foundations for optimum health and well-being from conception to adulthood. Thus, this is the important role health visitors play in optimising the health and well-being of children, maximising this contribution and ensuring it remains effective and evidence-based. This standard of practice was recommended within the National Service Framework for Children, Young People and Maternity Services,[43] and interpreted as,

> *The health and well-being of all children and young people is promoted and delivered through a co-ordinated programme of action, including prevention and early intervention wherever possible, to ensure long term gain, led by the NHS in partnership with local authorities.* (p21)

The four commissioning governments within the UK have committed to implementing this standard and have developed regional programmes of action which provide an evidence-based framework for health visiting practice. This is referred to as the Healthy Child Programme[18] in England, Healthy Child, Healthy Future in Northern Ireland,[20] the Universal Health Visiting Pathway in Scotland[22] and the Healthy Child Wales Programme.[23] These programmes outline a universal public health approach which is delivered within the respective nations and focuses on preventative early intervention. This is implemented through a list of contacts that offers health surveillance, immunisations, developmental reviews, screening and health promotion that supports positive parenting and healthy choices.[18]

| TABLE 2.2 |
| --- |
| *Strong parent–child attachment and positive parenting, resulting in better social and emotional well-being among children.* |
| *Care that helps to keep the child healthy and safe.* |
| *Healthy eating and increased activity, leading to a reduction in obesity.* |
| *Prevention of some serious and communicable disease.* |
| *Increased rates of initiation and continuation of breastfeeding.* |
| *Readiness for school and improved learning.* |
| *Early recognition of growth disorders and risk factors for obesity.* |
| *Early detection and action to address developmental delay, abnormalities and ill health, as well as concerns about safety.* |
| *Identification of factors that could influence the health and well-being of families.* |
| *Better short- and long-term outcomes for children who are at risk of social exclusion.* [18:8] |

The expected outcomes of the programmes can be seen in Table 2.2:

Political investment in the success of these programmes was also reflected within the Health Visitor Implementation Plan 2011–2015,[44] which strived to increase the HV workforce in England to continue to improve accessibility and ensure all families have access to the practical support they need to reach their optimum health and development. All families should have access to this salutogenic approach, which demonstrates positive regard and works in accordance with families' individual needs and attributes. Although the differing child health programmes have differing models of assessment, intervention and mandated contacts, the evidence informing the programme remains the same and is underpinned by the recommendations within 'Health for All' (4th ed).[45] The principles underpinning the programme are therefore similar and will be explored individually from a four nations' perspective.

## PROPORTIONATE UNIVERSALISM

Health visiting practice has a fundamental vision to improve the health and well-being of children and families, with a particular focus on promoting health equity. A key challenge within this approach is the growing evidence of health inequalities, which result in unavoidable and unfair health differences between differing population groups. This concept is defined by the World Health Organisation[45] as,

*Differences in health status or in the distribution of health resources between different population groups, arising from the social conditions in which people are born, grow, live work and age* (p1)

These health differences occur due to the social circumstances in which families and communities live, such as having a low income, poor housing, lack of access to services and transport links. This is also referred to as the social determinants of health, which can directly influence or limit the lifestyle choices that are made in relation to health.[45] Children that are nurtured and growing up in families and communities which are experiencing potential social and economic deprivation are at risk of experiencing poorer outcomes in relation to their long-term health and developmental well-being. 'Fair Society, Healthy Lives: The Strategic Review of Health Inequalities in England' post-2010[27] recognised this steep social gradient to health outcomes and recommended an approach to preventative service delivery to reduce the gap between the rich and the poorer members of society. This approach is known as 'Proportionate Universalism', whereby there is universal provision of preventative services with a more targeted approach offered in response to identified need.[27] This has influenced how health visiting practice is organised and developed to support health equity and reduce this unfair social demographic gradient related to health. Health visitors are highly skilled in working with families and searching for health needs, with a particular focus on assessing the social and environmental circumstances, and how these are putting children and families at risk of experiencing poorer outcomes in relation to their health and well-being. Support and interventions are therefore provided to an intensity equivalent to the level of need or the evidence-based risk factors identified for poor health outcomes.[27]

## England

In England, the Healthy Child Programme[18] implements the 4-5-6 Model of Health Visiting Support,[46] refer to Figure 2.1.

This framework of service delivery advocates a schedule of five mandated health visiting contacts. These include an antenatal health promoting visit, new baby review, 6- to 8-week assessment, 1-year review, 2- to 2.5-year review. During each contact, the health visitor will work in partnership with families and utilise their skills in searching for health needs, with a particular

focus on identifying health risks related to the 'six high impact areas'. These include[46]:

- Parenthood and Early Years
- Maternal Mental Health
- Breastfeeding
- Healthy Weight
- Minor Illness and Accidents
- Healthy two-year-olds and getting ready for school

The individual needs which have been identified and measured against the six high impact areas will be translated into a level of service delivery which is appropriate and proportionate to the identified level of need. In other words, the

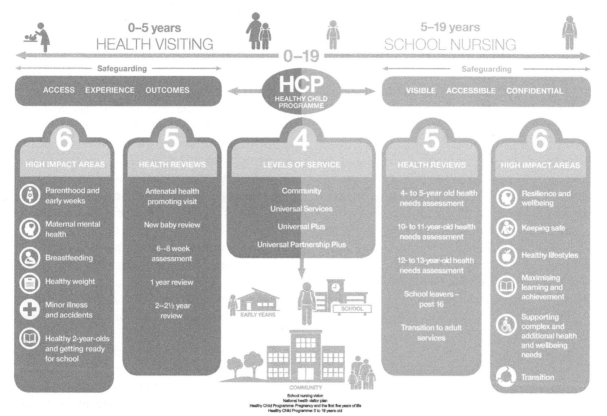

Figure 2.1 ▪ Healthy child programme[2] implements the 4-5-6 model of health visiting support. (Courtesy Public Health England.)

level of ongoing support and preventative intervention from the health visiting service will be planned and implemented in response to the individualised health risks identified within the family. The level of service and intensity is interpreted into four levels[47]:

**Community:** Community-based interventions to support and promote health and well-being, including parenting groups and baby massage groups.

**Universal Services:** The health visitor provides universal mandated contacts as part of the Healthy Child Programme and underpinned by evidence-based guidelines.

**Universal Plus:** More intensive support is provided from the health visitor to address identified needs in partnership with families: this could include breastfeeding support, weaning advice or positive parenting support.

**Universal Partnership Plus:** Ongoing support to address more complex needs and risk factors, which can include utilising the skills and expertise of other professionals and community services.

The assessment of need is a continual process within all mandated contacts, and the level of service provision required will be adapted in response to identified changing needs.

## Northern Ireland

The Healthy Child, Healthy Future early intervention programme in Northern Ireland[20] provides a framework of preventative intervention from pregnancy to 19 years. To capture this extended age range, an integrated and co-ordinated approach is foreseen between the health visiting service and the school nursing services to ensure intensive provision can be provided to children who may be looked after or requiring special educational provision. From the health visiting perspective, families can expect to receive five mandated health visitor contacts, including: a new baby review at home from 10–14 days, a 6–8 week review at home by the health visitor, a 14–16 week health visitor review at home, a 1-year review at home by the health visitor, a 2- to 2.5-year health review at home by the health visitor. During these contacts, health visitors will work in partnership with families to understand their individual circumstances and potential health needs in order to offer interventions to improve health and reduce the risk of poor outcomes. The level of need is interpreted through the application of the 'Understanding the Needs of Children in Northern Ireland, Thresholds of Need' model,[48] which offers a structured approach to interpret the level of targeted service provision that is required for each individual family. Service provision is categorised into four levels, refer to Figure 2.2. As interpreted in the 4-5-6 model, families can move between differing levels of service provision in response to positive service outcomes and their changing needs.

**Level 1: Base population**
Families independently access universal community and health visiting services through the universal mandated contacts.

**Level 2: Children with additional needs**
Families will be offered enhanced assistance from universal community and health visiting services in response to identified areas of vulnerability, including parenting support groups, breastfeeding support and postnatal emotional support.

**Level 3: Children in need**
Children who have been identified to meet the threshold to be classified under 'Article 18 of the Children Order (1995)[48] as 'Children in Need'. They will require community-based social care services to promote and safeguard their health and well-being.

**Level 4: Children with complex/acute needs**
These children have levels of health needs which are acute and complex due to disability

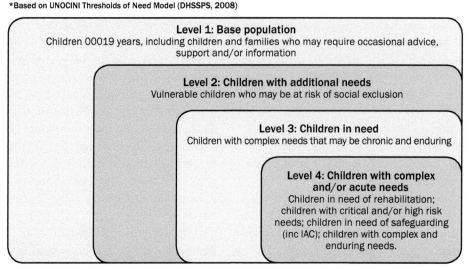

*Based on UNOCINI Thresholds of Need Model (DHSSPS, 2008)

**Level 1: Base population**
Children 00019 years, including children and families who may require occasional advice, support and/or information

**Level 2: Children with additional needs**
Vulnerable children who may be at risk of social exclusion

**Level 3: Children in need**
Children with complex needs that may be chronic and enduring

**Level 4: Children with complex and/or acute needs**
Children in need of rehabilitation; children with critical and/or high risk needs; children in need of safeguarding (inc IAC); children with complex and enduring needs.

*Varied model due to the age range up to 19 years as opposed to 18 years within UNOCINI

Figure 2.2 ■ Understanding the needs of children in northern ireland, thresholds of need model.[12] (Courtesy of Public Health England.)

or vulnerability due to their family circumstances. They require support and intervention from a multi-disciplinary perspective to protect their physical, social and emotional health and well-being.

## Scotland

The Universal Health Visiting Pathway in Scotland[22] strengthens the philosophy and importance of a person-centred approach to practice by integrating the 'Named person role'. All families are therefore allocated a named health visitor who is available and responsive to the changing needs of their allocated families, and work in partnership to provide information, advice and access to services that will promote and safeguard their health and well-being. The programme offers 11 mandated contacts, refer to Figure 2.3. Eight are provided in the first year of life and three child health reviews between 13 months and 4 to 5 years. The family's individual circumstances and the wider context in which they live remain at the centre during each contact, through the implementation of what is called a 'Triad of interconnected core

practice'.[22:7] This includes the development of a therapeutic relationship through home visiting and an individualised health needs assessment. It could be argued that, due to the extensive number of contacts within the first year of life, health visitors in Scotland can truly focus on early intervention and be highly responsive to the needs of families during this vulnerable stage in a child's life when the foundations for health and well-being are being established. It is anticipated that the high number of contacts will support the development of a therapeutic family/HV relationship, which will promote trust in families and facilitate the engagement and uptake of services that may be necessary to address identified needs. Thus, it is instrumental in reducing health inequalities by providing a gateway for families that may be difficult to reach or have difficulties accessing traditional services.

## Wales

The Healthy Child Wales Programme[23] was instrumental in developing a core set of universal contacts to ensure all children received equality

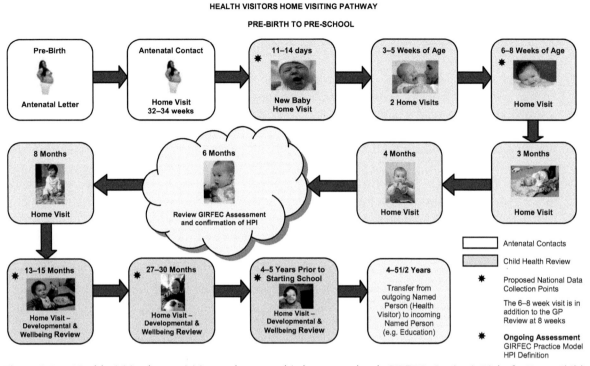

**HEALTH VISITORS HOME VISITING PATHWAY**

**PRE-BIRTH TO PRE-SCHOOL**

Figure 2.3 ■ Health visiting home visiting pathway pre-birth to pre-school. GIRFEC, Getting it Right for Every Child; GP, General Practitioner; HPI, Health Plan Indicator. (Courtesy of Public Health England.)

of access to preventative services and early intervention. Families are provided with nine mandated contacts, an antenatal visit, a birth visit within 14 days, a growth assessment at 8, 12 and 16 weeks, 6, 15, 27 and 3.5 months. It is anticipated that health visiting intervention may be increased according to the level of vulnerability and health need. The programme is proactive in recognising the impact of poverty and working in partnership with families to recognise their circumstances that put them at risk of health inequalities. The health visitor's assessment of need will include a professional assessment of family resilience. This activity encourages professionals to consider the wider context in which children live and identify and addresses the possible social economic and environmental determinants that increase the risk of poorer health outcomes. The 'Family Resilience Assessment Instrument Tool' (FRAIT) is used to measure these negative family

influences in conjunction with the factors that would have a protective influence.[23] An individualised family-centred plan of care is developed to address these potential areas of concern by working to strengthen protective factors and the overall family's resilience.

The Welsh health visiting service is particularly unique, as it delivers an intensive model of targeted service provision in identified areas of high economic and social disadvantage. The service is referred to as Flying Start. It is implemented through a collection of intensive targeted services, which aims to support a child's overall development, including language, cognitive, social, emotional and physical.[49] This is achieved by supporting parents to provide the environment and resources that will empower their children to reach their full developmental potential by facilitating access to practical support and positive parenting advice.[50] A four-entitlement approach is used to deliver this overall service which consists of evidence-based practice demonstrated to be effective. These four elements include[49]:

- *Enhanced Health Services: Increased health visiting support.* A family's health needs are assessed by their named health visitor and empowered to access the services within the programme to address their individual needs.
- *Parenting Programmes*: Supporting parents in their role and assisting them to acquire new parenting skills if necessary.
- *Childcare Provision*: Free part-time nursery provision for 2-year-olds, providing these children with a stimulating play environment that will assist in their learning processes and overall development. Parents are able to use this free time for respite or to enter employment or training.
- *Intensive support* for speech, language and communication development.

The main aim of Flying Start is to enhance a child's future health and developmental well-being, particularly to enhance their school performance by aiming to tackle and reduce the adverse effects of economic deprivation that influence a child's life chances and experiences.[50] The service is built on the philosophy that if parents access support through the services of Flying Start to provide the resources necessary to positively nurture their children, it can assist in reversing the negative effects of economic disadvantage. The service is targeted at families residing in geographical areas with a high prevalence of households receiving welfare provision. These defined areas are identified by postcode, and all families residing within these localities will have universal access to the Flying Start services. This unique selection process has tried to ensure the programme operates in areas of increased economic and social deprivation. However, as this selection process is not based on families' specific

needs, it could be argued that there is a potential risk of the service not reaching all families experiencing economic disadvantage. Flying Start teams consist of multi-disciplines from health, education and the local authority recognising that a multi-agency approach is required to address the diverse needs of families.[49] Health visitors, however, drive the service by signposting families to the unique support and interventions provided within the programme in response to their individual level of need. Families will receive the same health visiting provision outlined within the universal programme with full access to the Flying Start service entitlement. Flying Start health visitors have smaller caseload numbers, which enable them to provide more intensive individualised support.

## THINKING SPACE

Compare the UK's home nations health visiting core programme to the country you practice within. What are the main differences?
   Are you able to deliver a full core programme?

## EARLY INTERVENTION

The proposed framework of health visiting practice, within all the differing child health programmes across the four nations, is investing in the philosophy which supports the importance of early intervention. Early intervention involves supporting and empowering parents to provide a secure and loving environment for their child so that strong foundations for health and well-being can be built within the most influential stage of development. This approach to service provision has been driven by the expanding evidence base focusing on the principles of neuro development during early child development. When children are born, their developing brain is only at 25% capacity, and they experience a period of rapid neurological development during the first few years of life to achieve 80% capacity by the age of 3.[51–53]

This rapid development is heavily influenced by the parenting and experiences that are encountered during this crucial stage of development. The Harvard University Center on the Developing Child[52–54] and the Early Years Foundation[55] have continually documented how early experiences can influence long-term development and even alter gene expression. A child's genetic structure and the bodily expression of said genes are operated by a system known as epigenome. The epigenome is highly responsive and adapted to the child life experiences, and this will determine how the genes are activated and expressed within the body, particularly how they influence brain and behavioural development. The facilitation of a positive and stimulating environment has the capacity to unlock the epigenome's capacity for effective learning long term. Alternatively, exposure to negative experiences, which increases the stress response activation has the potential to change the chemistry of the genes and alter how they function and build capacity for effective learning.[52–54] These experiences could include unresponsive care due to parental mental health, high parental conflict or social and economic deprivation. Powell[20] also recognised how the social and economic circumstances in which people live can create social stress and influence the parental ability and available resources to provide a predictable and safe nurturing environment for children. This includes circumstances of unemployment, low income or homelessness. Prolonged exposure to a stressful environment can permanently alter an infant's brain architecture, making them more vulnerable to emotional and behavioural difficulties and physical ailments. Therefore, the early years are a pivotal stage when the brain architecture can be empowered to build a strong emotional and social structure to facilitate effective learning and future positive health outcomes.[51]

When infants are born, they have the capacity to learn and retain information, but they need to be exposed to positive experiences to build a firm foundation for their future health and well-being.[52,53] This can be effectively facilitated through a responsive care giving and supportive environment. When parents are emotionally responsive and attuned to their child's needs, thus including ensuring their basic care needs are met and their social and emotional needs are fulfilled through predictability, interaction and play.[54] This helps an infant to feel secure and build a strong attachment to their parents. This not only facilitates motivation to explore and build cognitive capabilities for lifelong learning but empowers the development of a firm social and emotional capacity, to manage their emotions and become resilient to unfamiliar situations and stressful experiences.[52–54] This positive care giving environment provides the right trajectory for social and emotional competence in later life and the ability to persevere and adapt to life challenges and experiences without adversity, thus becoming more socially and economically prosperous and productive in adulthood.[51] The National Institute for Health and Care Excellence (NICE)[56] has recognised the detrimental impact this aspect of development can have on the long-term health and well-being of children by stating,

*Good Social, emotional and psychological health helps protect children against emotional and behavioural problems, violence and crime, teenage pregnancy and the misuse of drugs and alcohol* (p7)

This crucial stage in a child's development is known as the first 1000 days, from conception to a child's second birthday.[57,58] Defined by Powell[59] as,

*The first 1,000 days, from a child's conception to age 2, is a critical period. During this time of heightened vulnerability, the foundations of a child's health and development (physical, cognitive, social and emotional and behavioural development) are laid and a trajectory is established* (p7)

Graham Allen, Member of Parliament (MP), was instrumental in guiding political direction towards the importance of considering this growing evidence base in his independent report, 'Early Intervention: The Next Steps' to the HM Government'.[51] This report outlined the importance of early intervention in supporting school readiness, ensuring it remained a public health priority. This philosophy underpins the preventative public health programmes across all countries of the UK providing a framework of health visiting service provision, which is directed by evidence-based early intervention within the first 1000 days of life. The health visiting service utilises this crucial window of opportunity to support and empower parents to provide the right conditions to promote their child's cognitive, social and emotional development. Health visitors have universal contacts with all families within this influential period of development commencing within the antenatal period and beyond. They are therefore in a unique position to support families to provide a supportive and nurturing environment that will encourage their children to meet their projected milestones in relation to their social and emotional development.

These contacts are also undertaken at an influential stage in family life when parents are highly responsive to health education and making lifestyle changes.[60] Through the implementation of the health visiting principles,[16] health visitors are highly skilled in searching for health needs and identifying children at particular risk of poorer outcomes in relation to the circumstances in which they live or through the experiences in which they have encountered. Health visitors are proactive in identifying vulnerability and motivating families to focus on their child's needs and engage in interventions and access available support services.[17] Through the use of individualised assessments, families who are trajected for poorer outcomes in relation to their children's social, emotional and cognitive development or dealing with social stresses, can be supported through evidence-based targeted interventions to promote their health and well-being. Ultimately, this approach will reduce health inequalities and ensure all children have access to the same opportunities or positive life experiences to achieve their optimum health and well-being. This has been further reiterated within Fair Society, Healthy Lives, the strategic review of health inequalities in England post-2010,[27] which reinforces the importance of this approach and the implementation of this service direction,

*Giving every child the best start in life is crucial to reducing health inequalities across the life course. The foundations for virtually every aspect of development – physical, intellectual and emotional, are laid in early childhood. What happens during these years (starting in the womb) has lifelong effects on many aspects of health and well-being (p22)*

## PUBLIC HEALTH PRIORITIES

A fundamental requirement within all four of the universal child health programmes is that health visitors have a responsibility to identify and address key public health priorities at each mandated contact. These public health priorities are guided by a measurement of the population's health needs through the collection of epidemiological data and the public health policy implementation that is developed to address the health needs, through evidence-based interventions and the allocation of resources. The public health approach and the allocation of resources will differ slightly across the UK in order to address and target the individual health needs influencing each nation. These can be reviewed in the public health strategies for each nation, which include Public Health Priorities for Scotland,[61] Public Health England Strategy 2020 to 2025,[62] Working to Achieve a Healthier

Future for Wales,[63] and Making Life Better.[64] All four strategies value the importance of early intervention and supporting families to promote a nurturing environment for their children to grow during the most influential stage of development, being the first 1000 days, thus laying the trajectory for their future health and well-being and their projected economic productivity long term. The Universal Child Health Programmes across the UK provide a framework of mandated contacts. Each mandated contact is a valuable opportunity, whereby key public health messages can be delivered by the health visiting service to motivate and empower families to make health enhancing choices that will have a long-term positive impact on the future health and well-being of their family.[23] These key public health priorities, assessed and reviewed at each mandated contact in accordance with the age and stage of development of the child, are detailed below[65]:

### Key public health priorities

- *Antenatal contact to lay the foundation for positive health behaviours and choices and identify potential risk factors in relation to social and environment circumstances prior to the baby's birth. Information and support will be provided regarding nutrition, breastfeeding, infant safe sleeping and the transition to parenthood.*
- *To promote the initiation and continuation of breastfeeding as the main source of infant nutrition from birth to 6 months of age.*
- *The promotion of a responsive and highly attuned parenting style, which supports the development of bonding and a secure attachment to develop.*
- *To support the facilitation of a healthy and safe nurturing environment, whereby a child is free from second-hand smoke exposure and has a safe sleeping environment to reduce the risk of sudden infant death syndrome.*
- *To promote the uptake of the immunisation programme and the national screening programme.*
- *The promotion of parental emotional health and well-being and the ability to provide a re-sponsive care giving environment. This will include the identification of potential risk factors, such as postnatal depression, domestic abuse and offering individualised emotional support, signposting to support services and promoting resilience.*
- *Providing evidence-based information on healthy weaning practices and the promotion of a healthy balanced nutrition to promote healthy weight gain and reduce the risk of obesity.*
- *Encourage age-appropriate physical activity to promote a healthy weight, but ultimately the development of gross motor skills.*
- *Promote the development of speech, language and communication through the facilitation of learning opportunities that provide stimulating activities, such as reading, attendance at group activities.*
- *Reduce the risk of unintentional injuries by promoting parental awareness of safety risks within the home and in the wider community.*
- *Promote the importance of a healthy oral hygiene routine and dental attendance.*
- *Encourage social engagement and attendance at available parenting support services to support families to access social support and facilitate a successful transition to parenthood.*
- *The safety and welfare of the child is paramount, and the local safeguarding procedures are adhered to if a child is identified as at risk of experiencing significant harm.*

During mandated contacts, health visitors will address these identified public health priorities by adopting an individualised approach in partnership with each family and target the advice and support provided to their individual needs and circumstances. They achieve successful outcomes through the development of a therapeutic and trusting relationship with families. Health visitors use effective communication skills, which project respect, humility, genuineness and empathy.[60] They develop goals in partnership with families, which positively reinforces their knowledge and strengths. This enables parents to feel valued and secure to express their situation more openly and build confidence and self-efficacy to respond to advice and address their individual needs.[65] However, as health inequalities exist across the population, this can influence the choices families have the capacity to make in relation to their health. Therefore, the provision of information or advice alone may not be effective without the adoption of an ecological approach and exploring the wider social and environmental factors that could be influencing attitudes, health choices and behaviours. Only then can targeted and individualised support and advice be provided to address the individual circumstances that may influence healthy choices. This approach is highly valued by parents, as the Institute of Health Visiting[47] has undertaken a review of the health visiting service from a parental perspective and identified that,

> *Mothers valued being treated as an individual, with a personalised service that was responsive to their individual circumstances and needs, rather than a 'one-size-fits' all approach* (p7)

Health visiting practice is continually evolving and adapting in response to growing evidence and political direction. For example, the Institute of Health Visiting[24] has recognised the need to review the 'Healthy Child Programme' in England to consider the updated evidence published within 'Health for all Children (5th edn)'.[61] Recommendations have been communicated to direct the government to increase the number of mandated contacts to eight and increase the priority high impact areas from six to 15 to ensure the service remains contemporary and evidence-based.

## INTEGRATED SERVICES

The principle of 'proportionate universalism', which encourages the targeting of skills and expertise to identified levels of needs, requires the professionals of the wider multi-disciplinary team to work in partnership to meet the diverse needs of families and communities.[27] All health care professionals have a public health role and responsibility to promote the health and well-being of families and communities. The health visiting service is proactive in addressing the health needs of families and communities by working collaboratively with community support services and members of the multi-disciplinary team. This predominantly includes professionals from primary care services, including general practitioners (GPs) and practice nurses, as well as midwives and school nurses, to ensure there is appropriate information-sharing so that children and families can transition effectively from maternity services, to health visiting services and finally to school nursing provision.[65] Health visitors are highly skilled in working in partnership with other services and professionals within the community and will signpost families to the skills and expertise of these resources when appropriate. This could include the community dental services, speech and language services, social services and the voluntary sector services, which provide parenting support.

The Flying Start programme in Wales is a good example of how services work within a co-ordinated and integrated approach to address the potential health needs and reduce health inequalities within communities. It comprises a range of professionals, including midwives, speech and language therapists, dieticians and nursery nurses. The Welsh government[65] promotes and recognises that,

> *The development of a multi-agency approach to Flying Start is key to the effectiveness of the programme and is instrumental in supporting both children and families, enabling early identification, assessment and referral* (p7)

Health visitors utilise their assessment skills and tools to search for health needs and identify potential risk factors for poor health outcomes and empower families to access the resources and expertise that are available within the Flying Start programme. This could include a referral to a speech and language therapist for a targeted intervention or attendance at the free childcare provision to optimise a child's social interaction and learning opportunities.

## CONCLUSION

We have explored the history of health visiting including reviewing how the role is presented across some countries of the world. There are many variations of the early years nurse with varying names associated with the role, and differences in the delivery of a universal and/or targeted programme for children. There are some similarities with the UK health visiting service, which has been in place for over 150 years. Since its inception, the health visiting service over the last decade has undergone many changes in response to the changing political landscape and changing public health priorities of families. However, the philosophy of the service has remained the same, with a clear goal to promote health, prevent disease and safeguard the health and well-being of future generations.

### KEY LEARNING POINTS

In summary: the key points of learning from this chapter are:
- How the health visiting service has evolved over the last 150 years;
- Identification on the essential role of health visiting in today's society as specialist practitioners, experts in health promotion, public health, health protection and safeguarding of children and families emotional and physical well-being;
- The ongoing relevance of the principles of health visiting;
- The variation in delivery of key public health priorities across the UK;
- The role of the health visitor as 'health creators' working with families, searching and addressing health needs in partnership with families and communities, influencing policy that affects health, with the aim of always placing families at the heart of their practice.

## FURTHER RESOURCES

1. Whitaker, K. A., Malone, M., Cowley, S., Grigulis, A., Nicholson, C., & Maben, J. (2015) Making a difference for children and families: an appreciative inquiry of health visitor values and why they start and stay in post. *Health and Social Care in the Community*. doi:10.111/hsc.122307 p1-11.
2. Cowley, S., Whitaker, K., Malone, M., Donetto, S., Grigulis, A., & Maben, J. (2017). What makes health visiting successful or not? 1. Universality. *Journal of Health Visiting*, 6(7), 352–360.
3. Cowley, S., Whitaker, K., Malone, M., Donetto, S., Grigulis, A., & Maben, J. (2018). What makes health visiting successful or not? 2. The service journey. *Journal of Health Visiting*, 6(8), 404–412.

## REFERENCES

1. Plunket Strategy. (2016). Plunket Strategy 2016–2021. *The journey towards generational change*. https://www.plunket.org.nz/assets/Plunket-Strategy/Plunket-Strategy-2016-2021_3Feb2017.pdf. Accessed 23 December 2021.
2. Nurse Family Partnership. https://www.nursefamilypartnership.org/about/. Accessed 24 February 2020.
3. Institute of Health Visiting. Health visiting across the World. www.ihv.org.uk/our-work/international/. Accessed 24 February 2020.
4. Nursing and Midwifery Council. (2004). *Standards of proficiency for specialist community public health nurses*. NMC: London.
5. JISC Archives Hub. Manchester and Salford Ladies Sanitary Reform Association. https://archiveshub.jisc.ac.uk/search/archives/b489e047-e6b1-3992-aaa3-5e40e2147729?component=4826dcba-24ff-3804-8c72-e42a7fcd8a43. Accessed October 25, 2019.
6. Adams, C. (2012). The history of health visiting. *Nursing in Practice: The Journal for Today's Primary Care Nurse*. Sept-Oct (68) p3. www.nursinginpractice.com/article/history-health-visiting. Accessed 25 October 2019.
7. Queens Nursing Institute (2020) Papers of Queens Nursing institute. Nursing Notes 1911. https://archiveshub.jisc.ac.uk/search/archives/86b36979-ec67-3141-96b9-a1814d1cb3f4. Accessed 24 December 2021.
8. Kings College London. https://www.kcl.ac.uk/aboutkings/history/famouspeople/florencenightingale.aspx. Accessed 12 November 2019.
9. Notification of Births Act. (1907).
10. Notification of Births Act. (1915).

11. Maternity and Child Welfare Act. (1918).
12. Dingwall, R. (1977). Collectivism, regionalism, and feminism: health visiting and British social policy 1850–1975. *Journal of Social Policy, 6*(3), 291–315.
13. Malone, M. (2000). A history of health visiting and parenting in the last 50 years. *International History of Nursing Journal, 5*(3), 30–43.
14. Cormack, U. (1959). The Younghusband report on Social Workers. *Public Administration, 37*(3), 299–302.
15. Jameson Report. (1959). *Report of the working party on the field, training and recruitment of health visitors.* London: Department of Health.
16. Council for the Education and Training of health visitors (CETHV). (1977). *An Investigation into the Principles of health visiting.* London: CETHV. https://discovery.nationalarchives.gov.uk/details/r/C93. Accessed 8 May 2019.
17. Cowley, S., & Frost, M. (2006). *The Principles of Health Visiting: opening health visiting into the 21st century.* Community Practitioners and Health Visitors Association (CPHVA).
18. Department of Health. (2009). *Healthy child programme.* London: Department of Health. London.
19. Department of Health. (2011). *Health visitor implementation plan 2011–2015: a call to action.* London: Department of Health.
20. Department of Health. (2010). Social services and public safety. Healthy child, healthy future: A framework for the child health promotion programme in Northern Ireland. https://www.health-ni.gov.uk/sites/default/files/publications/dhssps/healthychildhealthyfuture.pdf. Accessed 14 February 2020.
21. Welsh Government. (2009). A Vision for health visiting in Wales. www.gov.default/files/publications/2019-03/a-vision-for-health-visiting-in-wales.pdf. Accessed 9 March 2020.
22. The Scottish Government. (2015). Universal health visiting pathway in Scotland. Pre-birth to pre-school. https://www.gov.scot/publications/universal-health-visiting-pathway-scotland-pre-birth-pre-school/. Accessed 14 February 2020.
23. Welsh Government. (2016). *An overview of the Healthy Child Wales Programme.* Cardiff : Welsh Government.
24. Institute of Health Visiting. (2019). *Health visiting in England: A vision for the future.* London: Institute of Health Visiting.
25. Department of Health. (2015). Public health grant: proposed target allocation formula for 2016–2017. London: Department of Health.
26. Marmot, M., Allen, J., Boyce, T., Goldbatt, P., & Morrison, J. (2020). Health equity in England: The Marmot Review

10 years on www.instituteofhealthequity.org/the-marmot-review-10-years-on. Accessed 18 March 2020.
27. Marmot, M., Goldbatt, P., Allen, J., et al. (2010). *Fair Society healthy lives (The Marmot Review).* http://www.instituteofhealthequity.org/resources-reports/fair-society-healthy-lives-the-marmot-review/fair-society-healthy-lives-full-report-pdf.pdf. Accessed 18 March 2020.
28. Cowley, S., Whitaker, K., Malone, M., Donetto, S., Grigulis, A., & Maben, J. (2015). Why Health Visiting? Examining the potential public health benefits from health visiting practice within a universal service: A narrative review of the literature. *International Journal of Nursing Studies, 52*(1), 465–480.
29. Public Health Wales. (2020). The first 1,000 days collaborative. http://www.wales.nhs.uk/sitesplus/888/page/96062. Accessed 20 January 2020.
30. Lindstrom, B., & Erikkson, M. (2005). Salutogenesis. *Journal of Epidemiology Community Health, 59*(6), 440–442.
31. Antonovosky, A. (1979). *Health, stress and coping.* San Francisco: Jossey-Bass.
32. Sidebotham, P. (2013). Authoritative child protection. *Child Abuse Review, 22*, 1–4.
33. Center on the Developing Child. (2019). Brain Architecture. https://developingchild.harvard.edu/science/key-concepts/brain-architecture/. Accessed 8 March 2020.
34. Center on the Developing Child. (2019). What is Epigenetics? https://developingchild.harvard.edu/resources/what-is-epigenetics-and-how-does-it-relate-to-child-development/. Accessed 8 March 2020.
35. Bellis, M., Ashton, K., Hughes, K. E., Ford, K., Bishop, J., & Paranjothy, S. (2016). *Adverse childhood experiences and their impact on health—Harming behaviours in the Welsh adult population.* Wales: Public Health Wales NHS Trust.
36. Health Service Executive. https://www.hse.ie/eng/about/who/healthwell-being/our-priority-programmes/child-health-and-well-being/nationalhealthychildhoodprogramme/national-healthy-childhood-programme.html. Accessed 18 September 2019.
37. Public Health Wales Making Every Contact Count. http://www.wales.nhs.uk/sitesplus/888/page/65550. Accessed 18 February 2020.
38. Bellis, M., Hughes, K. E., Ford, K., Bishop Hardcastle, K. A., Sharp, C. A., et al. (2018). Adverse childhood experiences and sources of childhood resilience: A retrospective study of relationships with child health and educational attendance. *BMC Public Health, 18*(792), 1–12.

39. Antonovosky, A. (1987). *Unravelling the mystery of health. How people manage stress and stay well.* San Francisco: Jossey-Bass.

40. Rogers, C. (1980). *The way of being.* New York: Houghton Mifflin.

41. Bronfenbrenner, U. (1986). Ecology of the family as a context for human development: Research perspectives. *Developmental Psychology, 22*(6), 723–742.

42. Bradshaw, J. (1972). Taxonomy of Social Need. In G. McLachlan (Ed.), *Problems and progress in medical care: Essays on current research. Seventh series* (pp. 71–82). London: Oxford University Press.

43. Department of Health. (2004). *National service framework for children, young people and maternity services: Core standards.* London: Department of Health.

44. Hall, D., & Elliman, D. (2006). *Health for all children* (4th ed.). Oxford: Oxford University Press.

45. World Health Organisation. (2017). Ten facts on health inequities and their causes. https://www.who.int/features/factfiles/health_inequities/en/. Accessed 19 February 2020.

46. Public Health England. (2018). Overview of the six early years and school—Aged years high impact areas. Health visitors and school nurses leading the healthy child programme. https://dera.ioe.ac.uk/32487/1/overview_of_the_6_early_years_and_school_aged_years_high_impact_areas.pdf. Accessed 23 December 2021.

47. Institute of Health Visiting. (2020). What do parents want from a health visiting service? Results from a Channel Mum survey. London: Institute of Health Visiting.

48. The Children (Northern Ireland) Order. (1995). http://www.legislation.gov.uk/nisi/1995/755/contents/made. Accessed 19 February 2020.

49. Welsh Government. (2017). Flying start health programme guidance https://gov.wales/sites/default/files/publications/2019-07/flying-start-health-programme-guidance_0.pdf. Accessed 14 February 2020.

50. Cardiff Council. (2020). Welcome to Flying Start https://www.flyingstartcardiff.co.uk/. Accessed 14 February 2020

51. Allen, G. (2011) Early intervention: The next steps. Available from: https://assets.publishing.service.gov.uk/government/uploads/system/uploads/attachment_data/file/284086/early-intervention-next-steps2.pdf. Accessed 14 February 2020.

52. National Scientific Centre on the Developing Child. (2010). Early experiences can alter gene expression and affect long-term development: Working paper no. 10. http://www.developingchild.net. Accessed 14 February 2020.

53. National Scientific Centre on the Developing Child. (2016). Applying the science of child development in child welfare system. https://www.ddcf.org/globalassets/child-well-being/16-1013-center-on-developing-child_childwelfaresystems.pdf. Accessed 19 February 2020.

54. National Scientific Centre on the Developing Child. (2018). Understanding motivation: Building brain architecture that supports learning, health, and community participation. Working paper no. 14. www.developing-child.harvard.edu. Accessed 14 February 2020.

55. Early Intervention Foundation. (2020). What is early intervention? https://www.eif.org.uk/why-it-matters/what-is-early-intervention. Accessed 1 March 2020.

56. National Institute for Health and Care Excellence. (2008). Social and emotional well-being in primary education. https://www.nice.org.uk/guidance/ph12/resources/social-and-emotional-well-being-in-primary-education-pdf-1996173182149. Accessed 14 February 2020.

57. House of Commons Health and Social Care Committee. (2019). First 1,000 days of life. London: House of Commons.

58. European Foundations for the Care of Newborn Infants. (2020). Why the first 1,000 days of life matter. https://www.efcni.org/wp-content/uploads/2018/05/2018_04_23_EFCNI_1000Tage_Factsheet_web.pdf. Accessed 14 February 2020.

59. Powell, T. (2019). Early intervention. Briefing paper number 7647. London: House of Commons Library.

60. Emond, A. (2019). *Health for all children* (5th ed.). Oxford: Oxford University Press.

61. Scottish Government. (2018). Public health priorities for Scotland. https://www.gov.scot/publications/scotlands-public-health-priorities/. Accessed 14 February 2020.

62. Public Health England. (2019). Public Health England strategy 2020 to 2025. https://assets.publishing.service.gov.uk/government/uploads/system/uploads/attachment_data/file/831562/PHE_Strategy_2020-25.pdf. Accessed 14 February 2020.

63. Public Health Wales. (2018). Working to achieve a Healthier Future for Wales. http://www2.nphs.wales.nhs.uk:8080/PHWPapersDocs.nsf/public/6CC37E0D6AB576F7802582FA004C85E7/$file/7.1.260718%20App%201%20-%20Long%20Term%20Strategy%20Draft.pdf. Accessed 14 February 2020.

64. Department of Health. (2015). Making life better https://www.health-ni.gov.uk/topics/health-policy/making-life-better#toc-0. Accessed 14 February 2020.

65. Welsh Government. (2012). Flying start: Strategic guidance. https://gov.wales/sites/default/files/publications/2019-07/flying-start-strategy-guidance-for-local-authorities.pdf. Accessed 14 February 2020.

# PROFESSIONAL PRACTICE AND PRACTITIONER WELL-BEING

RACHEL STEPHEN ■ ROBERT NETTLETON

## CHAPTER CONTENTS

INTRODUCTION

WELL-BEING AND WORK

THE TRANSITION FROM STUDENT TO HEALTH VISITOR

SUPPORTING THE INDIVIDUAL

SUPERVISION

PRECEPTORSHIP AND MENTORING

HEALTH VISITING TEAM

CASE STUDY

INEQUALITY

ORGANISATIONS AND PRACTITIONER WELL-BEING

DEALING WITH REALITY

CONCLUSION

## LEARNING OUTCOMES

*To:*

- identify the contribution of work to well-being
- increase your awareness of impact of professional practice on well-being as a student and a qualified health visitor
- understand the factors that influence well-being arising from practice and the organisational context
- how to make use of preceptorship, mentoring and supervision to support personal effectiveness and well-being at work
- develop awareness of strategies that can build individual well-being
- reflect on your contribution to well-being in the workplace for yourself and the people you work with

## INTRODUCTION

Professional practice is what health visitors engage in through their day-to-day work – it's their job as well as their profession. Our work occupies a huge proportion of our time and energy and therefore affects our well-being. The relationship of work to well-being is double-sided: it makes demands of us and can also contribute to our well-being. The reasons *why* we work are many and extend beyond the crucial element of pay or 'earning a living'. This is particularly the case when we consider 'professional practice'. To practise a profession means to act out of obligations and motivations, a 'professional mission' that extends beyond the business of a particular employer. It means that we have obligations and motivations that belong to the profession – that we belong to and 'profess' in the public realm as a member of society in general, and specifically to our client base consisting, in the case of health visiting, of children, families, their community and the many agencies that also are important to them. Finally, 'well-being' is not a peripheral or second-order issue for health visitors, but is rather our core concern as health visiting is all about promoting and supporting the health and well-being of those we work with: it is our 'special subject', so to speak. In this chapter we wish to keep the focus on well-being but to move our attention to ourselves as professional practitioners. In doing so, we will acknowledge that the issues hinted at in this introductory paragraph do not necessarily align well but can and do give rise to tensions and contradictions that work against practitioner well-being and, thereby, professional effectiveness.

Well-being at work is a topic that is important in all occupational spheres as our occupational health nurse colleagues can tell us. In this chapter we will draw on some wider perspectives on work and well-being, but with a central focus on professional practice. A review of 25 years of health visiting scholarship and research[1] distilled a distinctive 'orientation to practice' with three components:

(i) A 'salutogenic' (i.e. health-creating) approach: proactive, identifying and building strengths and resources (personal and situational) and solution-focused.

(ii) Demonstrating a positive regard for others (human valuing), through keeping the person in mind and shifting (the health visitors') focus to align with parents' needs, recognising the potential for unmet need, actively seeking out potential strengths, maintaining hope.

(iii) Recognising the person-in-situation (human ecology) through a continuing process, always taking account of the individual and their personal and situational circumstances, whether acting in the client's space, the community or the workplace.

Throughout this chapter we suggest that these components structure your reflection on your own experience of and engagement with work as they have informed our reflection on writing this chapter:

(i) Is my experience of practising as a health visitor 'salutogenic' for me and for my colleagues? Am I proactive in identifying and building strengths and resources for me as a person and in my situation with those who share my work situation as colleagues? Am I solution-focused or part of 'the problem'? Do I foster resilience for myself and others?

(ii) Do I demonstrate a positive regard for those I work with (human valuing)? Do I recognise colleagues as persons (not just job roles), through keeping the person in mind and shifting my focus to align with their human needs, recognising the potential for unmet need, actively seeking out potential strengths, maintaining hope?

(iii) Do I recognise the person-in-situation (human ecology) through a continuing process, always taking account of the individual and their personal and situational circumstances, applying this both to myself and to colleagues within the organisation and other agencies that I work with? Do I recognise and take seriously the constraints and micro-politics of everyday working life as well as the bigger policy picture? Is my work context toxic to well-being or supportive?

## WELL-BEING AND WORK

Well-being refers to the subjective component of health as broadly and positively conceived in line with the World Health Organisation (WHO)'s constitutional definition of health as 'a state of complete physical, mental and social well-being and not merely the absence of disease or infirmity'. The WHO further defines well-being as: 'a state of mind in which an individual is able to realise his or her own abilities, cope with the normal stresses of life, can work productively and fruitfully, and is able to contribute to his or her community.'[2]

This perspective on health and well-being sees them as resources for living, including the capacity to work. However, the relationship between well-being and work can be seen as reciprocal. Work also affects our well-being. Emotional well-being can be linked to:

- Improved learning and academic achievement
- Reduced absence from work due to sickness
- Reductions in risk-taking behaviours like smoking
- Improved physical health
- Enhanced relationships
- More effective working practices
- Happy staff are more compassionate and provide safer care.[3:2]

The benefits of work are broadly based on the following:

- Employment is generally the most important means of obtaining adequate economic resources, which are essential for material well-being and full participation in today's society;
- Work meets important psychosocial needs in societies where employment is the norm;
- Work is central to individual identity, social roles and social status;
- Employment and socio-economic status are the main drivers of social gradients in physical and mental health and mortality;
- Various physical and psychosocial aspects of work can also be hazards and pose a risk to health.[3:2]

At the most general level, Wadell and Burton suggest, 'There is a strong evidence base showing that work is generally good for physical and mental health and well-being. Worklessness is associated with poorer physical and mental health and well-being. Work can be therapeutic and can reverse the adverse health effects of unemployment' (p. 3). However, not all work is equally beneficial. Schwartz argues that what motivates people in their work are those factors that maximise job satisfaction that contribute to well-being.[4] These include:

*Autonomy* – when employees are given independence and responsibility, and are given decisions to make, they take more pride in what they do, as well as feeling more trusted and respected.

*Investment* – employees feel more valued if their employer invests in developing their skills, whether it be time, money or effort.

*Mission* – employees should feel that they are contributing to a powerful, overarching mission, that permeates their everyday tasks so they feel as though they are part of something bigger than themselves.[4]

The unifying thread here is the sense that, as workers, we matter and what we do, our 'professional mission', also matters: it 'makes a difference'. Professional mission aligns well with Schwartz's conclusion that the holy grail for motivated employees is for them to see their 'work as a calling' or vocation – traditionally associated with the caring professions. Within this chapter we will explore the transition from student to health visitor identifying the challenge and rewards of change on the context of current policy and practice. As we do so, we will offer insights and resources for you to sustain your sense of professional mission and well-being in the workplace, for yourself and the people you work with as colleagues and families in the community.

## THE TRANSITION FROM STUDENT TO HEALTH VISITOR

Making the transition from student to qualified health visitor working autonomously in the community can be both exhilarating and anxiety-provoking. Many practitioners are moving from a setting in which they had a strong sense of professional identity, expertise, status and credibility. It can be challenging to step from such a position into one which at first seems to be so removed from the settings and roles left behind. However, although perhaps not at first apparent to the fledgling health visitor, the training and experience that nursing – with all its different specialities – demands provides some of the foundations for health visiting practice. Nurses provide care for people in their most vulnerable moments, whether that be birth, illness, trauma, death or loss. This position of immense responsibility and privilege equips us with the skills and confidence to reach out to people who are suffering despite our own inner fears and feelings of inadequacy. In addition, the nurse's ability to quickly assess a patient's condition and needs (in often the most challenging of situations), is a useful platform on which to build the needs assessment skills required to lead and deliver child and family public health programmes. However, what is central and universal to nursing, midwifery and health visiting is the capacity to form compassionate relationships with others. Universally it is the quality of the relationship that the nurse, midwife and health visitor forms with the patient/family that makes the real difference to every aspect of care from client experience, satisfaction to outcomes and financial expedience for the organisation and society.

There are, however, a number of specific challenges that the newly qualified health visitor faces. Health visiting requires a shift of professional orientation from a clinical setting, where the team is central to care, to a relatively autonomous role which can feel alien and isolating. Support and strategies that were once depended on for emotional well-being are no longer there. New coping strategies have to be developed and this can take time and resources.

There are also personal characteristics and personality types that may make the transition even harder. Health visiting requires practitioners to embrace a very wide range of issues within unstructured environments. It involves the capacity to respond to needs in a personalised way whilst also meeting performance indicators set by the organisation. Individuals who are used to a more immediate sense of completion from a task or care episode (especially if they have perfectionist tendencies) sometimes find that the often-relentless demands and unpredictability of the work can have a negative impact on their well-being. Hill and Curran found that the rates of burnout are higher in individuals with perfectionist thought patterns.[5] Perfectionists are more likely to berate themselves for not completing work to their exacting standards and find it harder to find that sense of satisfaction completion of something that meets their self-expectations brings. Health visiting, by the very nature of the work, is rarely complete; constant competing demands and priorities can frequently derail a planned workday. The 2018 staff survey of NHS trusts and foundation trusts reported that only 34% of health visitors had felt able to meet the competing demands on their time over the previous 12 months.[80]

### What may help?

- Focusing and drawing satisfaction from completing smaller episodes of work rather than focusing on work or goals that are incomplete or unachievable.
- Reframe episodes of care to notice what was achieved rather than what wasn't. For instance, *'The family have so many problems I don't know where to start and most of them seem so complicated, I just feel it's hopeless'* can be reframed to *'The family have a lot of difficulties but I listened*

*to them and made sure they knew that I understood that they are suffering. I can help them to think about what is important to them and we can think together about the first few steps'.*

- Concentrate on actions that you have control over and things you can influence. Don't waste energy worrying about or changing the things you can't control. Take small positive actions to give you a sense of moving forwards.
- In addition, self-compassion skills can help us to accept that we are 'doing the best we can' and exchange our own critical and judging thoughts about ourselves with compassionate and kind thoughts. Dr Kristen Neff, who has researched self-compassion for many years, suggests 'we give ourselves the same kindness and care we'd give to a good friend'.[6]

For many years there have been theoretical discussions around the drive to heal, care for or 'make others better'. Carl Jung's philosophical work expanded the concept of the wounded healer.[7] One of Jung's basic assumptions was that every individual has experienced some sort of trauma in life. He suggested that both conscious and unconscious factors, derived from personal experiences, drive human behaviour and encompass all individuals. In more recent times Conti-O'Hare wrote on her beliefs that individuals are often led to specific professions, such as nursing, by their desire to relieve the suffering of others after experiencing or witnessing traumatic events in their own lives.[8] These events may include witnessing physical or mental illness in our own family members, experience of loss or other emotional suffering.

Although this is an area that requires further study, research by Barr found that 73.9% of mental health professionals she surveyed believed their wounding experience(s) had led them to their chosen career.[9] Acute medical and surgical settings depend on this drive in health professionals to heal others in order to provide the best care for patients. Nurses can gain a great deal of personal and professional satisfaction when

a patient's wound begins to heal or a stroke patient begins to regain their speech and movement. However, as health visitors, we are not providing care for acute episodes of physical illness but are instead supporting families with all the individual complexities and unpredictability that relationships, mental/physical well-being, economic and environmental life experiences can bring. It is this that is most rewarding but also, for some, perhaps most challenging. During the process of learning and adaptation the health visitor learns skills that support families and in doing so will be required to suppress or dampen down the urge to 'fix' others by having the answers or solutions to their problems. Instead, skills such as providing a listening presence, wondering and curiosity, mastering the 'not knowing' stance, holding families in mind, using family's strengths to build and observing relationships are all encompassed in the art of health visiting. This is a seismic shift in focus for many of us and requires skills that are developed over time. Students coming from areas such as mental health, or indeed those who have already been working in health visiting teams, may find this less of a challenge.

### What can help?

- Good quality **preceptorship** and **supervision**[10] can help individuals with this process of change and provide space for the health visitor in training to think about her own feelings and needs.
- Sometimes just taking some time to talk to ourselves with a reassuring voice. Using statements like the ones below can be enough to calm the strong feelings in ourselves and help us accept that we do not always have the power to fix others.

*I feel so badly for this mother right now and I really want to make everything okay for her but I know I don't have the power to do that.*

*I'm doing the very best that I can, there is nothing more that anyone could do.*

*I really want to just tell this parent what they should do to make things better but I know that's not going to help.*

*Listening and bearing her suffering with her is enough right now.*

- Embracing ongoing learning and development opportunities which help us to master our craft, building our confidence and self-esteem.
- Develop skills in mindful listening:
  - Simplify your surroundings and mute any devices
  - Take a minute to clear your mind and think about how you're feeling before meeting someone
  - Listen to the other person with empathy and validate what they say. You don't have to agree but you can accept their perspective
  - Listen carefully and attentively. Pay complete attention to the other person, and don't let other thoughts – like what you are going to say next – distract you or make you feel anxious
  - Notice any thoughts, feelings and physical reactions that you are experiencing. These can be anxious thoughts or thoughts such as "I don't know the answer or what to say that will help" or it could be a judging thought about the other person. Just notice these with interest, acceptance and without judgement of yourself
  - Notice when your mind wanders and consciously let the thought go and gently bring your attention back to the person you are with
  - Accept that sometimes you won't have the answer and sometimes you might experience difficult feelings

Shafir suggests mindful listening can potentially have physical and psychological benefits. Shafir likens focusing on another person to stroking a pet – you forget about yourself, your blood pressure drops, and you feel calmer. The other person feels attended to, contained and held by you.[11]

Many new health visitors might notice that they do not get thanked as much as they used to or receive as many gifts as a memento of gratitude for their care. This might be experienced as a loss and it takes time to build our own internal positive feedback mechanisms that provide us with professional satisfaction. Aaron Beck developed the model of cognitive behavioural therapy (CBT) from his theory of selective abstraction.[12] This theory demonstrates that as humans we often notice only part of what we are looking at and that part is often the negative part. Our early ancestors would have found this life saving as they were able to scan the unpredictable world for threats that would become imprinted in their memories. Now that we live in a safer and more predictable world many of us have to train our brains to see the positive, which as health visitors can help us to adapt to a role where we are not receiving as frequent positive feedback or such obviously tangible results from our care.

### What can help?

- Noticing the tiny embryonic changes in a family's situation or the relationship between an infant and their carer is a crucial skill that not only enhances our own well-being (by providing us with positive feedback) but is the bedrock of **strengths-based models of working**.
- Emmons and McCullough demonstrated that we can **retrain our brains to notice more of the positive** by journaling for just 21 days, 3–5 things a day that have gone well for us.[13] They urge us to notice the small moment's such as a father who makes eye contact with you for the first time; or the moment when a mother and infant who are avoidant of making eye contact with each other, briefly meet each other's gaze. In doing this we can train our brains to find strengths, hope, kindness, comfort and beauty even in situations that seem full of pain, disconnection and hopelessness. Moreover, we can utilise these insights therapeutically to support families to enhance their own confidence, sensitivity and self-efficacy.

It is perhaps only in the last decade that we have come to recognise that a significant component of the health visiting role is grounded in infant, maternal and family mental health. In the past we have neatly sealed off mental health into mental health teams. We now recognise mental health as 'Everyone's Business' a phrase coined by the Maternal Mental Health Alliance. There is more evidence than ever that in pregnancy and the first year of our infant lives that we are more vulnerable to mental health problems and emotional disorders than at any other time in our lives. If we combine this with the existing vulnerability of the families targeted for health visiting intervention the emotionally demanding nature of the work becomes abundantly clear. Frequent environmental stress associated with human pain and distress in the workplace can impact on the physical and mental well-being of health professionals and result in burnout and, in some cases, traumatic stress-like symptoms.[14] The idea of emotional toil or labour has also been recognised: 'The concept of emotion work involves the management of emotions by an individual in order to conform to the demands of the particular social situation'.[15:156] Emotional labour is central to health visiting.[16] There have been no studies looking at the prevalence of vicarious trauma in health visiting however we know that nurses working in mental health are a particularly vulnerable group.[17] This work leaves health visitors vulnerable to stress and burnout particularly in times when the service is under pressure from increased demands and/or diminished resources. There are various terms and definitions in the literature for practitioner trauma that include secondary traumatic stress, post-traumatic stress disorder and vicarious trauma. Burnout is another frequently used term in the literature to describe the impact of work stressors. The NHS staff survey found that 44% of health visitors said that they had felt unwell over the last 12 months due to work related stress.[18] However, 57% said they had come to work despite feeling they were not well enough to carry out their duties. In addition to this only 28% of health visitors agreed there were enough staff to do the work and only 34% said they were able to meet the conflicting demands on their time.

The following lists may help us to recognise excessive stress or trauma in ourselves or others.

## Recognising the signs and symptoms of vicarious trauma

This is not an exhaustive list, but it covers some of the common signs of vicarious trauma[19]:

- Invasive thoughts of client's situation/distress
- Frustration/fear/anxiety/irritability
- Disturbed sleep/nightmares/racing thoughts
- Problems managing personal boundaries
- Taking on too great a sense of responsibility or feeling you need to overstep the boundaries of your role
- Difficulty leaving work at the end of the day/noticing you can never leave on time
- Loss of connection with self and others/loss of a sense of own identity
- Increased time alone/a sense of needing to withdraw from others
- Increased need to control events/outcomes/others
- Loss of pleasure in daily activities

The effects of vicarious trauma vary from person to person. For some people, there may be a wide range of signs and symptoms, while others may experience problems in one particular area of their lives.

## Recognising the signs and symptoms of burnout

This is not an exhaustive list, but it covers some of the common signs of burnout[19]:

- Physical and emotional stress
- Low job satisfaction

- Cynicism
- Feeling frustrated by or judgmental of families
- Feeling under pressure, powerless and overwhelmed
- Not taking breaks, eating on the run
- Unable to properly refuel and regenerate
- Frequent sick days or 'mental health days'
- Irritability and anger
- Feeling disassociated from families or that you don't care

Each and every one of us as human beings have mental health just as we have physical health. The most common causes of depression and anxiety in NHS staff are high perceived workload, the growing intensity and complexity of the work, rapid change within healthcare, low control and support and personal experiences of bullying and harassment.[20]

Stigma around mental health which has existed for many years makes it difficult for professionals to be authentic about their own. Perhaps we believe that strong, predictable and stable individuals do not suffer from mental health problems and fear the judgement of others, particularly within the professional context. However, the truth is that we all experience emotional disturbance, it's part of being human, many of us will also experience mental health disorders at some time in our lives. Dr Brene Brown, a renowned research professor, has written extensively on shame and vulnerability, she came from a social work background and found accepting her own vulnerability excruciating. She believes that vulnerability is basically uncertainty, risk, and emotional exposure. She also believes that it is the key to connection with others, but the thing we are least likely to show. Brene Brown writes about the courage it takes to be vulnerable and to share our emotions with others in an authentic way. However, she believes that courage is contagious and writes, 'Every time we choose courage, we make everyone around us a little better and the world a little braver'.[21] If we are to truly end the stigma of talking about mental health as health professionals we must find the courage to lead the way. It is important to ensure good staff well-being by encouraging conversation in the workplace.[22] Perhaps we also need to reframe mental health problems and think about the strengths of those of us with lived experience:

*I've got these conditions, anxiety, depression, addiction – and they almost killed me. But they are also my superpowers. The sensitivity that led me to addiction is the same sensitivity that makes me a really a good artist. The anxiety that makes it difficult to exist in my own skin also makes it difficult to exist in a world where so many people are in so much pain – and that makes me a relentless activist.[23]*

### What can help?

- Seeking out individuals and groups where we feel safe to be emotionally authentic
- Finding the courage to be vulnerable and accepting that difficult feelings are a normal part of the human experience and what connects us
- Doyle suggests telling ourselves, 'This is difficult, but we can do difficult things'.[23]
- Developing awareness of our own internal world and noticing when we are suffering. **Mindfulness practice** can be particularly helpful.
- Seeking out and accepting support for our own mental health when we need it without shame, remembering emotional sensitivity is also a 'superpower'. What we perceive as our weakness may actually be what makes us a truly great health visitor.

Finally, many health visiting students have come from settings where an episode of care is complete at the end of a working shift. However, as a health visitor accountability for families and worries that we have missed something often seem like a heavy bag that we just can't put down. When we are acting in an 'apprentice' role, we are strongly influenced by organisational culture and our supervisors/role models.[24] We pick up quickly on the fears of the organisation and the people working within it. In some organisations 'there can be an atmosphere of "fear", in particular fear of investigation and associated uncertainty relating to investigation, blame and prosecution'.[24] It is not difficult to understand why this may have arisen within health visiting when we have witnessed through high profile media reporting the impact that child death or serious incidents can have on society and the far reaching and traumatising effects for practitioners and organisations. There is nothing more abhorrent and unbearable to any of us than the suffering of an innocent child. Consequently, health visitors whose practice has been criticised following such incidents can struggle to cope with the intolerable burden this places on them. There is currently much debate around the fairness of individual practitioners being held responsible for what are often complex multi-system failures in families, organisations and society.[25] During the NHS staff survey 40% of health visiting staff surveyed reported feeling they were treated fairly after an error or near-miss, demonstrating that although progress has been made there is still much work that needs to be done.[18]

### What can help?

- Accept that you will be faced with choices where there is no right answer and you may make mistakes.
- When faced with difficult situations, constantly replaying the situation in your mind is not helpful. Instead, remind yourself what you did achieve and what you learnt from it.
- Responsibility must sit firmly with employing organisations to develop systems and supports that protect practitioners from the devastating effects of avoidable death or serious injury

within their caseloads whilst remaining accountable and open to learning.

An example of this comes from the 'just and learning' culture at Merseycare NHS Foundation Trust which is a **restorative practice approach** that recognises that in an untoward incident caregivers can be victims too. This significant shift in organisational culture came at the culmination of a journey, advanced in part by trade unions concerned at what seemed to be an unfair and distressing process for managing adverse incident investigations and human resources policies and processes.[24] Merseycare's approach comes from the concept that investigations often tend to see human factors as the cause of mistakes, seeing people as the problem, assuming that because we have policies and procedures in place things won't go wrong and if they go wrong people are blamed. Internal research found that this culture created barriers to transparency including fear, blame and shame. Their new approach is based on established academic works, in particular by Professor Sidney Dekker 'Just Culture'. Merseycare's work to embrace a **'Just and Learning Culture'** has centred on the desire to create an environment where staff feel supported and empowered to learn when things do not go as expected, rather than feeling blamed.[26] This is a culture that instinctively asks in the case of an adverse event: 'what was responsible, not who is responsible?'. It is not finger pointing and not blame-seeking. However, they also clearly point out that 'it is not the same as an uncritically tolerant culture where anything goes – that would be as inexcusable as a blame culture'.

## SUPPORTING THE INDIVIDUAL

There is much that can be done by individual practitioners and the organisations they work for to maintain well-being at work. Developing self-awareness and noticing the signs of stress are key to being able to act to prevent them from impacting on our mental health. Drawing on what works for us as individuals to help us to maintain our own emotional well-being. Table 3.1 shows some

| TABLE 3.1 | |
| --- | --- |
| **Supports and threats to mental well-being at work** | |
| **Supports** | **Threats** |
| Having a good team to share experiences, debrief, talk things through, have fun and look after one another | Mobile working |
| Laughter and humour | Staff leaving |
| Family and friends | Being a perfectionist |
| Exercise | Unrealistic demands from managers |
| Mindful activities and being self-aware | Not feeling listened to or valued |
| Being in nature and walking | Tensions in the team |
| Enjoying working with families and getting a sense of job satisfaction | Administration and record keeping |
| Outside activities such as music/singing/dancing or gardening | Feeling overwhelmed by demands |
| Faith | Having a child with special needs |
| Professional development – learning and mastering new skills and expertise | Balancing demands of home and work |
| Supportive mangers and leadership | Unqualified staff being used to undertake part of the role of the health visitor |
| Exercise | Not being able to switch off from the fear that something will happen |
| Hobbies such as gardening, sewing, art, choir | Elderly/sick parents or relatives |
| Learning not to take work home | Feelings of not being able to get job satisfaction or build good relationships with families due to competing pressures |
| Getting the professional help needed | Having an anxious personality |
| Self-compassion | |
| Focusing on what has worked or gone well (even if it seems very small) | |
| Agenda matching with families and being clear and boundaried about the length of the visit | |

of the threats to mental well-being and some of the supports frequently cited by health visitors during the delivery of the Institute of Health Visiting's resilience training delivered over the last 5 years.

## SUPERVISION

Supervision is considered good practice now across a range of professional disciplines and has a number of forms. In general, it consists of practitioners meeting regularly with another professional, not necessarily more senior, but normally with training in the skills of supervision, to discuss casework and other professional issues in a structured way. This is often known as clinical, safeguarding or restorative supervision or consultation. The function of supervisor and team support is to help individuals restore emotional equilibrium and adapt to a challenging work environment. In psychodynamic terms, this interpersonal process is similar to emotional containment.[27] It is agreed that emotional equilibrium needs to be recovered before employees can cognitively engage in problem solving to perform competently at work.[28] Rimé's psychological research found that talking to others helps individuals process emotions (making sense of their feelings), restores equilibrium and facilitates understanding.

Clinical supervision has been part of health visiting for many years and its value in combating stress and improving practice is acknowledged by many in the field.[29,30] Currently within health visiting in the UK the picture is complex and supervision is carried out at various levels and in several different guises. Scotland has taken action to ensure supervision becomes a part of practice. The Nursing 2030 Vision published by the Scottish Government considers supervision to be an essential part of support for nurses and has provided the opportunity to adopt a refreshed approach to supervision in practice.[31] NHS Education for Scotland has developed an online training resource for supervisors and supervisees which is being rolled out.[76]

Pollock et al carried out a systematic review of evidence relating to clinical supervision for nurses, midwives and allied health professionals these demonstrated an absence of convincing empirical evidence and lack of agreement over the nature of clinical supervision.[32] Nineteen primary studies were included and these highlighted a lack of consistency and large variations between delivered interventions. However, many state that clinical supervision has been an integral part of successful interventions in health visiting.[33–37] Colthart et al found that support and clinical supervision can benefit staff and service users.[38] This report points to inquiries which have highlighted lack of support and clinical supervision as potential contributory factors for adverse care events. They suggest that for support and clinical supervision to be embedded effectively, leaders and managers must value and promote them in their organisations.

Sloan and Watson (2002, cited by Ref. [39]) found that Proctor's model in 1986 is the most commonly used model. However, they also contest that one model does not fit all aspects of nursing, and a 'one fit for all' philosophy should not be sought; individual organisations and supervisors should choose a model that suits them and their service. In recent years there has been a growing interest in the restorative function of supervision in health visiting. This form of supervision contains elements of psychological support including listening, supporting and challenging the supervisee to improve their capacity to cope, especially in managing difficult and stressful situations.[40] Hunter and Warren who carried out a study of

resilience in midwifery suggest that, whereas traditional clinical supervision has focused on clinical competency, recommendations from the literature also encompass the need for interventions aimed at enhancing personal confidence and self-efficacy, and addressing stress management techniques (Gillespie et al, 2007; Arvidsson et al, 2008 – cited by Ref. [41]). Hunter and Warren suggest that, to date, there has been limited research that has tested the hypothesis that interventions such as restorative supervision enhanced resiliency in midwives or nurses.[41] This is an area where independent research is very much required. However, although there is a lack of empirical evidence to support the effectiveness of restorative supervision, when asked to describe models of support that foster health visiting resilience, restorative supervision was frequently mentioned as being helpful in the 2014 'State of Health Visiting Survey' carried out by the Institute of Health Visiting.

The Institute of Health Visiting's Vision for the Future report recommends that plans are put in place to develop leadership capabilities within the health visiting workforce.[43] This should include a robust strategy for supervision. Health Education England have initiated a review of educational supervision which has cross-system support and will be applicable to all healthcare learners and their educators.

## PRECEPTORSHIP AND MENTORING

It has long since been accepted as standard practice that newly qualified health visitors enter a period of preceptorship. The Nursing Midwifery Council (NMC) suggests a period of preceptorship when moving to a new and different role for all registrants. McInnes developed the National Preceptorship Framework for Health Visiting – the first two years.[10] This document recommends that the preceptee receive support in the form of regular and planned meetings with the preceptor for 12 months and a final, closing meeting at the end of that period. It is also recommended that the preceptor have a minimum of one year's post registration (ideally two) experience as a health visitor in their current role and keep themselves up to date with current health visiting theory and evidence as well as new ways of working.

Preceptorship in nursing and health visiting refers specifically to a support and development role to facilitate transition into a new area of professional practice. However, mentorship is a support and development relationship that can be accessed at any time within a professional career. 'Mentors are guides, they lead us along a journey of our lives. We trust them because they have been there before. They embody our hopes, cast light on the way ahead, interpret arcane signs, warn us of lurking dangers, and point out unexpected delights along the way'.[42:17] This view of mentorship is rather different from the role of mentor that has, until recently, been a feature of nursing education by which mentors have typically been allocated to learners in the practice learning environment often having a significant role in assessment. The broader view of mentorship described by Daloz suggests an opportunity for practitioners to identify for themselves a supportive and developmental relationship from a respected and trusted peer to champion their professional journey, which may include taking account of their health and well-being.

Health Education England continue to debate the role and functions of such supportive and developmental relationships and recognise that there are some fundamental questions.[24] They suggest that acknowledging and understanding the implications of generational differences between supervisors and postgraduate learners is critical to defining the optimal trainer–trainee relationship. The impact that generational differences have on supervision and mentorship may not be equivalent. For example, is peer-to-near peer mentorship more desirable for postgraduate learners, or

is it preferable to have a supervisor from a different generation with a wealth of knowledge and experience? The iHV, in their recent document Health Visiting in England a Vision for the Future, recommend that to strengthen health visiting leadership new health visitors should undergo a two-year preceptorship period supervised and mentored by senior health visitors who might be Fellows of the iHV.[43] On completion they could be given the status of 'chartered' health visitor or similar, in line with many other professions.[43]

What is accepted is that the preceptor/mentor offers a space for reflective practice; 'a window through which the practitioner can view and focus herself within the context of her own lived experience in ways that will help her confront, understand, and work towards resolving the contradictions within her practice between what is desirable and actual practice'.[44:34] Remember, 'We do not learn by doing but by doing and realising what came of what we did'.[45:367] This process of building confidence in what we are doing and sharing our concerns about families or anything related to the work environment and our own well-being (when done well) is a fundamental platform from which the health visitor can thrive. New practitioners need a safe base to be open and honest. Research suggests that learners most value the interpersonal skills of a mentor when in practice. These skills can often make the difference between a practitioner staying or leaving.[46] Whilst completing research in the field for the DOH, Corkan found that several new health visitors reported the transition from training to being qualified was difficult since the SCPHN programme prepares students for health visiting in an ideal world, yet the reality has often been different.[47] This is not new: in 1974 Kramer spoke about the 'reality shock' for newly qualified nurses. In addition, she found that working with colleagues who have low morale and/or high levels of stress is very difficult for newly qualified health visitors.

In all areas of industry and business it has been established[48] that mentoring 'fosters talent' in the organisation, increases productivity, improves communication, and improves retention. McInnes also recommend that there is a restorative element to preceptorship (although the preceptorship should not replace supervision) to explore the emotional impact of practice.[10] The opportunity to explore feelings and name stress can foster hope, which is essential to resilience.[49]

Supervision, mentoring and preceptorship, when effective, can start the real journey of learning from novice to expert. In addition, they can offer space to make sense of our own feelings and emotions through the mind of another. This is important when we think of the different aspects of practice, organisational culture, office politics and families' stress and trauma that newly qualified health visitors are bombarded with.

## HEALTH VISITING TEAM

In all of this we must not forget the value of the team in supporting novice health visitors. In an iHV online survey in 2015, health visitors were asked 'How do you get support with pressure and stress at work?' The most frequently reported source was 'informal support from colleagues sharing an office' (n = 1002, 85%). This underlines that regardless of any formal support measures, peer support is well established within the professional culture of health visiting. There is also a body of work that shows that positive social interactions also lead to both physical and mental health benefits, for example,

*When I think of the support I have been lucky enough to receive from my team, I think of the cups of tea, the kind comments and the 'How was that visit?' conversations we have had. These are the opportunities for reflection and expressing my feelings that are meshed inextricably with my everyday practice. I also*

*think of the relationships I am beginning to build with colleagues – the social events and work and casual conversations about life outside the office.[50:13]*

Support such as this provides a 'safe base' from which the novice can learn and develop; its worth is immeasurable. It is to be hoped that, with the increasing popularity of 'mobile working', this form of predictable, accessible and safe support does not become eroded. Little is known today about the impact of remote, mobile and flexible working on employee health and well-being. Even less is known about the impact it could have on the well-being of health visitors. Can social media ever replicate this support? There are examples of social media support such as the 'Tea and Empathy group', which aims to foster a compassionate and supportive atmosphere throughout the NHS.[23] Could models such as these be effective at team level?

## CASE STUDY

Emma had worked in a surgical gynaecology unit. She was in a senior position in the unit and felt confident in her role. Emma decided to train as a health visitor after having children of her own and finding the relationship that she had with her own health visitor supportive.

Having qualified as a health visitor Emma was working in an inner-city area with a demanding caseload. Most of her work seemed to be focused on families with complex needs which seemed unsurmountable. Poverty, loneliness and despair seemed to be key features and Emma felt unprepared for the relentless demands on her and the never-ending workload. She felt herself going through the motions filling in the forms, asking the questions, writing records but never feeling that she had made a real difference to the lives of families whose situations were unrecognisable compared to her own. She frequently felt frustrated that families seemed unwilling or unable to take the advice that she gave them.

Emma looked back on her time in her old role and remembered the thank you's and the positive feedback that she got on a daily basis from patients. She yearned for that feeling of walking away at the end of a shift and leaving her patients in the hands of colleagues who would care for them. Emma felt a creeping fear every time she thought about her families and worried constantly that something would go terribly wrong and she would be to blame. Sometimes she would wake up early thinking about everything that could go wrong and dread going to work.

Emma had developed a good relationship with her mentor Marion and told her how she was feeling. Marion could recognise many of the feelings that Emma had from when she first qualified. She shared with Emma her experience of extreme anxiety around work that eventually led to her seeking help from her GP. She also spoke to Emma about her discovery that she was extremely self-critical and that developing self-compassion skills had helped her to recognise when she was overwhelmed or suffering and soothe herself.

Six months later Emma started on a training programme that focused on building parent–infant relationships. Emma's interest in the area grew and she developed a passion for this work. Emma learned to look for the tiny strengths in family relationships instead of feeling overwhelmed by the deficits. This became her starting point; she realised that the training in looking for the good and focusing on what is possible translated to other areas in her life. Several case conference chairs commented on Emma's detailed observations and insights into the parent–infant relationships. She also realised that when you find a way to help families feel good about themselves everything changes. Emma's confidence grew and with it the satisfaction she got from the work.

Emma began to accept that risk would always be a part of the job but that she wasn't alone with that. She listened out for that voice within her that doubted herself or warned her of everything that she hadn't done. Each time she heard it she listened calmly and then spoke to herself in the way that Marion spoke to her. She reminded herself that she was doing the very best she could and that no one could do any better. Emma discovered the little things in life that brought her joy and calm. Walking her dog in nature, cuddling her children, watching a plant in the garden grow and change over time, laughing with colleagues, watching a box set with her partner in front of the fire. She tried to notice these moments, feel grateful for them, and allow herself to enjoy the warm feelings that they brought even briefly.

As her confidence as a practitioner grew so did her tenacity and skill in influencing within her organisation in a positive way. Emma set up an Emotional Well-being group for colleagues where they shared difficult feelings, explored well-being strategies, laughed, cried and supported one another.

## INEQUALITY

In 2020 the Black Lives Matters movements and the inequalities revealed by COVID-19 shone a light on racism and the treatment of black and minority ethnic (BAME) communities across the globe. A large-scale study carried out in July 2020 by the Health and Care Women Leaders Network of the NHS Confederation found that, in addition to the stress of responding to the crisis, the COVID-19 pandemic had amplified alleged bullying, sexism and racism on the part of managers. This was especially true for staff from BAME backgrounds, who also reported feeling traumatised by the disproportionate impact of the virus. Ross et al carried out research looking at the lived experience of BAME staff working within the

NHS.[51] She found that they did not feel they had equal opportunities to progress in their careers, that they had been denied developmental opportunities that appeared to come readily to their white counterparts. Very few people at the most senior levels of the NHS reflect them. On top of that, each working day can bring a range of micro-aggressions from other colleagues. When we take the time to listen to the voices of colleagues from BAME communities it is not difficult to understand why these repeated experiences over many years have a devastating impact on mental well-being.

Adebowale and Rao found that BAME medical students are resigned to the likelihood that nothing will be done if they report a racial incident, so they don't bother.[52] Instead, they internalise the humiliation and prepare for a career where discrimination is commonplace, 'no doubt affecting their self-esteem and their ability to perform'. They state that they are firmly in agreement with Harvard professor David Williams, who suggests that to bring about the scale of organisational change the NHS needs, 'It takes commitment and deliberate concerted action to change an organisation's culture and make a difference'. Williams says 'The rhetoric must be matched by behaviour and policies that have teeth and the authority to implement change'.

Ross et al looked at the effectiveness of approaches taken by NHS organisations to address workforce race inequalities and develop positive and inclusive working environments, such as[51]:

- establishing staff networks
- ensuring psychologically safe routes for raising concerns (specifically by appointing Freedom to Speak Up Guardians)
- enabling staff development and career progression.

They concluded that approaches to race equality and inclusion are not 'one size fits all'. There is a lack of proven interventions and it is down to individuals and organisations making a concerted effort at a local level to iterate the approach that 'works' for them. Addressing inequalities and inclusion needs to be an ongoing, 'moment-by-moment' activity that engages with and responds to people's lived experiences.

One of the complex issues that has been voiced strongly by the Black Lives Matter movement is the idea that the white dominant society is complicit in the failure to create change and develop an inclusive culture. Doyle talks about the process of unlearning what we think we know about how inclusive the world we inhabit actually is.[23] She says that after really listening to the experiences of marginalised groups she became 'increasingly uncomfortable as the truth agitated my comfortable numbness'.

In addition to racism, we must not forget other groups that experience inequality, such as lesbian, gay, bisexual and transgender communities. Repeated negative experiences can lead to fear, shame, isolation and unnecessary suffering. Inclusion and acceptance are at the heart of well-being and a basic human right that each and every one of us deserves. If this is not a core value at the centre of the organisations that we work for it is difficult to see how it can translate to the families and communities that we work with.

It is going to be an enormously complex journey and will involve strong and committed leadership and each of us listening with open hearts and a willingness to make this wrong right. There is no place for inequality and prejudice in the NHS or society as a whole of this we must be certain.

The NHS People Plan 20/21 introduces health and well-being conversations for all staff which should include equality, diversity and inclusion, to empower people to reflect on their lived experience, support them to become better informed on the issues, and determine what they and their teams can do to make further progress. Health

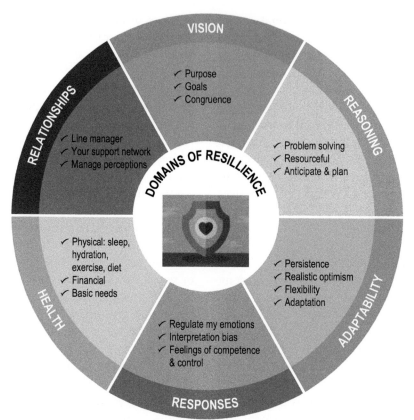

**Figure 3.1** ■ Domains of professional resilience (Ref. [52], cited in 'Health and well-being conversations – support for facilitators. https://people.nhs.uk/guides/health-and-wellbeing-conversations-support-for-facilitators/steps/the-6-domains-of-resilience/. Reproduced with permission, Wallbank, S., 2020. http://www.restorativesupervision.org.uk/.)

and Well-Being Conversations should focus on the six domains of resilience below:

## ORGANISATIONS AND PRACTITIONER WELL-BEING

During the past two decades there has been increasing recognition that the NHS must address the well-being of staff as a matter of urgency. With increasing demands on time, resources, and energy, in addition to poorly designed systems of daily work, it's not surprising health care professionals are experiencing burnout at increasingly higher rates, with staff turnover rates also on the rise.[54] The institute for Healthcare Improvement recognises that joy in work is more than just the absence of burnout or an issue of individual wellness, it is a system property. It is generated (or not) by the system and occurs (or not) organisation-wide. Joy in work – or lack thereof – not only impacts individual staff engagement and satisfaction, but also patient experience, quality of care, patient safety, and organisational performance.[54]

Organisations that prioritise staff health and well-being perform better, with improved patient satisfaction, stronger quality scores, better outcomes, higher levels of staff retention and lower rates of sickness absence.[55] Where staff report poor well-being, the evidence is clear that there are poorer financial outcomes and patient outcomes.[24,56,57] Staff well-being is the strongest predictor of service performance and therefore needs to be the key indicator of organisational performance, positioned firmly at the heart of the NHS and organisations working within it.

What is clear from the literature is that compassion sits firmly at the centre of the solution to many of the issues around practitioner well-being. In his writing of the forward to the HEE report Towards Commissioning for Compassion[58] the Experience, Participation & Equalities Director for NHS England, Dr Neil Churchill, stated that 'High quality patient experience cannot be achieved – ethically or sustainably – at the expense of staff'. He points out that many healthcare systems around the world are therefore working to balance two global phenomena: the growing demand, intensity and acuity for healthcare and the associated risks of staff experiencing stress, burnout and compassion fatigue. Compassion involves the ability to notice, feel or perceive another person's pain, and to be with them or act to alleviate that person's suffering.[59] Evidence demonstrates that compassion breeds compassion: cooperative behaviour can cascade in human networks, with those treated kindly wanting to extend generosity towards others.[60] Certainly, compassion needs to be at the core of each and every human relationship, from the parent and the infant, parent and health visitor, health visitor and manager, commissioner and manager to the executive board and politicians. Breakdown in compassion at the top of this chain is likely to result in breakdown at the other end. Each and every one of us needs to feel heard, seen, valued and safe to enable us to thrive.

There is a clear case that poor staff health and well-being has a significant impact on the performance of NHS organisations (West, 2018 cited in the Ref. [22]). It is now recognised that the well-being of staff is so integral to the delivery of good care that there should be commitment and leadership at the highest level to champion and navigate the needs of staff.

NHS Scotland is making efforts to improve the experience of those working in the NHS using iMatter. Integral to the model is the ability of individuals and teams to shape the action which is taken in response to the feedback. iMatter Scotland is a *staff experience continuous improvement tool* designed with staff in NHS Scotland to help individuals, teams and Health Boards understand and improve staff experience. An independent evaluation of iMatter and Dignity at Work, carried out by Strathclyde University in 2018–2019 (cited in Ref. [61]) found that staff, managers and trade unions viewed iMatter as an effective tool for promoting staff engagement,

*We began to think about mental health and well-being within the workplace, understanding how to deal with it positively and how to support each other.*

In 2014 research was commissioned by NHS England which resulted in the report Building and Strengthening Leadership – Leading with Compassion.[62] This research also identified that compassion applies to everyone. At an individual level people need to develop routine habits to stay balanced, keep rooted to their core purpose, and plan ahead for situations where work is personally depleting, and notice the signs when they have to activate those plans. The role of the manager/leader is pivotal. He or she must be able to notice and respond to need, while connecting. The Commission heard that there has been a steady erosion in the provision of psychologically safe and confidential staff-only spaces in many NHS settings.[24] They also concluded that it is important to note that the culture and environment at the organisational level has the potential to trump other determinants: good people in corrosive or toxic environments have been known to collude in undesirable behaviour. There has for many years within the psychotherapies been a strong emphasis on the research of Menzies Lyth and others who have further developed her original ideas.[49] She suggested that nurses defend themselves against feeling overwhelmed by guilt, anxiety and uncertainty. Indeed, these defences were viewed as having been developed by the organisations and systems within which the nurses were operating to ultimately defend the organisation. In more recent years Christine Bidmead found such defences still exist within health visiting.[63] Whilst home visiting with health visitors during her PhD research she found that some health visitors ignored the 'emotional cues' of mothers during visits (personal communication with the researcher). When interviewed afterwards the health visitors said that they were focused on giving information that the organisation expected them to give to the family. It was also clear that they would not be supported to carry out follow-up visits to families who did not meet the threshold criteria for targeted visiting. There is a great deal of feeling within health visiting currently that staff are rewarded for 'ticking boxes'. These behaviours could fall into the categories identified by Menzies Lyth that undermine relationships.[49] They include depersonalisation, categorisation, denial of the individual's significance, detachment and denial of feelings, ritual task-performance and reducing the impact of responsibility by delegating decision-making to superiors. Understanding how a social institution functions with this social defence system can provide a starting point for change. Leadership is central to developing healthier organisational cultures that protects and develops resilient organisations, staff and families. Social defence systems serve to disconnect relationships. In contrast Bidmead et al reported the role the organisation plays in facilitating the purposeful nature of the health visiting process based on relationship-building and partnership-working.[64] The data revealed the importance of organisations in supporting an approach that provided continuity of care, clinical supervision, manageable caseloads, time for home visiting and simplified record-keeping.

Building resilience in staff has recently been a popular approach to building staff well-being. However, there is a risk that the focus on helping individuals to develop their own resilience is unlikely to be effective if there is not also work undertaken to develop both team and organisational resilience. Resilience should not be about helping people to cope with intolerable situations. Rather it is about helping people cope, and even transform, adversity through addressing the systems which are contributing to sustaining it.[65] The Health Education England NHS Staff and Learners mental Well-being Commission found that the perceived use of resilience to shift responsibility from the organisation to the individual has resulted in some practitioners feeling that the term 'resilience' has negative connotations, implying that they are emotionally weak.[24] There is also some academic contention regarding the term. Asking individuals to improve their resilience without acknowledging that the system they work within can seem almost designed to foster poor mental health may worsen the relationship between postgraduate learners and their employers. This is because organisations may interpret resilience as individuals having the tools to self-care, therefore abrogating the organisation of further responsibility.

In terms of whether training for staff can enhance well-being there is little doubt that this should be an important component of organisations' 'Mental health at work plans'. However, this needs to be accessed by staff at all levels from board down and should not be a stand-alone initiative but part of a broader plan. An independent study by Krekel et al found that a course called 'Exploring What Matters', developed by Action for Happiness, enhances well-being, reduces symptoms of mental ill-health and encourages pro-social action in the general population.[66] The course consists of eight consecutive weekly sessions lasting between 2 and 2.5 hours each. Each of these sessions builds on a thematic question: for example, what matters in life, how to find meaning at work, or how to build happier communities. Each of these questions, in turn, is rooted in scientific evidence on mental well-being and pro-sociality based on an extensive, internal review of the literature, which is summarised in King,[67] as well as insights from evidence on motivation and group learning styles.

### 10 Keys to happier living[67]

Giving
Relating – connect with people
Exercising – taking care of your body
Awareness – living life mindfully
Trying Out – keep learning new things
Direction – have goals to look forward to
Resilience – find ways to bounce back
Emotions – look for what's good
Acceptance – be comfortable with who you are
Meaning – being part of something bigger

The programme has been evaluated by academics from the London School of Economics and Oxford University using a randomised controlled trial. Baldwin et al 2020[81] and Baldwin et al 2021[82] have demonstrated that a mixed model Emotional Wellbeing Group for health visiting teams found improvements accross a range of scales and subscales used to measure mental well-being, percieved stress, compassion satisfaction, burnout and secondary trauma. The results show that, compared to a control group, the course delivers large and statistically significant benefits in terms of:

■ Improvements in subjective well-being
■ Reductions in symptoms of depression and anxiety
■ Enhanced levels of compassion and social trust

'Thriving at work', the review of mental health and employers,[68] looked at how employers can better support all employees, including those with poor mental health or well-being, to remain in and thrive at work. Included within the recommendations were six 'core mental health standards' that include, amongst others, implementing a mental health at work plan, developing mental health awareness, encouraging conversations about mental health, improved working conditions and monitoring employee mental health and well-being. All the recommendations were accepted by the UK Government in their Work, Health and Disability paper, 'Improving Lives'. This was followed by a guide published by MIND one year later. It is designed to help employers to understand and implement the standards and actions that *Thriving at Work* recommends.[75] There are good examples around the country of organisations that are implementing their own solutions to enhance well-being at work. For example, the Taunton initiative, HALT (hungry, angry, late, tired) campaign, which has featured training sessions about removing the barriers to taking a break at work.

In 2020 the World was blindsided by the global pandemic of COVID-19. This created much stress and suffering with the inevitable effects on well-being. However, it also brought into sharp focus the emotional demands on front line staff including the health visiting workforce. In response there has been an upscaling at pace of research, resources, technology, interventions and policies aimed at supporting the well-being of NHS staff. Examples include:

**Scottish Government**: Launched a National Well-being Hub for people working in health and social care.

**Northern Ireland Health and Social Care Public Health Agency**: developed the TAKE 5 and #InItTogether resources for staff

**Health for health Professionals Wales:** Expanded their free, confidential service making it available to all Health Professionals and Healthcare Students working in NHS Wales.

**NHS England**: Developed the NHS people's promise which is a promise they want NHS staff to make to each other[77] – to work together to improve the experience of working in the NHS for everyone. From 2021 the annual NHS Staff Survey will be redesigned to align with Our People Promise.

It is crucial that the momentum that the crisis has created is sustained and built on. It is not difficult to see why investment and energy devoted to nurturing the well-being and development of health visiting teams will have wide reaching effects for children and families and indeed the health of the nation.

## THINKING SPACE

Workplace compassion and culture is embodied in the interpersonal actions and behaviours of colleagues, from taking the time to make a drink for a colleague, to appreciation of the wider context of a staff member's personal circumstances. In this regard, compassion towards staff, like compassion towards patients, has a significant interpersonal behaviour component. Workplace compassion exists in the details of policies and procedures but is enacted interpersonally between staff, and not solely in interactions with staff in hierarchical positions of authority and power. (Towards Commissioning for workplace Compassion[69]). Consider the above quotation with your colleagues.

Can an 'organisation' be compassionate?

Do you experience compassion in your day-to-day work environment?

How do you experience this? In other words what specific behaviours or actions can you recall that manifest compassion?

Is this exceptional or normal within your experience?

When it comes to building a culture of compassion do you think that your colleagues would consider you a 'giver' or a 'taker'?

Think: 'If I wasn't here, would this workplace be experienced and more or less compassionate by my colleagues?

## DEALING WITH REALITY

It is commonplace to complain that there are gaps between 'theory and practice' or between 'policy and practice'. This disjuncture is a topic worth investigation in itself, suffice to say that the motivations for work in a professional field such as health visiting include ideals embodied in theory and policy that are routinely open to challenge from the day-to-day demands of 'reality'. In this chapter we have explored the factors that on the one hand a) impact upon the well-being of practitioners arising from practice itself, such as the needs of children and families in their communities as well as from the organisational and service context; and, on the other hand, b) how we each personally respond and contribute to these challenges.

In a major study of factors affecting the recruitment and retention of health visitors, Whittaker et al found that the sense of being able to 'make a difference' to children and families was an overriding factor in whether health visitors joined and remained within the profession.[70] They identified that how services were organised, both structurally and culturally, could support or hinder practitioners' sense that they could 'make a difference'. This does not mean, however, that practitioners are helpless victims of their workplace environment. On the contrary, 'making a difference' is the way that practitioners can exercise their agency, that is, can actively contribute through their actions and attitudes to their work environments. Indeed, a principle of health visiting is 'influencing policy affecting health', which can be applied not only to our clients but to the well-being of ourselves and colleagues. That is not to say that this is easy.

The profound interplay between the 'subjective' experience of work (in general) and the 'objective' reality of work has been explored in depth by the French psychoanalytic philosopher Christophe Dejours as the psychodynamics of work. Dejours builds upon the earlier work of Lyth-Menzies and others to develop a more widely applicable theory of work and working that nevertheless has resonance for the particularities of health visiting. 'Work' he suggests is 'defined as what the subjects (i.e. each of us as workers) must *add* to the orders (e.g. the requirements of the job), or alternatively, what they must add of themselves in order to deal with what does not function (everyday reality) when they limit themselves to a scrupulous execution of orders'.[71:47]

An example of how this sheds light on working as a health visitor is the impact of the mandate of five child and family health reviews translated into Key Performance Indicators (KPIs) for the providers of health visiting services in England. A 'Vision for Health Visiting', published by the Institute of Health Visiting,[43] refers to 'Ticking the box and missing the point'.

*Mandating the five universal reviews has skewed prioritisation of resources to achieving targets for numbers of universal contacts achieved at the expense of personalised support for families with identified needs, or with any regard to quality. What gets measured gets done – A focus on process outcome measures, often mean the delivery of statutory and mandatory functions are protected to the detriment of early intervention and prevention services.*[43:11]

*This does not at all imply that these universal reviews are unimportant, but that this selective focus on KPIs has a distorting effect on the service received by families and on health visitors' practice. It circumscribes the autonomy of practitioners to practise effectively. It diminishes the three conditions for motivation in work identified by Schwartz 4 by reducing autonomy; reducing the perception that the employer invests in staff by indicating that*

*the organisation is only interested in 'ticking the box' to measure KPIs; and undermining a sense of 'mission' because the KPIs, on their own, ignore or devalue the comprehensive professional mission to 'make a difference'.*

Dejours [71] points out that,

*It is impossible to achieve quality if the orders (e.g. KPIs) are scrupulously respected. Indeed (all) ordinary work situations are rife with unexpected events, breakdowns, incidents, operational anomalies, organisational inconsistency and things that are simply impossible to predict, arising from the materials, tools, and machines as well as from other workers, colleagues, bosses, subordinates, the team, the chain of authority, the clients and so on… [t]here is always a gap between the prescriptive and the concrete reality of the situation. Working thus means bridging the gap between prescriptive and concrete realities.*[70:47]

**(Ref. [71]: 47. Original italics).**

This characterisation of the psychopathology of work may well be recognisable to health visitors, but is not a counsel of despair from Dejours. Indeed, he suggests that 'working well' implies violating the described constraints of organisational conditions through creative and skilful intelligence: a kind of blending of the art and science of practice that is sensitive to the context of everyday realities for ourselves, and those we work with as colleagues and clients. The fact that the KPIs leave 'gaps' between what is prescribed and 'reality' therefore leaves space within which we, as practitioners, can take a critical but creative stance by enacting and articulating the 'art of the possible'. An example of this can be found in the case studies of how the Institute of Health Visiting's aspirational 'Vision of health visiting' is already being realised.

## THINKING SPACE

God, grant me the serenity to accept the
things I cannot change,
Courage to change the things I can,
And wisdom to know the difference.
The Serenity Prayer. Attributed to the
theologian, Reinhold Niebuhr.

Reflect on how this well-known prayer prompts us to explore the gap between the ideal and the real and how we can survive, thrive and even transform the reality of our working lives.

'Survive, thrive and transform' is the motto of the WHO Global Strategy for Women's Children's and Adolescents' Health 2015–2030. Can you apply this to your work-place?

Revisit the health visiting 'orientation to practice' applied to your work experience,

   (i) Is my experience of practising as a health visitor 'salutogenic' for me and for my colleagues? Am I proactive, identifying and building strengths and resources for me as a person and in my situation with those who share my work situation as colleagues? Am I solution-focused or part of 'the problem'? Do I foster resilience for myself and others?
  (ii) Do I demonstrate a positive regard for others (human valuing) I work with? Do I recognise colleagues as persons (not just job roles), through keeping the person in mind and shifting my focus to align with their human needs, recognising the potential for unmet need, actively seeking out potential strengths, maintaining hope?
 (iii) Do I recognise the person-in-situation (human ecology) through a continuing process, always taking account of the individual and their personal and situational circumstances, applying this both to myself and to colleagues within the

organisation and other agencies that I work with? Do I recognise and take seriously the constraints and micro-politics of everyday working life, as well as the bigger policy picture? Is my work context toxic to well-being or supportive?

## CONCLUSION

In this chapter we have explored the relationship between work and well-being, focussing further on professional practice in health visiting. We have also explored how the distinctive context of health visiting practice brings its own challenges for student health visitors experiencing role transition; but we have also noted the way in which the health visiting orientation to practice provides resources for actively reflecting and supporting well-being for ourselves as practitioners as well as for those we work with. An organisational perspective has helped us to identify how the workplace can be configured to support well-being or to erode it. However, we have also seen that at the level of the team and the individual there are insights and practices that we can adopt in order to exercise our agency, influencing the climate within which we work, expressing core values of compassion and sustaining relationships that affirm our human worth.

### KEY LEARNING POINTS

- Practicing gratitude and learning to notice the small moments when things go well can help our brains focus less on threats
- Focus and draw satisfaction from completing small episodes of work
- Developing self-compassion skills can help us to notice when we are suffering and to act to sooth and nurture ourselves
- Good quality preceptorship and supervision can help individuals with the process of change

- Embracing ongoing learning and development opportunities helps us to master our craft, building our confidence and self-esteem
- Seek out and accept support for our own mental health when we need it without shame
- Organisations that prioritise staff health and well-being perform better
- Evidence demonstrates that compassion breeds compassion
- Focus on helping individuals to develop their own resilience is unlikely to be effective if there is not also work undertaken to develop both team and organisational resilience

## FURTHER RESOURCES

Actionforhappiness.org.

Developing Self Compassion. https://self-compassion.org.

How are you feeling at work? https://www.nhsemployers.org/retention-and-staff-experience/health-and-wellbeing/taking-a-targeted-approach/taking-a-targeted-approach/how-are-you-feeling-today-nhs-toolkit.

https://www.mentalhealthatwork.org.uk.

Mental health in the workplace. https://www.nhsemployers.org/retention-and-staff-experience/health-and-wellbeing/taking-a-targeted-approach/taking-a-targeted-approach/mental-health-in-the-workplace.

Northern Ireland Health and Social Care Public Health Agency. (2020). Supporting the well-being needs of our health and social care staff during COVID-19: A framework. https://www.publichealth.hscni.net/sites/default/files/HSC_Regional%20Staff%20Wellbeing%20w.

Our NHS People. Supporting our people, helping you manage your own health and wellbeing whilst looking after others. https://people.nhs.uk.

Scottish National Wellbeing Hub for people working in health and social care. https://www.promis.scot.

Stress and its impact on the workplace. https://www.nhsemployers.org/retention-and-staff-experience/health-and-wellbeing/taking-a-targeted-approach/taking-a-targeted-approach/stress-and-its-impact-on-the-workplace.

Whatworkswellbeing.org.

## REFERENCES

1. Cowley, S., Whittaker, K., Grigulis, A., Malone, M., Donetto, S., Wood, H., et al.(2013). *Why health visiting? A review of the literature about key health visitor interventions, processes and outcomes for children and families.* National Nursing Research Unit, King's College London. http://www.kcl.ac.uk/nursing/research/nnru/publications/index.aspx.

2. WHO. (2001). *Strengthening mental health promotion.* Geneva: World Health Organisation. (Fact Sheet, No. 220). https://www.who.int/mental_health/evidence/en/promoting_mhh.pdf.

3. Wadell, G., & Burton, A. K. (2006) *Is work good for your health and wellbeing. An independent review of the evidence on the relationship between work, health and wellbeing.* Department of Work and Pensions. https://www.gov.uk/government/uploads/system/uploads/attachment_data/file/209510/hwwb-is-work-good-for-you-exec-summ.pdf.

4. Schwartz, B. (2015). *Why we work.* New York: TED Books, Simon and Schuster.

5. Hill, A., & Curran, T. (2016). Multidimensional perfectionism and burnout: A meta-analysis. *Personality and Social Psychology Review, 20*(3), 269–288.

6. Neff, K., & Dahm, K. (2015). Self-compassion: What it is, what it does, and how it relates to mindfulness. *Handbook of Mindfulness and Self-Regulation,* 121–137.

7. Newcomb, M., Burton, J., Edwards, N., & Hazelwood, Z. (2015). How Jung's concept of the wounded healer can guide learning and teaching in social work and human services. Advances in Social Work and Welfare Education. 17, 55–69.

8. Conti-O'Hare, M. (2002). *The theory of the nurse as a wounded healer: From trauma to transcendence.* Sudbury, MA: Jones and Bartlett Publishers.

9. Barr, A. (2006). *An investigation into the extent to which psychological wounds inspire counsellors and psychotherapists to become wounded healers, the significance of these wounds on their career choice, the causes of these wounds and the overall significance of demographic factors.* Glasgow: (Unpublished dissertation). University of Strathclyde.

10. McInnes, E. (2015). *A national preceptorship framework for health visiting: The first 2 years.* London: Institute of Health Visiting.

11. Shafir, R. (2000). *The zen of listening – Mindful communication in the age of distraction.* Quest Books.

12. Beck, A. T. (1967). *Depression: Causes and treatment.* Philadelphia: University of Pennsylvania Press.

13. Emmons, R., & McCullough, M. (2003). Counting blessings versus burdens: An experimental investigation of gratitude and subjective well-being in daily life. *Journal of Personality and Social Psychology, 84*(2), 377–389.

14. Stamm, B. H. (2010). *The concise ProQOL manual* (2nd ed). Pocatello. ID: ProQOL.org.

15. Bendelow, G. (2009). *Health, emotion and the body*. Oxford: Polity Press.

16. Pettit, A., & Stephen, R. (2015). *Supporting health visitors and fostering resilience – Literature review*. London: Institute of Health Visiting.

17. McCann, I. L., & Pearlman, L. A. (1990). Vicarious traumatisation: A framework for understanding the psychological effects of working with victims. *Journal of Traumatic Stress, 3*(1), 131–149. https://doi.org/10.1007/BF00975140.

18. NHS Staff Survey. (2018). https://www.nhsstaffsurveys.com/Page/1064/Latest-Results/2018-Results/.

19. The Lookout. (2019). *Vicarious trauma and burnout*. https://www.thelookout.org.au/family-violence-workers/self-care-family-violence-workers/vicarious-trauma-burnout.

20. Kinman, G., & Teoh, K. (2018). Society of occupational medicine report: What could make a difference to the mental health of UK doctors? A review of the research evidence. https://www.som.org.uk/sites/som.org.uk/files/What_could_make_a_difference_to_the_mental_health_of_UK_doctors_LTF_SOM.pdf.

21. Brown, B. (2010). In *The gifts of imperfection: Let go of who you think you're supposed to be and embrace who you are* (pp. 30). New York: Simon and Schuster.

22. NHS Employers Strategy and Innovation Directorate. (2019). *Workforce health and development framework*. https://www.nhsemployers.org/-/media/Employers/Publications/Health-and-well-being/NHS-Workforce-HWB-Framework_updated-July-18.pdf.

23. Doyle, G. (2020). *Untamed - stop pleasing, start living*. UK: Penguin Random House.

24. Health Education England. (2019). *NHS Staff and Learners Mental Wellbeing Commission: How to engage staff in the NHS and why it matters*. The Point of Care Foundation.

25. McNicoll, A. (2017). Ten years on from baby P: Social Work's Story. *Community Care*. https://www.communitycare.co.uk/2017/08/03/ten-years-baby-p-social-works-story/.

26. Dekker, S. (2016). In *Just culture: Restoring trust and accountability in your organization,* (3rd ed.). Oxford: Taylor and Francis.

27. Bion, W. (1962). *Learning from Experience*. London: Heinemann.

28. Rimé, B. (2009). Emotion elicits the social sharing of emotion: Theory and empirical review. *Emotion Review, 1*(1), 60–85.

29. Palsson, M., Hallberg, I. R., Norberg, A., & Bjorvell, H. (1996). Burnout empathy and sense of coherence among Swedish district nurses before and after systematic clinical supervision. *Scandinavian Journal of Caring Sciences, 10*(1), 19–26.

30. Walsh, K., Nicholson, J., Keough, C., Pridham, R., Kramer, M., & Jeffrey, J. (2003). Development of a group model of supervision to meet the needs of a community health nursing team. *International Journal of Nursing Practice, 9*(1), 33–39.

31. Scottish Government. (2017). Nursing 2030 vision. www.gov.scot/publications/nursing-2030vision-9781788511001/.

32. Pollock, A., Campbell, P., Deery, R., Fleming, M., Rankin, J., Sloan, G., & Cheyne, H. (2017). A systematic review of evidence relating to clinical supervision for nurses, midwives and allied health professionals. *Journal of Advanced Nursing, 73*(8), 1825–1837. https://doi.org/10.1111/jan.13253.

33. Davis, H., & Spurr, P. (1998). Parent counselling: an evaluation of a community child mental health service. *Journal of Child Psychology and Psychiatry, 39*, 365–376.

34. Barlow, J., Stewart-Brown, S., Callaghan, H., Tucker, J., Brocklehurst, N., & Davis, H. (2003). Working in Partnership: The development of a home visiting service for vulnerable families. *Child Abuse Review, 12*, 172–189.

35. Brocklehurst, N., Barlow, J., Kirkpatrick, S., Davis, H., & Stewart-Brown, S. (2004). The contribution of health visitors to supporting vulnerable children and their families at home. *Community Practitioner, 77*, 175–179.

36. Davis, H., & Tsiantis, J. (2005). Promoting children's mental health: The European Early Promotion Project (EEPP). *International Journal of Mental Health Promotion, 7*, 4–16.

37. Barnes, J., Ball, M., Meadows, P., Howden, B., Jackson, A., Henderson, J., & Niven, L. (2011). *The family nurse partnership in England*. Department of Health.

38. Colthart, I., Duffy, K., Blair, V., & Whyte, L. (2018). Keeping support and clinical supervision on your agenda. *Nursing management (Harrow), 25*(5), 20–27. doi: 10.7748/nm.2018.e1804.

39. Botham, J. (2013). What constitutes safeguarding children supervision for health visitors and school nurses? *Community Practitioner, 86*(3), 28–34.

40. Proctor, B. (1986). Supervision: A co-operative exercise in accountability. In M. Marken, & M. Payne (Eds.), *Enabling and ensuring – Supervision in practice*, Leicester, UK: National Youth Bureau, Council for Education and Training in Youth and Community Work.

41. Hunter, B., & Warren, L. (2013). *Investigating resilience in midwifery: Final report*. Royal College of Midwives.

42. Daloz, L. A. (1986). *Effective teaching and mentoring: realizing the transformational power of adult learning experiences*. Wiley.

43. Institute of Health Visiting. (2019). *Health visiting in England: A vision for the future*. London. Institute of Health Visiting. https://ihv.org.uk/news-and-views/press-releases/ihv-launches-health-visiting-in-england-a-vision-for-the-future/.

44. Driscoll, J. (2003). Practicing clinical supervision: A reflective approach. In S. Hinchcliff, S. Norman, & J. Schober (Eds.), *Nursing practice and health care* (4th ed.). London: Arnold.

45. Dewey, J. (1938). *Experience and education*. Macmillan: New York.

46. Petty, G. (2004). In *Teaching today* (3rd ed.). Cheltenham: Nelson Thornes.

47. Corkan, L. (2012) A health visiting career, DOH. https://assets.publishing.service.gov.uk/government/uploads/system/uploads/attachment_data/file/216557/dh_134574.pdf.

48. Clutterbuck, D. (2004). In *Everyone needs a mentor; fostering talent on your organisation* (4th ed.). Chartered Institute of Personnel and Development (CIPD).

49. Menzies Lyth, I (Ed.) (1988). The functioning of social systems as a defence against anxiety: A report on a study of a general hospital. In *Containing anxiety in institutions; Selected essays*. Free Association Books, London, Originally published in 1959 in *Human Relations*, 13: 95-121, reprinted in 1961 by Tavistock Publications and in 1970 as part of the Tavistock Institute of Human Relations pamphlet series.

50. Dobson, A. (2017). Newly qualified health visitor: Support during transition to practice. *Journal of Health Visiting*, 5(1), 2017.

51. Ross, S., Jabbal, J., Chauhan, K., Maguire, D., Ranfhawa, M., & Dahir, S. (2020). Workforce race inequalities and inclusion in NHS providers. The Kings Fund. https://www.kingsfund.org.uk/publications/workforce-race-inequalities-inclusion nhs.

52. Adebowale, V., & Rao, M. (2020). Racism in medicine: Why equality matters to everyone. *British Medical Journal*, 368, m530. doi: 10.1136/bmj.m530. pmid:32051166.

53. Wallbank, S. (2017). *The restorative resilience model of supervision: An organisational training manual for building resilience to workplace stress in health and social care professionals*. Pavillion Publishing.

54. Perlo, J., Balik, B., Swensen, S., Kabcenell, A., Landsman, J., & Feeley, D. (2017). *IHI framework for improving joy in work*. IHI White Paper. Cambridge, Massachusetts: Institute for Healthcare Improvement.

55. Lown, B. (2018). Mission critical: Nursing leadership support for compassion to sustain staff well-being. *Nursing Administration Quarterly*, 42(3), 217–222.

56. Scottish Government. (2011). Safe and well at work: Occupational health and safety strategic framework for NHS Scotland, Scottish Government.

57. NHS Wales. (2014). Caring for staff: The NHS Wales staff psychological health and well-being resource. An online resource for leaders, managers and teams, supporting you to increase and promote staff psychological health and well-being in your organisation. http://www.nwssp.wales.nhs.uk/sitesplus/documents/1178/Caring%20for%20Staff%20%2D%20The%20NHS%20Wales%20Staff%20Psychological%20Health%20and%20Well-being%20Resource.pdf.

58. Health Education England. (2018). *Towards commissioning for workplace compassion – A support guide*. https://www.england.nhs.uk/wp-content/uploads/2018/10/towards-commissioning-for-workplace-compassion-a-support-guide-v2.pdf.

59. Poorkavoos, M. (2017). *Towards a more compassionate workplace*. www.roffeypark.com/wp-content/uploads2/Towards-a-more-compassionate-workplace-in-the-events-and-hospitality-sector.pdf.

60. Fowler, J., & Christakis, N. (2010). Cooperative behavior cascades in human social networks. *Proceedings of the National Academy of Sciences of the United States of America*, 107 (12) 5334–5338; https://doi.org/10.1073/pnas.0913149107.

61. A Healthier Scotland – Scottish Government. (2020). Everyone matters 2020 – Workforce vision – Health and social care staff experience report. https://www.shb.scot.nhs.uk/board/foi/2020/03/2020-099a.pdf.

62. NHS England. (2014). *Building and strengthening leadership – Leading with compassion*. https://www.england.nhs.uk/wp-content/uploads/2014/12/london-nursing-accessible.pdf.

63. Bidmead, C. (2013). Health Visitor/parent relationships: A qualitative analysis. Appendix 1. In S. Cowley, K. Whittaker, A. Grigulis, et al. (Eds), *Appendices for Why health visiting? A review of the literature about key health visitor interventions, processes and outcomes for children and families*. National Nursing Research Unit, King's College London. Pp. 1–59. https://www.kcl.ac.uk/nmpc/research/nnru/publications/reports/appendices-12-02-13.pdf

64. Bidmead, C., Cowley, S., & Grocott, P. (2016). The role of organisations in supporting the parent/health visitor relationship. *Journal of Health Visiting*, 4(7).

65. Diprose, K. (2015). Resilience is futile. *Soundings*, 58, 44–56.

66. Krekel, C., De Neve, J. E., Fancourt, D., & Layard, R. (2020). *A local community course that raises mental wellbeing and pro-sociality*. Discussion Paper, Centre for

Economic Performance: London School of Economics and Political Science.

67. King, V. (2016). *10 keys to happier living: A practical handbook for happiness.* Headline Publishing Group.

68. Stevenson, D., & Farmer, P. (2017). *Thriving at work: The independent review of mental health and employers.* Department of Work and Pensions and Department of Health and Social Care.

69. NHS England. (2018). *Towards commissioning for compassion: A support guide.* Publications Gateway Ref No. 08058, https://www.england.nhs.uk/wp-content/uploads/2018/10/towards-commissioning-for-workplace-compassion-a-support-guide-v2.pdf.

70. Whittaker, K. A., Malone, M., Cowley, S., Grigulis, A., Nicholson, C., & Maben, J. (2017). Making a difference for children and families: An appreciative inquiry of health visitor values and why they start and stay in post. *Health Soc Care Community, 25*, 338–348.

71. Dejours, C. (2006). Subjectivity, work and action. *Critical Horizons, 7*(1), 45–62.

72. Department of Health and Department of Work and Pensions. (2017). *Improving lives the future of work, health and disability.* https://assets.publishing.service.gov.uk/government/uploads/system/uploads/attachment_data/file/663399/improving-lives-the-future-of-work-health-and-disability.PDF.

73. Department of Health. (2009). *Healthy child programme: Pregnancy and the first five years of life.* DOH. https://assets.publishing.service.gov.uk/government/uploads/system/uploads/attachment_data/file/167998/Health_Child_Programme.pdf.

74. Health and Care Women Leaders Network, NHS Confederation. (2020). *COVID-19 and the female health and care workforce – Survey of health and care staff for the Health and Care Women Leaders Network, NHS Confederation.* https://www.nhsconfed.org/-/media/Confederation/Files/Networks/Health-and-Care-Women-Leaders-Network/COVID19-and-the-female-health-and-care-workforce-FINAL2.pdf.

75. Kramer, M. (1974). *Reality shock: Why nurses leave nursing.* USA: C V Mosby.

76. MIND UK. (2018). *How to implement the thriving at work mental health standards in your workplace.* https://www.mind.org.uk/media/25263166/how-to-implement-the-thriving-at-work-mental-health-standards-final-guide-online.pdf.

77. NHS Education for Scotland. (2020). *TURAS clinical supervision resource.* https://learn.nes.nhs.scot/3580/clinical-supervision.

78. NHS England. (2020). ***WE ARE THE NHS****: People Plan 2020/21 – Action for us all.* https://www.england.nhs.uk/publication/we-are-the-nhs-people-plan-for-2020-21-action-for-us-all/.

79. Ross, S. (2020). *A hopeful moment? Addressing race inequalities in the NHS workforce.* https://www.kingsfund.org.uk/blog/2020/07/addressing-race-inequalities-nhs-workforce.

80. Scottish Government. (2013). Everyone matters: 2020 health workforce vision.

81. Baldwin, S., Stephen, R., Bishop, P., Kelly, P. (2020). Development of the Emotional Wellbeing at Work Virtual Programme to Support UK health Visiting teams, *Journal of Health Visiting,* Vol. 8, No. 12.

82. Baldwin, S., Stephen, R., Bishop, P., Kelly, P. (2021). Evaluation of an emotional well-being at work programme for supporting health visiting teams during COVID-19, *Primary Health Care,* doi; 10,7748/phc.2021.e1741.

# 4

# SOCIAL POLICY, CONTEXT OF PUBLIC HEALTH AND THE ORGANISATION OF HEALTH VISITING SERVICE PROVISION

ALISON HACKETT ■ KATHLEEN CLARKE ■ JOYCE WILKINSON

## CHAPTER CONTENT

INTRODUCTION

THE NATIONAL APPROACH TO PUBLIC HEALTH WITHIN THE UNITED KINGDOM

SOCIAL POLICY

ORGANISATION OF HEALTH VISITING SERVICE PROVISION

CONCLUSION

## LEARNING OUTCOMES

*To:*

- identify and critically appraise relevant public health and social policy
- apply local and national approaches to protect and support the health and wellbeing of children and families
- practice safely and effectively reflecting evidence within local contexts

## INTRODUCTION

Across the United Kingdom (UK), protecting and improving the health and wellbeing of the public and reducing inequalities in health are key priorities for each of the four countries.[1-4] However, how this is achieved varies, as each of the devolved countries has its own public health body, their own public health strategy and social policies. Nonetheless, a key theme running throughout the public health strategy in each nation is the need to ensure that children and young people achieve their full potential and have the best start in life. There is a growing evidence base linking early intervention with improved outcomes for children and young people. For example, Growing Up in Scotland (GUS) is a longitudinal Scottish government (SG) funded study which has been following the journey of two birth cohorts of children and their families since 2005.[5] Although the findings have highlighted that there are still inequalities between children and young people from the poorest backgrounds when compared to their more affluent peers, they also point to an improvement in the outcomes for vocabulary acquisition and problem-solving at 3 years of age and an improvement in maternal mental wellbeing scores.[5] Factors associated with these improvements included the provision of parenting support, early childcare, promoting and supporting the physical and mental health and wellbeing of mothers and promoting resilience; and the health visitor was found to play a key role.[5]

This chapter will consider the social policy context of public health with a focus on the early years; and provide an overview of the organisation of health visiting service provision within the UK. It should be read in conjunction with Chapter 1. The importance of early intervention and the key role health visitors play in improving the health and wellbeing of children, young people and families will be highlighted. In addition, it will argue for continued investment in health visiting education and a commitment from all devolved governments to maintain the focus on early intervention. To facilitate learning, this chapter includes a number of individual learning activities, which can also be tailored to group activities.

The chapter will begin with a brief overview of the national approach to public health in each of the devolved countries with a specific focus on the early years, before providing a critique of the social policy context and organisation of health visiting service provision.

## THE NATIONAL APPROACH TO PUBLIC HEALTH WITHIN THE UNITED KINGDOM

As stated previously, each of the devolved nations of the UK has devised their own approach to tackling inequalities in health, preventing disease and protecting and improving the health and wellbeing of the population. Over the last two decades, each of the devolved governments has acknowledged the need to address the wider socio-economic determinants of health in an effort to reduce health inequalities; however, recent mortality trends in Scotland and England have highlighted that, over the last decade, the rate of improvement in health has slowed and health inequalities are increasing.[6] It can be argued that the austerity policies implemented by the Coalition government in 2010 and continued by the current Conservative government have shown an impact.[6,7] For example, Loopstra et al[7] carried out an analysis of the number of new food banks opening between 2010 and 2013 in local authorities across

the UK. They found that the opening of a new food bank in a local authority area was associated with higher levels of unemployment rates, local spending cuts and cuts to welfare benefits.[7] Similarly, a mixed methods study designed to understand the extent of food bank use in Glasgow's deprived communities revealed that cuts to welfare benefits were associated with foodbank use.[8] Of particular note in MacLeod, Curl and Kearn's[8] study was a link between poor health, food poverty and foodbank use and the potential risk of exacerbating pre-existing health issues. The findings from these studies serve to highlight the need for public health strategies to tackle the wider socio-economic determinants of health.[6] This has become more evident during the coronavirus pandemic, which has highlighted that individuals, families and communities who experience the greatest deprivation are at increased risk from the impact of COVID-19 on their health and wellbeing outcomes.

This section will now provide an overview of the public health strategy and public health agency in each of the devolved nations and discuss the similarities and differences and any implications for health visiting service provision.

### Scotland

It is the ambition of the Scottish government that Scotland will be the best place for children to grow up and develop into: successful learners, confident individuals, responsible citizens and effective contributors. In addition, it is their vision that opportunities for children, young people and families at risk will be improved across the life course, the nation's inequalities will be addressed and people will be healthier and live longer. However, it is acknowledged that there are a number of public health challenges that need to be addressed, in particular, improving children's mental wellbeing, dental health increasing the numbers of babies and children with healthy weight and the COVID-19 pandemic.[9]

In 2017, 'A Fairer Healthier Scotland: A strategic framework for action 2017–2022' was published.[9] This document outlines the strategic priorities to improve the health and healthy life expectancy of the people of Scotland, as it is recognised that Scotland continues to be the 'poor man of Europe'. Five strategic priorities were identified, each underpinned by a rights-based approach and 'the principles of participation, accountability, non-discrimination, empowerment and legality (PANEL)'.[9:3] Priority Two is of particular relevance to health visiting, as it concerns the health and wellbeing of children, young people and families. The long-term outcomes to improve their health and wellbeing include the need for local and national policies and strategies to be evidence based to promote and build resilience, reduce poverty and adverse childhood experiences. In addition, it is anticipated that more parents, families and young people will use information and advice designed to improve their health and wellbeing.[9] Consequently, over the last 2 years, there has been a redesign of health information for parents informed by input from health visitors, academics and other health professionals. More recently, as part of the public health reform in Scotland, in response to the recommendations of the Christie Commission Report,[10] the Scottish government[11] published 'The Public Health Priorities for Scotland'. Six public health priorities for the next decade have been identified and agreed by the Scottish government and the Convention of Scottish Local Authorities (COSLA), in collaboration with a wide range of stakeholders.[11] These priorities are interconnected and link clearly to Dahlgren and Whitehead's[12] Rainbow Model, as they focus on targeting the determinants of health at the level of the individual, their social and community network and the economic, cultural and environmental level. For example: improving the places people live, work and play; ensuring children, young people and families flourish by getting the right support, in the right place at the right time; promoting good mental health and wellbeing and building resilience; reducing the harm caused by alcohol, tobacco and drug use; reducing the gap in income and wealth to promote a fairer, more inclusive economy; and promoting healthy eating, physical activity and a healthy weight.

As part of the public health reforms, the Scottish government and COSLA[11] set out their proposals for the creation of a new national public health body, 'Public Health Scotland' with the purpose of building on and strengthening public health assets, and facilitating more effective targeting of resources to improve the health and wellbeing of people in Scotland. Public Health Scotland was launched on the 1st April 2020, and it comprises of Health Scotland, Health Protection Scotland and National Services Scotland's Information Services Division. It is anticipated that, by amalgamating these agencies, the new national public health body will be more effective at addressing inequalities in health, improving the health of the people in Scotland and reducing pressures on the provision of health and social care.[11] However, achieving this will rely upon effective leadership, collaborative interagency working and information systems that 'speak to one another', something that is currently a challenge within health and social care. Nonetheless, this new public health body has the potential to streamline and deliver a whole systems approach to public health in Scotland to protect and improve the nation's health and wellbeing. Its success will be measured via how effectively it achieves the public health priorities and works collaboratively with the NHS, health and social care partnerships, national and local government, third and private sectors, higher education institutions and communities.[11]

## Northern Ireland

In Northern Ireland (NI), 'Making Life Better' is the strategic framework for public health.[4] This document sets out a 10-year plan from 2013 to 2023 to achieve the vision of the NI government to improve the health and wellbeing of the nation, reduce health inequalities and enable and support everyone to achieve their full potential. There is a clear focus on creating conditions where individuals, groups and communities feel empowered to take control of their own lives.[4] The strategic public health framework has been structured around the following six themes: giving every child the best start; equipped throughout life; empowering healthy living; creating the conditions; empowering communities and developing collaboration. Akin to Scotland, these themes are underpinned by a rights-based approach, highlighting an increasing awareness that everyone has the right to achieve their full potential, to be involved in decisions that affect their lives and to be treated equally.

The public health agency (PHA) is the public body responsible for protecting and improving the health and social wellbeing of the population of Northern Ireland and reducing inequalities in health. It was established in 2009, following radical reform of health and social care and their subsequent integration.[13] The 'Corporate Plan 2017–2021' outlines the long-term outcomes and actions that the PHA, in collaboration with a wide range of stakeholders, should achieve.[13] There are five broad outcomes and actions which are underpinned by a set of guiding principles. Of particular relevance to the public health role of health visitors are the following principles: effective communication, partnership working, building on and learning from good practice, making best use of evidence-based practice and contributing to the evidence base through participating in research. These principles are reflective of the current Nursing and Midwifery Council (NMC) Domains and Proficiencies for Specialist Community Public Health Nursing. In common, with the public health agencies operating in the other countries of the UK, the PHA advocates a whole systems and life course approach to achieving the strategic priorities.[4]

## Wales

The Welsh government have outlined their commitment to protecting and improving the health of the people of Wales within the document 'Our Strategic Plan 2019–2022'.[3] This strategic plan outlines the public health priorities for Wales for the next 3 years, and it forms part of their longer-term plans to improve the health of the population of Wales and reduce health inequalities over the next decade. Seven public health priorities have been identified, which target the determinants of health at the individual, social and community network and economic, cultural and environmental levels. As in Scotland, there is a significant focus on prevention and early intervention, improving mental wellbeing, building resilience and securing a healthy future for the next generation.[3] In common with Scotland, England and Northern Ireland, developing evidence-based policy and practice to improve health and wellbeing are regarded as important priorities in Wales.

The agency tasked with the responsibility for protecting and improving the health of the Welsh population is Public Health Wales. This agency supports a whole system, life course and assets-based approach and, similar to Scotland, its success will be measured in how effectively it achieves the public health outcomes and indicators outlined in the strategic plan.[3] What is inherently clear within the public health approach for Wales is the commitment of the Welsh government and Public Health Wales to address the determinants of health at all levels of influence and across the social gradient. This is in direct contrast to England, where the approach appears to be more targeted on vulnerable individuals, groups and communities.[1]

## England

The ambition of the UK government resembles that of Scotland, Wales and Northern Ireland, in that they want children and young people to have the best start in life.[1] In September 2019, the 'PHE Strategy 2020–2025'[1] was published. This document sets out the public health priorities for

England, of which there are 10, organised into four themes: healthier, fairer, safer and stronger. Similar to Scotland, there is a focus on promoting healthier diets and healthier weights across the life course; improving mental health, reducing the harm from tobacco and reducing inequalities in health. However, in contrast to Scotland and Wales, building resilience is not clearly articulated within Public Health England's (PHE) strategic priorities despite the growing evidence base linking resilience with improved health and wellbeing outcomes not only for individuals but also for communities.[14] Moreover, unlike Scotland and Wales government policy, England seems to contradict PHE's focus on reducing health inequalities; indeed, Marmot et al[6:125] are scathing of the government in England and contend that,

*Action on health inequalities has not been a priority for national government in England since 2010 and there has been no national strategy in the intervening period. This is despite stalling life expectancy and widening inequalities, as reflected in a steeper social gradient in health between socioeconomic groups and also widening health inequalities between regions.*

PHE, established in 2013, is the agency tasked with the responsibility of protecting and improving the health of the population in England and reducing health inequalities. Moreover, PHE has a key role in delivering the NHS Long Term Plan for England and the PHE Strategy for 2020–2025 in collaboration with a wider range of stakeholders. PHE is a single agency that supports a systems approach to health protection and improvement; akin to Scotland, effective and strong leadership and building relationships with partner agencies are identified as essential to achievement of the 10 national priorities.[1] This should come as no surprise, as it is widely acknowledged in health and social care that effective leadership and working in partnership with others are key to improving outcomes.[15] However, as previously argued in this chapter, austerity measures are one of the greatest barriers to the achievement of the public health priorities, and unless there is a change in policy direction, the gap between the least and most deprived individuals, families and communities will continue to widen.[6]

## THINKING SPACE

Consider the role of the health visitor in contributing to the public health priorities relevant to the nation in which you are currently practicing.

What are the implications for health visiting practice?

This chapter will now consider and critique social policy within the United Kingdom.

## SOCIAL POLICY

Social policy is the means by which measures relating to citizens' wellbeing and welfare is decided upon and promoted.[16] Evidence-based practice and policy is now an enduring theme on which policy is based, although the extent to which this actually occurs varies considerably.[17] In addition, the role of evidence in policymaking and delivery is not a straightforward one, and policy can often be seen as the driver of evidence, rather than evidence being the basis on which policy is formed. However, while these debates continue, professional practitioners and citizens are bound by the outcome of policymaking and implementation processes. It is they who have to work and work with policy, much of which has a significant impact on their lives. Social policy in the UK mainly concerns the welfare state, and as health visitors (HV), many of our clients – children and their families and wider care networks, are impacted by social policies. While much of social policy has been created by our governments, wider influences are also at play, those of international and global agencies who have a role in informing the basis by which more local and community policy plays out.[16]

Policy is generally considered to be implemented via a 'top-down' process; however, there is always scope for this to be influenced at local level and, as one of the tenets of Health Visiting is to influence policy, there is clearly a role for HV in this.

The nature of the UK as a single London-based, government entity, is changing, largely due to devolution and the creation of the devolved administrations in Scotland, Northern Ireland and Wales. In addition, there are greater moves away from centralised public policymaking and the welfare state, to take account of the creation of much more local government bodies,[16] even as far as neighbourhood level.

It is at this level that HVs are required to work, and therefore there is a need to understand the current policy landscape, and in particular, the impact of the welfare state on children and families.

While social policy is often seen as that provided by the state, there are other sources of social welfare that have a significant role to play in supporting children and families. These are friends and wider family, and in addition, non-governmental organisations including voluntary and charitable organisations. HVs have a clear role in working with families to recognise the support networks that are important to them and link them to local organisations which can provide practical and emotional support, particularly for parents.

Changing demographics in the UK and other developed countries demonstrate that the focus of social policy needs to take account of the ageing population and, increasingly, the numbers of the very elderly who need social welfare. In addition, there are simultaneous changes to mortality, fertility and migration[18] which have an impact, not only on family structures, but also on the composition of the home environment in which children live and grow. There is clearly a need for

the HV to understand and adapt to these changes. These manifest in the following:

- Decline in marriages
- Increase in cohabitation
- Increase in lone parent family numbers
- The later age of mothers at childbirth
- The numbers of teenage pregnancies (the UK has one of the highest rates in Europe)

The number of dependent children living in different family compositions has clear implications for the provision of welfare benefits and also for the ways in which HVs work with these families to support them in a changing policy environment.

One of the most significant and enduring issues relating to the welfare state is that of the shortfall between tax raising (income to the treasury) and spending on social welfare (provision of benefits for those who are eligible).[19] However, to have some sense of how much someone benefits from these is almost impossible to observe, as it relates to how much these mean to individuals and families.[20] This is further complicated by the provision of services that are often seen as 'free', such as education and healthcare, including that provided by HV. Analyses of the distribution of welfare would seem to suggest that lower income families gain more than those in higher income brackets, as they receive more than they pay at any one time. As noted above, there is an ageing population in the UK and this calls into question whether groups are being treated equally by the welfare state. The changing nature of family composition may mean that children with young parents may still be living 'at home' with their siblings and with relatively young grandparents, and these in turn, are caring for ageing parents. This can mean that the benefits families receive are often impacted on by this situation. In turn, this can make the HV role more complicated as they work with and care for whole families, rather than just babies, children and their parents. 'Informal welfare'[21] is the provision of care or support for families by other family members or those of a wider social network, such as friends and neighbours. This can manifest gender inequalities, as women take on the burden of care, and this leads to a dilemma for policymakers, as unpaid care and employment are largely incompatible. As there is a growing unpaid care gap, governments have toyed with the idea of providing paid services to those providing informal welfare, and this may become a reality at some point in the near(er) future. While it is not the main focus of the Health Visiting role, the health of carers remains a key concern, as there is substantial evidence showing that the health of carers is at risk, particularly their mental and psychological health.[21]

Children and young people are also known to be carers for a parent and/or younger siblings. This has a direct impact on their education and, subsequently, life chances and trajectory. Increasingly, there is a view from governments that this is detrimental to children, and as a result, they should be protected from either excessive or inappropriate caring responsibilities. HVs need to be aware that some children may be primarily cared for by siblings if there is parental ill health within the family.

The study of the welfare state and the benefits that individuals and families receive would seem to show that there are fundamental differences between social groups and the way in which they benefit from welfare income. These are differences between men and women; disabled and non-disabled people; and those of different socio-economic and ethnic groups, sexualities, nationalities, religions and ages. These differences are not straightforward and are often cross-cutting: some of these groups have clear needs that are readily met by social policy initiatives, while for others, these are less so. There are significant differences in life chances between these groups and one of the roles of the HV is to ensure (as far as is

possible) that babies and children are supported to have the very best life chances and experiences that they can have.

Those of different ethnic groups are at greater risk of unemployment and poverty[22] and, as a result, are disproportionately impacted by the welfare provision, which, in turn, has a direct influence on the life chances and health of children and families. This has become more apparent during the coronavirus pandemic, which has revealed that people from Black, Asian and minority ethnic communities are at an increased risk of dying from the disease.[23] The exact reason for this is not yet known, but it is thought that pre-existing health conditions and socio-economic factors are implicated.[23]

Poverty has been shown to be linked to social exclusion,[16] and both are on the increase in the UK. Of course, these are not problems that are exclusive to the UK, but poverty is an unacceptable reflection of life in the 21st century for many. HVs are meeting these issues for children and families on a daily basis.

As mentioned earlier, there is a shift to focus on the individual as having greater responsibility than ever for their own health and wellbeing, and thus absenting the welfare state from many of the ways in which it previously supported citizens. Healthcare is the principal aspect of the welfare state in which this comes to the fore. While the medical profession remains a powerful influence, increasingly, the views and experiences of service users, carers and the wider public are taking into account. HVs have a role in advocating for children and families, and therefore may well have a part to play in influencing local and national policy relating to health and health services. While large sums of money have been committed (and promised) to the NHS, a significant shortfall remains, leading to care inequalities and fiscal restraint in the provision of health services. As a result, there is a greater than ever focus on coalitions between the NHS, the private sector and voluntary and charitable organisations, to provide healthcare services and support.

As there is a greater focus on individuals taking responsibility for their health, to a degree this is clearly acceptable. However, in some situations (such as those discussed in the following part of this chapter relating to public health), individuals are limited in the extent to which they can influence policy and therefore its influence on them. In addition, the state's expression of compassionate support for individuals in need is impacted by this view.[24] Children, older people and those living with disabilities are those who are most vulnerable to poverty and yet are those who have the greatest need of health services. Effective healthcare requires the support of other aspects of the welfare state, such as housing and social care agencies. However, the working relationship between these has often fallen short, and this has led in some way to the integration of health and social care, but while this is seen as one way of dealing with former problems, it is not without its challenges and is not in any way a universal panacea.

As healthcare faces ongoing fiscal challenges, it has become ever more important to find interventions of proven effectiveness. Working with an evidence base for care is now the norm for all healthcare practitioners, and as a result, there is increasing pressure on them (including HVs) to be knowledgeable about which interventions are the most effective and who is likely to derive the most benefit from these. At the same time, HVs and other healthcare practitioners are required to involve patients/clients more than ever before in decisions about their own and their families' care. Not all individuals have the same ability to make their preferences known, and it is clearly important for HVs to advocate for children and families and work in close partnership with them.

As a result of these financial situations of the NHS, there is a greater emphasis on the prevention of ill health than previously, and HVs have a clear role in supporting children and families to achieve this, either through education or direct interventions.

While healthcare plays a crucial role in protecting the wellbeing of children and families, other aspects of social policy are also important. For example, housing policy and family policy, both have a clear impact on children and their families. Lack of council or affordable housing stock and the rise in the numbers of private landlords have a significant impact on the quality of life of families. Changes to welfare benefits have also hit some families particularly hard, with some having to make the choice between 'heating and eating' and having to prioritise rent over other costs of living.[25] In-work poverty is becoming a more substantial issue than it has previously been. One situation that is a focus of media attention and reflects the pressure on family budgets is that of the use of foodbanks. Often access to these relies on support or referral from HVs, and it is clearly important that HVs know which resources are available in the areas in which they work. Children are vulnerable to situations brought about by poverty, and these are often the result of lone parent families, unemployment or long-term illness or disability. The level of welfare provided by the state can be a crucial aspect of children's health, wellbeing and life chances.

Children are important recipients of welfare, and those growing up in the 21st century live increasing complex lives in a range of family compositions and settings. Children's rights have become more a focus in recent years, and as a result, child welfare policies are more fluid than ever before to reflect these changes. There is often an assumption by the state that children's best interests are the same as those of their families, but this is not always the case, and HVs will be very much aware of this. There are tensions between the responsibilities of the state and the rights and responsibilities of parents for their children. Related to these is the requirement for the state to intervene when children are believed to be 'at risk' and HVs play a key role as acting as both an intermediary and advocate for children in these situations. While is it completely right that the state has roles and responsibilities in the protection of children, and this is a key aspect of policy and practice, it is not without its challenges, as these often fall to several agencies and different professionals, and not the state alone.

The 2007–2008 recession, triggered by a global financial crisis and resulting austerity measures, has had an impact on lower income families, which has become a key concern for successive governments. This has led to further cuts in welfare benefits as one aspect of the government's response to this.[26] The extent to which women (in particular, mothers) can participate in the labour market while balancing the challenges of the costs and availability of childcare, makes this extremely challenging for families and policy-makers alike. The extent of provision of adequate welfare benefits for children and families has become, and remains, a key concern for governments as they try to balance their duties to provide for and protect children through the welfare state, whilst being mindful of the responsibilities of parents and families to do the same.

As the devolved administrations in Scotland, Northern Ireland and Wales take on a greater role in decisions about social policy and the provision of welfare benefits, the future is to some extent, unknown. The changes which are imminent as a result of exiting the European Union and further calls for Scottish independence bring further uncertainties. What remains is the greater than ever focus on individual responsibility for health, and to an extent, welfare, and the key role that HVs will have in this, going forward.

There is also a part for HVs to play in supporting children and families in changing individual behaviour, an increasing focus of social policy. Ensuring the health and wellbeing of individuals is passing responsibility for these away from government to individuals.[27] Preventing ill health

and promoting healthy behaviours and lifestyle is a key role for the HV. The public health agenda is easily as influential in children's lives as the welfare state and social policy.

### THINKING SPACE

Thinking locally, nationally and globally, how does social policy impact on your role as a Health Visitor?

The final section of this chapter considers the organisation of health visiting services.

## ORGANISATION OF HEALTH VISITING SERVICE PROVISION

The provision of health visiting services in the UK reflects the devolved government administrations within England, Scotland, Wales and Northern Ireland, specifying each administration's social policy and priorities to meet health ambitions; within the overarching directives from the Home Office.[28] More similarities than differences exist in service delivery, despite some variance in service models, governance, management and financial arrangements. At the heart of all four countries are prevention and early intervention strategies, which sit alongside human rights legislation to reduce inequalities and improve outcomes for future generations. Also, a move towards a more salutogenic approach, where an ecological, assets-based and solution-focused route to better health is being adopted. As yet, data are unavailable to make accurate comparisons between these different approaches and outcomes, as data collection across the four administrations is complex, due to multi-factorial elements influencing collection.[28] What is clear is that professional advancement has been limited as a result of a reduction in health visiting specialist roles, in turn causing frustration and disappointment and leading to a lowering of morale in the profession. Indeed, the deployment of health visitors to community and acute nursing services during the coronavirus pandemic has added to their frustration as families, especially the most vulnerable, were left with limited support.[29]

Where there has been a significant difference between the four nations is in grading of the health visitor post, where in Scotland alone, the Agenda for Change professional band has been raised from six to seven. This is in recognition of the attributes necessary to fulfil the complex demands of the HV role, including that of the named professional in national 'getting it right for every child' (GIRFEC) policy.[30] This has helped to improve morale especially in areas working to full capacity. Nevertheless, as with the other countries of the UK, challenges still exist where HV numbers are lower than that required to meet the ambitions of strategic plans, which impacts on morale irrespective of the banding, particularly when compromises to service delivery, where reduced contacts with families need to be made. For example, the antenatal visit may not be delivered.

This section provides a brief overview of the organisational arrangements across the UK for health visiting services. Two short case studies are included and activities are suggested to facilitate learning. It may be helpful to refer to the practice tools within your own Health Board/Trust area of practice to direct your activities.

## Scotland

The Universal Health Visiting Pathway[31] has been the model for health visiting service delivery in Scotland in recent years and which contributes to the early years programme 'getting it right for every child' (GIRFEC).[30] As set in legislation, Children and Young People (Scotland) Act 2014, the GIRFEC model is where all agencies working with children and young people share the same vision, language and processes to meet shared outcomes, taking a public health approach to reduce inequalities. The vision is for children to have the best start in life and grow to become responsible citizens. This requires joined up working for the wellbeing of children.

In this delivery model, HVs work with families where a first visit is undertaken in the antenatal period, and then from day 10 when new babies arrive. They have contacts with children and their families in the early years until school entry. Prevention and early intervention strategies are applied working in partnership relationships. This partnership working extends to other statutory agencies and the third sector. HVs ensure the voice of the child is central and families are included in decision-making. These elements are each essential to the success of the model. The Universal Health Visiting Pathway[31] facilitates 11 home visits to all families, eight within the first year of life, and three child health reviews between 13 months and 4 to 5 years. These core contacts are supplemented with additional contacts should the HV consider them necessary. The underlying principles for the pathway are person-centred and assests-based to promote the development of positive relationships from the antenatal period. This then forms the foundations for successful relationships throughout the early years and beyond. Being available to families in the early days after a new birth helps to cement those relationships, supporting families in their own homes and to plan ahead, which is important to promote, support and safeguard the future wellbeing of children.

Scotland has 14 NHS Boards, which are responsible for commissioning health visiting services and who also employ them. One exception is where NHS Highland commission services from Highland Council local authority area. This is where arrangements for integration of health and social care developed, with Highland Council taking responsibility to lead on children's services, and NHS Highland leading for adult services. In Argyll and Bute local authority area, HVs remain employed by NHS Highland.

Unique to Scotland as stated, HV posts have been uplifted from Band 6 to Band 7 under the Agenda for Change pay scale. The named person service was expected to progress within the Children and Young People (Scotland) Act 2014, but this was rescinded as a result of legal complexities with information sharing. The HV as named professional remains a key role in GIRFEC policy, however, and this new banding recognises the associated additional health visiting responsibilities.

### *Case study activity: Ahmad family*

You are a health visitor working in a rural community. The Ahmad family, a Syrian refugee family, has just arrived and been allocated to your caseload:

Male baby: Ali 6 weeks old
Female child: Mya (2)
Male child: Mohammad (4)
Mother: Mona (37)
Father: Mohammad (49)
Mohammad's parents:
Grandma Ahmad (72)
Grandpa Ahmad (80)

**Health visitor:**

Seek out your local policy re health care provision for refugee families.

What is your role?

What information do you need, and where will you get it?

When planning your family assessment, what additional questions might you ask related to the family being in refugee status? How will you support cultural and religious preferences?

What are the family health care entitlements?

Where can you access guidance and support?

Assess your own cultural knowledge. Are you working from an evidence base? Do you have gaps in your knowledge and understanding?

Where can you access education to address your needs?

## Northern Ireland

The child health programme for surveillance, immunisations, child health wellbeing and safety is a universal programme in Northern Ireland, captured in The Healthy Child, Healthy Futures programme, which begins in pregnancy through to 19 years of age. HVs are expected to undertake nine visits to a family before a child starts school. Similar to that in Scotland, one contact is made in pregnancy.[32] Services are commissioned by the Health and Social Care Board (HSCB), working alongside the Public Health Agency and five local commissioning groups or Trusts.[33] The Hardiker model underpins the service plan where four tiers of service are delivered dependent on assessed need: (1) Children aged 0 to 4 years in receipt of Child Health Promotion Programme; (2) Children and families with additional support from the HV; (3) Children identified as 'Children in Need' as defined within The Children (Northern Ireland) Order 1995; (4) The most vulnerable children, i.e. on the Child Protection Register and/or Children 'Looked After'. The Child Health Promotion Programme is the core service provision for all children and families with children under school age. Ongoing assessment is promoted, allowing for scope to move across the levels of service based on up-to-date information. Integrated working is promoted, working in partnership with parents, children, partner agencies and third sector to achieve the best outcomes. As with other UK countries, meeting the planned service provision is compromised where HV numbers are below that required.

HVs are employed in Trusts previously mentioned, their numbers are based on the Hardiker model and the intensity of their caseload. Recognition is given to the complexity of cases, HVs work in collaboration with their leaders to seek consensus on how to reach realistic caseload sizes. Some skill mix is incorporated.

## Wales

In Wales, to meet the needs for all children aged 0 to 7 a core programme of health visiting services follows the progressive universalism approach within The Healthy Child Wales strategy.[34] HVs make nine contact visits to families before the child is 4 years old, and this model works in conjunction with the universal provision of immunisation and screening services. A minimum set of interventions to all families with pre-school children, irrespective of need, is followed. Antenatal visits are carried out when a referral has been received.

Three strands of service are available and are tailored to need: Universal, the core minimum service intervention; Enhanced, additional interventions based on the assessment; Intensive, further interventions, where from continuous assessment and analysis, more intensive support has been identified. In addition, The Flying Start programme serves areas of most need, where HVs work to reduced caseload sizes of 110 maximum, as opposed to 250 with Healthy Child Wales.[34] Flying Start is offered universally to those within targeted geographical areas in each local authority, where the highest levels of households in receipt of income benefit are evident. Multi-disciplinary and multi-agency collaborative practice is essential to the success of the model to improve outcomes for children and families. Partnership working with local authorities, communities, education and the third sector facilitates collaboration intended to reduce health inequalities and child poverty. Emphasis is placed on the HV leadership role in making those collaborations successful, and within the Flying Start programme, it is expected that most HVs will be co-located with their agency partners to maximise opportunities for this way of working to be successful. The development of the Family Resilience Assessment Tool (FRAIT), a tool to assess family needs including protective factors, is being developed to support health visiting practice.

HV services are employed through health boards in Wales, of which there are seven, and these are tasked with commissioning responsibilities. As with other UK countries, the health boards are constantly challenged with recruiting numbers required for these reduced caseloads. In turn, HVs regularly manage many more cases than these programmes suggest for safe and effective practice. Skill mix is a feature within Wales to support and enhance service delivery, it is emphasised, not as a replacement for qualified HVs.[35]

The ambition for health visiting is 'In Wales there will be an empowered multi-disciplinary workforce led by HVs providing expert clinical leadership to a team that have the skills and competencies to meet the needs of service users and to deliver quality outcomes set by the Government'.[35]

### Case study activity: Barker family

Female child: Eve (4)
Female child: Sally (8)
Mother: Tyler (23)

Tyler is a lone parent of two children, and they all live on the sixth floor of an inner-city high-rise flat. Sally has asthma and Eve is not yet fully toilet trained. It is known that Tyler has mental health diagnoses of Obsessive Compulsive Disorder (OCD) and anxiety, which reduce her ability to relax and enjoy quality time with her children. This impacts on the children's wellbeing. She worries about hygiene, germs coming into the home from outside activities and other children coming to her home to play. She struggles taking children to appointments, to school and nursery, both regularly miss days of attendance.

*Health visitor:*

Undertake a search of the literature and identify two or three contemporary papers on the challenges of parenting with mental health diagnoses of OCD and anxiety, aiming to find evidence on the most effective strategies to minimise any actual or perceived risk to the children's health and wellbeing.

Outline a family action plan you would discuss with Tyler.

*Consider:*

Any appropriate referrals?

Any resources that could support this family?

To which contact pathway would you assign this family? What is your evidence for your decision?

## England

The Healthy Child Programme[36] is the current government policy in England, where HVs in leadership roles work alongside parents, families and communities in partnership relationships. Before this, following significant case reviews precipitated initially following the death of Victoria Climbié at the hands of her carers in 2000, policy was redesigned to encourage collaborative working, promoting the sharing of information between agencies for the protection of children. The aim with this new policy is to deliver key objectives to reduce inequalities and to minimise harm, in order to achieve the best outcomes for children and families. This is being promoted through traditional home visiting by heath visitors in the early years to identify and respond promptly to need.

This model consists of five contacts which are mandatory, targeted to areas of highest need and in alliance with safeguarding practice. It is recognised that this model based on universal principles lacks a person- or family-centred approach in many areas, with HVs being unable to provide a service based on need. This is intended to be addressed in the new vision for health visiting. This new vision promotes partnership working with families where, following a comprehensive assessment, a more tailored approach of intensive universal plus, or universal partnership plus support, can be delivered when the need for additional assistance is identified.

The Institute of Health Visiting[37:5] recommends a 'public health response with action based on the principles of proportionate universalism', in this new vision. Consisting of 'eight universal contacts and additional tailored support where needed, aligned primarily to fifteen High Impact Areas'. Furthermore, adopting an evidence-based approach for what works, this vision proposes a shift in relationships with families and communities to one where each will also contribute to the service model agreed locally. This promotes a collaborative association with key stakeholders to achieve the agreed goals. Good leadership both clinically and politically, together with proper funding, is recognised as essential to deliver on this new vision.

Before 2013, the NHS in England was responsible for the health visiting workforce, delivery and development of service. Since then, the health visiting service has been managed through a local authority public health model, where services are commissioned from a range of sources. Five commissioning support units governed by the NHS form the foundations for developing this public health driven service, with GPs at the forefront. This approach is intent on maximising a social and health integration model. For HVs though, they may find themselves employed in a local authority area in a Trust or a partnership where the HV works within a business model and new creative arrangements are in place, some of which are pilot projects and locally driven. This arrangement is part of a wider health and social services transformation where Vanguards, essentially integrated service clusters for whole systems redesign, are in the making.[38] Currently, there are similarities in service delivery, but consistency can vary across the country. This has a notable impact on staffing levels and quality of service, with a reduction in home visiting and other contacts in many areas. In these commissioning arrangements, HV contracts can be short term, have reduced staffing levels and poor administration systems. HVs can be unable to access continuing professional development. This provides the ideal cocktail for low morale and dissatisfaction in the profession in places where employers have little understanding of the health visiting service or of the consequences of diminishing services. Increasingly, HVs are depending on this new vision delivering what it intends through reigniting the profession with increased staffing levels and opportunities to fulfil the shared ambitions for improving children's futures.

## CONCLUSION

This chapter has provided a brief overview of the national approach to public health in each of the devolved countries of the United Kingdom, with a specific focus on the early years. It has also provided a critique of social policy and the organisation of health visiting service provision. The importance of early intervention and the key role health visitors play in improving the health and wellbeing of children, young people and families have been highlighted.

To ensure that all children have the best start in life and beyond, there is a need for continued investment in building the health visiting workforce and a commitment from the UK and devolved governments to maintain a focus on early intervention.

## KEY LEARNING POINTS

- Health Visitors respond to the contemporary evidence base for protecting and improving health and wellbeing outcomes for children and families
- Health Visitors will understand the extent to which social policy and the welfare state impact on and influence health visiting practice
- Health Visitors recognise the importance of keeping abreast of the changing landscape of local and national contexts in which they practice

## REFERENCES

1. Public Health England. (2019). *PHE strategy for 2020–2025*. London: Public Health England. https://www.gov.uk/government/organisations/public-health-england. Accessed 7 Mar 2020.
2. Scottish Government. (2018). *Public health priorities for Scotland*. Edinburgh: Scottish Government. https://www.gov.scot/binaries/content/documents/govscot/publications/corporate-report/2018/06/scotlands-public-health-priorities/documents/00536757-pdf/00536757-pdf/govscot%3Adocument/00536757.pdf. Accessed 7 Mar 2020.
3. Public Health Wales. (2019). *Our strategic plan 2019–2022*. Cardiff: Public Health Wales. https://phw.nhs.wales/about-us/our-priorities/long-term-strategy-documents/public-health-wales-strategic-plan-2019–2022. Accessed 7 Mar 2020.
4. Department of Health, Social Services and Public Safety. (2014). *Making life better: A whole systems strategic framework for public health*. Belfast: Department of Health, Social Services and Public Safety. https://www.health-ni.gov.uk/sites/default/files/publications/dhssps/making-life-better-strategic-framework-2013-2023_0.pdf. Accessed 7 Mar 2020.
5. Scottish Government. (2015). *Tackling inequalities in the early years: Key messages from 10 years of the growing up in Scotland study*. Edinburgh: Scottish Government.
6. Marmot, M., Allen, J., Boyce, T., Goldblatt, P., & Morrison, J. (2020). Health equity in England: The Marmot Review 10 years on. *British Medical Journal, 368, m693*.
7. Loopstra, R., Reeves, A., Taylor-Robinson, D., Barr, B., McKee, M., & Stuckler, D. (2015). Austerity, sanctions, and the rise of food banks in the UK. *British Medical Journal, 8*(350), 1775.
8. MacLeod, M. A., Curl, A., & Kearns, A. (2019). Understanding the prevalence and drivers of food bank use: Evidence from deprived communities in Glasgow. *Social Policy and Society, 18*(1), 67–86.
9. NHS Health Scotland. (2017). *A Fairer Healthier Scotland: A strategic framework for action 2017–2022*. Edinburgh: NHS Health Scotland.
10. Christie, C. (2011). *Commission on the future delivery of public services*. Edinburgh: Scottish Government. Public Services Commission.
11. Scottish Government COSLA. (2019). *A consultation on the new National Public Health Body 'Public Health Scotland'*. Edinburgh: Scottish Government.
12. Dahlgren, G., & Whitehead, M. (1993). *Tackling inequalities in health: What can we learn from what has been tried? Working paper prepared for the King's Fund International Seminar on Tackling Inequalities in Health*. London: King's Fund. Cited in: Dahlgren, G., Whitehead, M. (2000). *European strategies for tackling social inequities in health: Levelling up Part 2*. Copenhagen: World Health Organisation.
13. Public Health Agency. (2019). *Public Health*. Belfast: Public Health Agency. https://www.publichealth.hscni.net/directorates/public-health Accessed 7 Mar 2020.
14. World Health Organisation. (2017). *Strengthening resilience: A priority shared by Health 2020 and the Sustainable Development Goals*. Venice: World Health Organisation. http://www.euro.who.int/__data/assets/pdf_file/0005/351284/resilience-report-20171004-h1635.pdf?ua=1. Accessed 6 Mar 2020.

15. West, M., Armit, K., Loewenthal, L., Eckert, R., West, T., & Lee, A. (2015). *Leadership and leadership development in healthcare: The evidence base*. London: The Kings Fund. https://www.kingsfund.org.uk/sites/default/files/field/field_publication_summary/leadership-in-health-care-apr15.pdf. Accessed 6 Mar 2020.

16. Alcock, P. (2016). What is social policy? In P. Alcock, T. Haux, M. May, & S. Wright (Eds.), *The student's companion to social policy*. (5th ed., pp. 7–13). Oxford: Wiley Blackwell.

17. Boaz, A., Davies, H., Fraser, A., & Nutley, S. (Eds.). (2019). *What works now? Evidence-informed policy and practice*. Policy Press.

18. Falkingham, J., & Vlacharitoni, A. (2016). The demographic challenge. In P. Alcock, T. Haux, M. May, & S. Wright (Eds.), *The student's companion to social policy* (5th Ed, pp. 183–190). Oxford: Wiley Blackwell.

19. Farnsworth, K., & Irving, Z. (2016). The economic context. In P. Alcock, T. Haux, M. May, & S. Wright (Eds.), *The student's companion to social policy* (5th ed, pp. 191–198). Oxford: Wiley Blackwell.

20. Hills, J. (2016). The distribution of welfare. In P. Alcock, T. Haux, M. May, & S. Wright (Eds.), *The student's companion to social policy* (5th ed., pp. 212–219). Oxford: Wiley Blackwell.

21. Pickard, L. (2016). Informal welfare. In P. Alcock, T. Haux, M. May, & S. Wright (Eds.), *The student's companion to social policy* (5th ed., pp. 269–278). Oxford: Wiley Blackwell.

22. Kiess, J., Norman, L., Temple, L., & Uba, K. (2017). Path dependency and convergence of three worlds of welfare policy during the Great Recession: UK, Germany and Sweden. *Journal of International and Comparative Social Policy*, 33(1), 1–7.

23. Office for National Statistics. (2020). Coronavirus (COVID-19) related deaths by ethnic group, England and Wales: 2 March 2020 to 10 April 2020. https://www.ons.gov.uk/peoplepopulationandcommunity/birthsdeathsandmarriages/deaths/articles/coronavirusrelateddeathsbyethnicgroupenglandandwales/2march2020to10april2020?hootPostID=b229db5cd884a4f73d5bd4fadcd8959b. Accessed 30 June 2020.

24. Feldman, S., Huddy, L., Wronski, J., & Lown, P. (2019). The interplay of empathy and individualism in support for social welfare policies. *Political Psychology*. doi: 10.1111/pops.12620.

25. McKenzie, H., & McKay, F. H. (2018). Thinking outside the box: Strategies used by low-income single mothers to make ends meet. *Australian Journal of Social Issues*, 53(3), 304–319.

26. Beatty, C., & Fothergill, S. (2018). Welfare reform in the United Kingdom 2010–2016: Expectations, outcomes, and local impacts. *Social Policy & Administration*, 52(5), 950–968.

27. Pyckett, J. (2016). Changing behaviour. In P. Alcock, T. Haux, M. May, & S. Wright (Eds.), *The student's companion to social policy*. (5th ed., pp. 56–62). Oxford: Wiley Blackwell.

28. Black, M., Barnes, A. J., Baxter, S., Beynon, C., Clowes, M., Dallat, M., et al. (2019). Learning across the UK: A review of public health systems and policy approaches to early child development since political devolution. *Journal of Public Health*. https://academic.oup.com/jpubhealth/advance-article-abstract/doi/10.1093/pubmed/fdz012/5364180. Accessed 13 November 2019.

29. Adams, C. (2020). *Time to leave redeployments and return to the health visiting front line*. Institute of Health Visiting. https://ihv.org.uk/news-and-views/voices/time-to-leave-redeployments-and-return-to-the-health-visiting-front-line/. Accessed 30 June 2020.

30. The Scottish Government. (2017). Getting it right for every child. Edinburgh: The Scottish Government. https://www.gov.scot/policies/girfec/ https://www.gov.scot/policies/maternal-and-child-health/universal-health-visiting-service/. Accessed 22 February 2020.

31. The Scottish Government. (2015). *Universal Health Visiting Pathway in Scotland: PreBirth to Pre-School*. Edinburgh: The Scottish Government. http://www.gov.scot/Publications/2015/10/9697. Accessed 19 February 2020.

32. Department of Health Social Services and Public Safety. (2010). *Healthy child health future. A framework for the universal child health promotion programme*. Belfast: Department of Health Social Services and Public Safety. https://www.health-ni.gov.uk/sites/default/files/publications/dhssps/healthychildhealthyfuture.pdf. Accessed 22 February 2020.

33. Department of Health, Health and Social Care. (2017). *A policy framework for nursing and midwifery workforce planning in Northern Ireland delivering care phase 4 health visiting*. Belfast: Department of Health, Health and Social Care.

34. NHS Wales. (2016). *An overview of the Healthy Child Wales Programme*. Cardiff: NHS Wales. https://gov.wales/sites/default/files/publications/2019-05/an-overview-of-the-healthy-child-wales-programme.pdf. Accessed 22 February 2020.

35. Welsh Government. (2012). *A vision for health visiting in Wales*. Cardiff: Welsh Government. https://gov.wales/sites/default/files/publications/2019-03/a-vision-for-health-visiting-in-wales.pdf. Accessed 20 February 2020.

36. Public Health England. (2018). *The healthy child programme*. London: Public Health England. https://www.gov.uk/government/publications/healthy-child-programme-0-to-19-health-visitor-and-school-nurse-commissioning. Accessed 22 February 2020.
37. The Institute of Health Visiting. (2019). *Health Visiting in England: A Vision for the Future*. London: England. 7.11.19-Health-Visiting-in-England-Vision-FINAL-VERSION.pdf (ihv.org.uk).
38. NHS England. (2015). *New Care Models: Vanguards – developing a blueprint for the future of NHS and care services*. London: England. https://www.england.nhs.uk/wp-content/uploads/2015/11/new_care_models.pdf. Accessed 19 February 2020.

## RESOURCES (FURTHER READING)

Alcock, P., Haux, T., May, M., & Wright, S. (Eds.). (2016). *The student's companion to social policy* (5th ed.). Oxford: Wiley Blackwell.

# PART 2

# Fundamentals of Health Visiting Practice

## PART OUTLINE

5 HOME VISITING AND THERAPEUTIC RELATIONSHIP-BUILDING TO SUPPORT THE TRANSITION TO PARENTHOOD

6 ASSESSMENT

7 EVIDENCE-BASED PRACTICE AND EARLY INTERVENTION TO SUPPORT CHILDREN AND FAMILIES

8 LEADERSHIP SKILLS FOR LEADING HEALTH VISITING PRACTICE

9 TECHNOLOGY AND HEALTH VISITING PRACTICE

10 FACILITATING HEALTHY BEHAVIOUR – AN EMPOWERMENT APPROACH

# HOME VISITING AND THERAPEUTIC RELATIONSHIP-BUILDING TO SUPPORT THE TRANSITION TO PARENTHOOD

LIZ STURLEY ■ LYNETTE SHOTTON ■ BRIDGET HALNAN

## CHAPTER CONTENTS

INTRODUCTION

WHAT IS A THERAPEUTIC RELATIONSHIP AND WHY IS IT IMPORTANT?

HOW HEALTH VISITORS DEVELOP EFFECTIVE RELATIONSHIPS FOR PRACTICE

MOTIVATIONAL INTERVIEWING

AUTHENTICITY IN THERAPEUTIC RELATIONSHIPS

THERAPEUTIC RELATIONSHIPS AND SAFEGUARDING

TRUST

UNIVERSAL SERVICES AND THERAPEUTIC RELATIONSHIPS

HOME VISITING AND RELATIONSHIP-BUILDING

COMMUNITY WORKING AND RELATIONSHIP-BUILDING

RELATIONSHIPS AND INCLUSIVE PRACTICE

TRAUMA-INFORMED PRACTICE AND RELATIONSHIP-BUILDING

BUILDING RELATIONSHIPS WITH FATHERS

EQUALITY, DIVERSITY AND INCLUSION IN HEALTH VISITING

CONCLUSION

## LEARNING OUTCOMES

To:

- describe the features of a therapeutic health visiting relationship.
- define what skills can be used by the health visitor to establish a therapeutic relationship.
- appraise how home visiting can influence therapeutic health visiting relationships.

- critique the impact that trauma and experiences of inequality and uniformity have on developing therapeutic relationships.
- examine and reflect on the importance of building health visiting relationships with fathers.
- reflect on practice and identify any professional development needs.

## INTRODUCTION

The focus of this chapter is to consider the importance of building therapeutic relationships in order to support the transition to parenthood. The chapter will build on previous chapters and consider how the evolution of the health visiting service influences relationships with individuals, families and communities, as well as the response of the service to the changing nature of modern society.

## WHAT IS A THERAPEUTIC RELATIONSHIP AND WHY IS IT IMPORTANT?

It is widely accepted that health visitors need to be confident and effective in engaging with and building positive relationships with individuals, families, and communities in order to understand and work effectively together to support, safeguard, and promote behaviour change.[1] This is underpinned by key skills and qualities, which include the ability to demonstrate empathy and respect and to communicate effectively[2], emphasise the importance of working in partnership in the development of health visiting relationships and the need for reciprocity.

Reciprocity is, for health visiting, a fundamental term and connects with relationship-building on many different levels. Reciprocity, which in general terms means 'exchanging something for mutual benefit'[4] has been further defined as a 'sophisticated dance', one which involves initiation, regulation and termination of communication in such a way as to promote the well-being of the infant (Solihull cited in Refs. [5]). When these three things go well between adults/caregivers and children, this process results in a satisfying and fulfilling interaction where the child feels listened to, understood, and connected with, as does the adult. These principles are not dissimilar to the way that good relationship-building can work in health visiting. Here, the appropriate initiation, regulation and termination of communication in the relationship with the service user is imperative in developing trust and therefore, also serves to act as modelling behaviour. This can further support interactions between the parent/carer and child, and has been shown to produce improved outcomes for children, such as those found by Family Nurse Partnership programmes.[6] When positive relationships are established between health visitors and service users, this provides a mechanism whereby assessment and identification of risks and strengths and the following interventions are more successful, but furthermore, the relationship itself can also have a therapeutic effect.[2] This underpins work at both the community and individual level and will be discussed in more detail later in this chapter.

## HOW HEALTH VISITORS DEVELOP EFFECTIVE RELATIONSHIPS FOR PRACTICE

Establishing an effective relationship has been defined by Cowley et al as perhaps the most essential feature of an effective health visitor/parent relationship and Cowley describes this effective relationship as one that demonstrates partnership.[7] The ethos here is to work in partnership with parents and carers and to emphasise a strengths-based approach, including activities that promote salutogenesis.[67] Salutogenesis, first described by Antonovsky (1979), was cited by Mittelmark and Bauer [68] as the way that people view life, deal with stress in life and access available resources to manage stresses and challenges. Many parents value the sense of knowing and being known by a health visitor[8,69] and one element of feeling known could be argued to be that the individual feels that they, their strengths and abilities are recognised and valued. Public health bodies in the four United Kingdom nations have increasingly been recommending that these concepts should be embedded in educational training programmes, as well as for visiting practices to use strengths-based approaches when working with families, Department of Health and Social Care (2011).[9–11,70] Turnell and Edwards (1997) are amongst the pioneers talking about strengths-based working, particularly in relation to social workers working with child protection scenarios. Turnell and Edwards describe situations of working with families where family strengths were not recognised and the outcome created a bleak picture for families, focussing mainly on deficits. To address this, they developed a programme of working with families in child protection scenarios known as Signs of Safety, which is now used internationally and works on optimising individual and family strengths.[11] David Olds also researches and writes about the use of family strengths and it is this, as well as other research, that the Family Nurse Partnership is based upon.[72,73] Therefore, the act of recognising family and individual strengths has been evidenced as an effective way of increasing the safety of vulnerable children.[74] Although much evidential work focusses on strengths-based working in relation to safeguarding and child protection scenarios, working in such a way supports all families to feel capable and effective in the way that they care for their children. The Family Nurse Partnership model uses motivational interviewing to support the delivery of strengths-based working[12] by enabling the individual's ability to verbalise their own motivations to achieve their goals or changes to their life. Motivational Interviewing (MI) is a skilled approach and does not work in all practitioner/client interactions and is not necessarily easy to teach effectively.[13] Miller and Rose identified that motivational interviewing

does improve client outcomes[13] and is, therefore, worthwhile in developing as a practitioner skill. Health coaching uses elements of motivational interviewing and can be used by nurses, such as health visitors, to support the individuals they work with to recognise and realise their own capacities to change their lifestyles, using and developing the individual's confidence, skills and knowledge. These types of health-enhancing conversations use asset-based models of health care, rather than a deficit model,[14] and have been used in work such as The Family Partnership Model (Quinn 2011) where focus on individual and family well-being, and the reduction of social and psychological disadvantage, is enhanced by the development and use of the practitioner's skill in developing positive, enabling relationships.[71]

## MOTIVATIONAL INTERVIEWING

Although MI has been described earlier as a difficult skill, there are distinctive activities practitioners undertake when engaging in conversations that use MI. The basic fundamental activities used in MI use the acronym OARS; Open ended questions, affirmation, reflection and summaries.[75] At times practitioners may use directing conversations, perhaps where a parent asks what the evidence tells us. However, practitioners use guiding and following to elicit shared conversations.[76] Here, the practitioner is looking to use open questions to encourage discussion and will encourage the client to recognise their strengths and offer honest and truthful affirmation, including times the client has succeeded. The practitioner will reflect back to the service user/client their words, allowing the conversation to develop, and summarise effectively using, when possible, the service users/clients conversational change talk.

MI is underpinned by four fundamental processes. These are collaboration, evocation, acceptance and compassion.[15] Collaborative conversations are not directed, rather the practitioner takes part in a conversation about behaviour change where the client feels that there is not a power imbalance in favour of the practitioner. It is important to note that the practitioner is not telling the client how to change or what they should do. In collaborative scenarios the practitioner uses summarising skills to present the challenge back to the client and can suggest them considering together options or solutions to the situation. Evocation creates a mood where the client can realise a connection between their desired change and their own values. This can be created by 'eliciting' the client's perspective, why they wish to change, how they perceive this could be achieved, what their own values and aspirations are, and also why they may want to maintain equilibrium by not changing and staying the same. Acceptance means that the circumstances that the client brings to the conversation are accepted, that the person has value and ability to change whomever they are. The practitioner demonstrates a desire to understand the client's situation. The practitioner respects the clients desire to self-govern and recognises and offers affirmation in a truthful manner of the client's strengths, ability and success; this may acknowledge activities the service user/client finds hard. This can be a difficult concept for some health visitors to manage due to anxieties that present with child safety concerns. However, not demonstrating acceptance can create a sense of judgement, which we know service users/clients do not appreciate and, as demonstrated by the work of Turnell and Edwards (1997)[11] which has been further developed by Roberts et al. (2019).[16] Equally, when a strategy is followed that implements appropriate safety mechanisms in high risk families and accepts an individual's ability to self-govern, recognises strengths and is honest about risk, then safer outcomes for children and young people can found.[16] Compassion

is described as 'an authentic, emotional response when perceiving others' suffering and results in a desire to help' (Seppala 2013 cited in [77]). It is important that practitioners do not pity or feel sorry for their service users/clients and do not, unless asked, act as an expert and avoid a desire to find 'right' situations, known as the 'righting reflex'.[76]

## AUTHENTICITY IN THERAPEUTIC RELATIONSHIPS

Developing person-centred, therapeutic relationships requires training, practice and skill and some health visitors may be unsure of their skills and competence in developing these types of relationships.[17] Koloroutis and Trout (2013) explain that when we decode the elements of successful moments in relationships involving a practitioner, such as a health visitor and client, we see certain qualities. These are that the practitioner is actively available for the person and tuned into them as a human being. We 'suspend conclusions' whilst enquiring and spend careful time listening to what is shared; this is where we listen to understand and not assume the answer. We follow the verbal and nonverbal cues displayed by the individual, becoming quieter perhaps in response or more animated, mirroring the clients communication. We may either literally or figuratively hold the person and undertake actions that demonstrate that we are there to care for them.[17] This type of relationship is described as an authentic relationship. Authenticity is described by Hinojosa et al. (2014)[18] as a situation where the practitioner has an understanding of themselves including their motivations, feelings and bias and aims to create compatibility between these feelings and behaviours and the actions and behaviours that they display; this is sometimes described as congruence. Rogers considered congruence in his work examining the theory of therapeutic relationships and asserted that unconditional positive regard and empathy were important aspects of successful congruent behaviour and therapeutic relationships.[78] Unconditional positive regard can be a challenging perspective for health visitors when working with families due to our unconscious bias. Bias can be a difficult status to manage, as the brain is naturally inclined to categorise situations as part of our evolved mechanisms to help us make sense of our world quickly through the use of 'cognitive shortcuts' (Teal et al. 2012).[79] Therefore, taking part in activities, such as supervision, can help us to see when bias may be becoming unhelpful in developing relationships (Low et al. 2018). Johnston (1999) suggests that unconditional positive regard may be even more difficult to achieve when working in challenging situations and it is widely accepted that the daily work of a health visitor involves working with some of the most vulnerable families and children in society (Parker-Radford 2014).[20,79-82]

## THERAPEUTIC RELATIONSHIPS AND SAFEGUARDING

Developing congruence with health visiting clients contributes to a sense of harmony and satisfaction in the way that interactions play out. Perhaps one of the best definitions of relationships that are satisfying was made by Bowlby where he says 'human beings of all ages are happiest and able to deploy their talents to best advantage when they are confident that, standing behind them, there are one or more trusted persons who will come to their aid should difficulties arise.'[83] Therefore, successful health visiting relationships are ones that families feel that their health visitor is a trusted person that they can turn to when a difficulty arises and so should be able to feel some contentment and trust with the relationship.

Relationships that demonstrate the previous qualities and help facilitate beneficial change for the client can be described as therapeutic relationships and from a health visitors perspective this is what we seek to achieve in order to create better health and well-being for the child and carers. True therapeutic relationships are ones which the practitioner does not need to receive reward from the interaction,[17] however, it would be fair to describe such conversations as satisfying within the work role. There are simple actions that can be undertaken in order to develop therapeutic relationships, such as introducing yourself, ensuring you know your client's name and explaining your role.[21] However, developing therapeutic relationships also requires the practitioner to develop relational expertise and an ability to inquire in a manner that does not leave the client feeling vulnerable. Within health visiting there are times that relational care and the instrumental elements of care could come into conflict especially when child safeguarding concerns are a significant aspect of care Koloroutis and Trout (2013).[17] argue that these factors are intrinsically linked, and that care cannot be therapeutic if one element is removed. In work that involves safeguarding, beneficial change for the child and family is at the core of most work; therefore maintaining a relational relationship is equally important to adhering to policy; however there is skill in balancing the two aspects of care. This is not easy, therefore, developing the skills required does require practice. Rollnick and Miller describe particular characteristics of effective conversation and explain as previously stated, that directive conversation can be appropriate at times; however generally guiding and following conversations facilitate more effective conversations than when we tell people what to do.[76] Such conversations can support the client's ability to cope with their experiences either through active listening skills, providing evidence-based guidance or referrals to appropriate services, whilst also just being available to the person within the constraints of the service. Further to these aspects, the successful therapeutic relationship supports families to develop their own strategies to gain autonomy of their circumstances.[17] Power in health visiting relationships should lie with the family, rather than the health visitor and perhaps in situations where families feel that they have no autonomy, they then begin to withdraw from services.[22] Safeguarding situations are perhaps examples when families feel powerless and this is where they are most likely to feel betrayed by services and relationships can be broken.[2] This presents a challenge for health visitors; in these contexts it is vital that the skills for building a therapeutic relationship are used and the strengths-based approach, outlined earlier, is adopted.

## TRUST

Developing trust is an essential element of therapeutic health visiting relationships. Trust is built on a number of factors many of which demonstrate that the professional is reliable, evidenced through explaining service provision, keeping to this service offer, attending appointments at appointed times, being open and honest about knowledge or lack of knowledge, about their situation and gaining consent when making referrals.[22] At times situations arise, such as child safety concerns, where consent is not required. However, health visitors still have a duty to inform their client that a referral must be made and the rationale for this. This is a fundamental aspect of honesty and developing trust with service users/clients and an underpinning value of working in a trauma-informed manner.[23] This will be further explored later in this chapter. These situations can create challenges in building trust[2,24] and potential safety concerns for the health visitor; therefore, the practitioner does

need to consider the safest manner to share such information Bidmead et al. agree that, in order for parents to be able to build trust they must have some element of control in the relationship – the relationship must be a partnership. Day and Harris further support this:[85] parents with long-standing difficulties in particular describe that health visitors need to pay attention to their feelings, beliefs and their own communication skills – such as empathy, understanding, humility, acceptance and respect – in order for therapeutic relationships with families to work. Scripting is to some extent undertaken within health visiting contacts due to the expectations of each contact, for example, depending on national requirements. Key Performance Indicators (KPIs) in England or national indicators in Scotland may demand certain key contacts or information to be conveyed. For example, depending on national policy and guidance an average birth visit will require certain actions to be undertaken that may include the physical examination of the child, weighing, questions about feeding, sharing of information, such as how to reduce the risk of sudden infant death and an assessment of the mental health of the parents. These activities, due to the previously described constraints on health visiting service provision, do often need to be completed within a maximum time limit. Seminal work by Jourard[86] cited in Ref. [17] considers the impact that this type of scripting has on the relationships that practitioners develop with the clients. He proposes that this type of scripting can be used to protect the practitioner when time is a factor, and this is particularly of concern in contemporary health visiting where contacts and time frames for visits are usually set by a service provider. Programmes such as the Family Nurse Partnership allow visiting patterns with longer and more frequent visits, and there is good evidence that the therapeutic relationships that develop are strong and effective to support client change.[87]

| | |
|---|---|
| 1. Motivational Interviewing | Incorporates OARS:<br>▪ Open ended questions<br>▪ Affirmation<br>▪ Reflection<br>▪ Summary |
| 2. Authenticity | Incorporates the ability to be:<br>▪ Actively available<br>▪ Suspend conclusions<br>▪ Actively listen<br>▪ Attend to verbal/non-verbal cues<br>▪ Aware of unconscious bias<br>▪ Availability |
| 3. Trust | Incorporates skills and attributes including:<br>▪ Open and honest<br>▪ Reliable<br>▪ Communicate clearly<br>▪ Client/service user autonomy<br>▪ Tune into client/service user need<br>▪ Awareness of previously experienced trauma<br>▪ Compassionate resilience |

## UNIVERSAL SERVICES AND THERAPEUTIC RELATIONSHIPS

Universal home visiting services are being implemented by many countries around the world, directed at improving parent and child well-being, with recognition that an infant's future health and well-being is influenced by experiences in pregnancy and the first years of life, from conception to age two[25,88] (Enhancing the provision of home visits, especially for children in low-income families, has been noted as a key priority for future governmental investment.)[9,25]

Within the United Kingdom, services use a range of universal and proportionate universalism with the provision of a structured core offer of home visits, which is generally understood and socially accepted.[26] Cowley et al., suggest that universalism provides an equitable service, ensuring all families receive a basic minimum of health visiting contact and also allows individuals who experience greater need a way to access more support.[8] However, note that this is not without problems. Whilst emphasis has been placed on providing antenatal contact for all prospective parents, this is often not a service that new parents request and indicate that many may be initially ambivalent about this, particularly in the case of the health-promoting aspects of the contact, which may call into question health beliefs and practices of parents and carers. However, it is important that this is considered an opportunity to build a relationship, and here the skill of the health visitor is paramount in establishing rapport and paving the way for a therapeutic relationship, which is key in relation to searching for health needs and, as such, remains one of the four domains of health visiting set out by the Nursing and Midwifery Standards.[27]

Cowley et al,[7] narrative review examined the public health benefits from health visiting practice within a universal service. A planned programme of home visiting is considered essential in helping to develop effective relationships, but this is only possible if health visitors are able to offer regular support and are thus viewed as the first point of contact for support in relation to children's health and well-being. One of the challenges the current system of health visiting in many areas presents is that families do not see the same health visitor for each contact. Whilst this is not always possible to achieve, Jespen and Hardie[28] suggest that effort is needed to minimise the number of staff changes. Women who have a health visitor they know and trust are much more likely to seek help and support and also to report domestic violence and abuse, mental health issues and disclose personal histories and changing circumstances.[25] On this basis, there have been increased calls to focus on continuity of care, and so far as possible to ensure that each family sees the same health visitor for each appointment.[25] Equally, where families require support from a range of services, this must be managed carefully, and it is here where health visitors are in an ideal position to act as lead professional; in all four nations a named health visitor is ideally the focus of services.

## HOME VISITING AND RELATIONSHIP-BUILDING

Home visiting is the most common form of contact a health visitor will have with families and children.[7] For any relationship to be built there needs to be a clear understanding of the rights of parents in relation to home visiting. When visits are undertaken within the home it is important to understand the rights of clients. The European Court of Human Rights' Guide on Article 8 of the European Convention on Human Rights[103] states that 'Everyone has the right to respect for his private and family life, his home and his correspondence…. There shall be no interference by a public authority with the exercise of this right except such as is in accordance with the law and is necessary in a democratic society in the interests of national security, public safety or the economic well-being of the country, for the prevention of disorder or crime, for the protection of health or morals, or for the protection of the rights and freedoms of others' (European Court of Human Rights 2019). Therefore, any contact made by a health visitor or similar service within the family home must only be made with consent and prior arrangement. Parents have a legitimate right to refuse a visit and a right to choose not to engage with health visiting services. This point of law has been emphasised when the Supreme Court[104] found that Parts 4 and 5 of the Children and Young People (Scotland) Act 2014[77] did not meet the criteria set out within Article 8 of

the European Convention on Human Rights,[103], with the result that the Scottish Government have been required to repeal these elements; a particular concern was identified in relation to information-sharing. This important legislation[73] identified the health visitor and schoolteacher as key contacts in the delivery of public services to children and young people in Scotland as a 'Named Person'. However, parents and parent groups objected in the strongest terms, labelling the legislation a 'state snoopers charter'.[29] This legal case emphasises parental influence in the way that services engage with their client group.

The home setting is considered to be the optimum place for relationship-building and it is suggested that parents are often more likely to open up in their own home.[7] This is perhaps linked to feeling more relaxed in this environment, but also this shifts the balance of power, as the health visitor is a guest in the family's home. However, in the early part of establishing a relationship, Cowley et al[7] recognise that care must be taken and there is a need for negotiation and a long-term approach to introducing the health visiting service and establishing a therapeutic relationship. Indeed, Brooke and Salmon[3] conclude from their own work that there is evidence that insensitive initiation of service, or delivery of services which do not meet clients' needs, fractures the health visitor/client relationship. Whilst home visiting offers a unique insight into family life and circumstances and offers potential opportunities for health promotion, focusing only on activities known to compromise health and well-being and over-looking strengths may inhibit the therapeutic relationship. This is perhaps to some extent a fundamental characteristic of the health visiting role and the origins of the profession are inherently linked to surveillance or 'policing'.[30] Indeed, whilst the early home visiting initiatives are not well documented, they are thought to have stemmed from religious and philanthropic concerns, as well as borrowing on the principles and developments within the nursing profession.[31] In the United Kingdom the work of health visitors has been associated with different forms of surveillance. Indeed, the key proficiency of 'searching for health needs' embedded in the principles of health visiting first introduced by the Council for the Education and Training of Health Visitors in 1977[32] continues to feature highly in current NMC standards for education and training,[27] being mapped to the key public health principle – surveillance and assessment of the population's health and well-being.

The history of health visiting, and how this has influenced contemporary health visiting practice, is further explored within other chapters of this book, and the authors would encourage readers to review these sections and consider how history has influenced relationship-building. These developments paved the way for the health visiting service as we know it today, where the emphasis continues to be on providing universal and practical support to parents, with home visiting still a core feature of health visiting provision in order to engage in preventative work, identify needs and ensure early intervention.

The building of relationships with clients/families starts before health visitors enter the family home, therefore the way health visitors make initial contact is important. However, the way that health visitors choose to communicate whilst in the family home also influences relationship-building. In relation to home visiting there is little written about the etiquette of how to undertake a home visit other than local policy and guidance that is specific to localities and even less is written about home visiting in relation to fathers, which will be explored later in the chapter. Generally, as practitioners, health visitors have been guided during their health visiting education regarding how best to undertake this work.

Due to the lack of health visiting literature available for this subject matter, examples from social work are often considered. Winter and Cree (2016) consider that for social workers the issue of power imbalance is a significant factor when undertaking home visits. This is also true for health visitors, and whilst health visitors do not have the same powers as social workers, Peckover[30] identifies the power discourse that is inherent in health visitor/client relationships and that this does impact on the quality of that relationship. Winter and Cree (2016) also note the historical aspect of home visiting, referring to a 'friendly lady visitor', whom they describe as middle-class ladies. Here, they note the value-laden premise on which the role was established, whereby middle-class ladies were employed to survey and impose their superior values upon a subject group who were deemed lacking in knowledge of parenting or in unsatisfactory circumstances. Peckover[30] found that, although additional challenges face health visitors when undertaking work that involved child welfare and safety or domestic abuse (intimate partner abuse), productive, beneficial relationships could still be developed that allowed individuals to be kept safe. However, Peckover[30] emphasised that, for health visitors to develop these beneficial relationships they were required to develop their practice and understanding of the differences between lay, professional and sociological aspects of the health visitor role. This can be facilitated by engaging in opportunities for reflection and supervision, as well as through informal discussions with peers. Here practitioners can reflect on the challenges of their role, but also identify opportunities for developing practice, as well as personal resilience and emotional insight.[2] It is also important to note that relationships with service users change over time and context, but also that where there is a need to reconnect with families, this requires a combination of respect, honesty, and for health visitors to listen to and acknowledge individual feelings. Here, in situations where a relationship has been affected by challenging circumstances, there is potential for families to understand professional responsibilities and to be assured that professionals are acting in the best interests of their child and family.[2]

Luker and Chalmers proposed that health visitors felt the need for an excuse to enter the family home, quoting referrals from a General Practitioner or hospital or offering the universal service that families were entitled to. It is perhaps not surprising that delivery of a service that families may feel they do not need will not foster helpful relationships. This is noted as one of the specific barriers to effective health visiting and one that can be further compounded by poor relationships. Indeed, some of the parents in Donetto and Maben's[105] study cited the long-lasting effects of unsatisfactory experiences with their health visiting service and this included feeling judged about life-style choices and approaches to parenting. Bennett[106] emphasises the importance of listening to parents to support the improvement of health visiting services; in a survey undertaken in the South of England, 98% of feedback from parents was positive when health visitors made clients/service users feel relaxed, listened to, unjudged, empowered and the health visitor was helpful to them. Cowley et al[7] recognise that successful health visiting services demonstrate certain traits, including delivering person-centred, human-valuing services that revolve around the service user and their situated environment. Equally, offering choice and flexibility about how service users engage is important and this may challenge the traditional reliance on home visiting.

### Case study 1

You visit Mandy for her antenatal contact. Mandy is 19 and this is her first baby. She has not heard of a health visitor before and had not expected contact from any services other than her midwife until after her baby was born. Mandy has what she describes as an on/off relationship with the baby's father. She is living with her mother and brother and is currently on maternity leave from her job in a local supermarket. When you visit the home, the environment is smoky, and Mandy indicates she has cut down but has been unable to give up completely. Mandy shows you some of the preparation she has made for her new baby, including formula milk and sterilising equipment.

Thought point: How would you use this visit as an opportunity to establish rapport with Mandy?

## COMMUNITY WORKING AND RELATIONSHIP-BUILDING

Whilst historically home visiting has been central to the work of health visitors, there has been increasing recognition that this is not always the best model for all service users. Indeed, Donnetto and Maben[105] emphasise the importance of parental autonomy in choosing how and where individuals and families wish to engage with the health visiting service; this is underpinned by providing a service which offers a range of options that include out-of-home-based activities. Community or group activities delivered by health visiting services can be enhanced by promoting the parent as the expert, and such work as that delivered in London where a reorganisation of service allowed remodelled relationally based baby clinics to be established. In these clinics the baby is the focus and activities are oriented around play with the baby. Consequently, this has shown an enhanced engagement with families as well as observation of improved outcomes for children.[33] Community-based work such as this, and the offer of other community-based services, provides the potential for parents and carers to meet a range of professionals, which may allow them to self-select practitioners with whom they have greater rapport and trust. These settings also offer opportunities for peer support and the formation of reciprocal relationships with others in their community, which can have a meaningful and important impact on health and well-being.[105] Arguably, this is facilitated and enhanced by the health visiting service.

A recent scoping review by Cowley et al[8] points to the value of health visiting outside the home and contacts in a range of local venues, including children's centres, well-baby clinics and through the delivery of support groups, was valued by parents. Whilst the value of these activities is not well-researched, Cowley et al[8] suggest that these community out-of-home health visiting activities are so important, they should be considered part of the core practice of health visiting provision. Indeed, historically health visitors have been considered to be the eyes and ears of the community.[20] Whilst home visiting is vital to working with children and their families and carers, out-of-home support is often considered a safety net and in-between home visits provide reassurance that help and support can be accessed as needed. Such unplanned and needs-based availability of services can enable contacts with vulnerable families who might otherwise fall through the net of service provision, but also acts as an important hub for the community.[8] This is a valuable feature of embedding relationships with the service at local level and ensuring that parents and carers feel that the health visiting service is the first point of contact for advice and support. The changing nature of service provision and the removal of children's centres and community clinics in many areas, described in other chapters, means there have been significant changes to how parents engage and seek knowledge about caring for their child, including increased reliance on peer support, the internet and private groups facilitated by social media.

Whilst having a specific base has historically been a feature of how health visiting is located within a particular community, arguably the rapid expansion of the service (driven by the Health Visitor Implementation Plan[10] in England) brought about challenges in relation to availability of office space, parking and the demand for an IT infrastructure, contributing to the emergence of new ways of working.[34] One such change has seen the introduction of mobile working. This refers to the use of a mobile device, enabling professionals to access clinical IT systems and record-keeping systems outside of a physical/organisational base. This process is supported by mobile telephones. Arguably mobile working can provide benefits from an organisational perspective, which include the need for less office space, reduced travelling time between community locations and a base, increased paper-light record keeping and contemporary record-keeping.[34] However, what is essential in this model is that health visitors remain visible within the community and not only have IT access and access to office space at various locations within the community – such as in General practitioners (GPs) surgeries, health centres and child and family centres – but also that members of the community know how to contact them in the absence of a single, defined space.

This concern is outlined in a recent publication by Bryar et al[35] based on a recent survey of health visitors in England by the Institute of Health Visiting. Here, the authors note concerns about the relationships health visitors have with other members of the primary care team, particularly GPs. Whilst there is great variability, a third of health visitors reported seeing a GP one to two times per month and 33% less frequently or hardly ever. The concern here is that, with the erosion of community bases and increased mobile working, health visitors are becoming less visible not only to service users, but also to key members of the primary care team. Effective primary care is based on trusting relationships, not only with service users, but also between professionals and it is here where interprofessional communication provides an opportunity to share information, learn from each other and ensure that individuals receive the best care and that professionals work together to safeguard those at risk.[35] This will address concerns that our vital role as the eyes and ears of the community is being diminished and help us work effectively with other community colleagues and our service users to preserve this.[20]

One of the positives of models of health visiting based on mobile working is that health visitors report being able to work more efficiently, and consequently have more time to spend on actual face-to-face contacts with service users.[34] The immediate access to the internet provides professionals with access to information to support health visiting contacts, removing the need to carry around written resources, which date quickly. This can provide an opportunity to stimulate discussion and encourage parents and carers to participate in accessing and reviewing health-related sources.[34] However, this does rely on internet connectivity and the skill of the professional in facilitating this interaction. Indeed, it is noted that there is a gap in relation to what is known about how using a mobile device during a health visiting contact impacts on the relationship-building between the health visitor and the service user/s.[36] One concern is that the use of a laptop or mobile device may produce a physical barrier or become a distraction that impacts on the ability to engage in meaningful relationship-building, and it is here where skilled communication and the ability to manage mobile technology is essential.

In 2020 the outbreak of the coronavirus disease (COVID-19) pandemic[37] initiated a radical change in the way that health and social care services were able to interact with their service user groups. Health visiting contacts across the four UK nations were impacted by the temporary stopping of some services or the use of non–face-to-face contacts, such as using telephone and text or video services.[38] In Scotland initiatives to use technology services employing remote consultation, such as NHS Near Me,[39] have been deployed, which has allowed the social distancing requirements of COVID-19 to reduce infection, but has also been noted to improve accessibility of services and appointments and also reduce the environmental impact of travel.[40] The use of

remote consultation is well established in countries where distance and geography can be a barrier to accessing health care, such as Canada, Australia and Scotland. Jelle van Gurp et al[41] identified that teleconsultations allowed health care professionals to develop a unique insight into the lives of service users and that over the long term a trusting close relationship could be established. Service users identified that teleconsultation could fit into their domestic life with some ease and allowed a visual contact that created the feeling of physical proximity, though challenges with service user privacy were identified due to the potential for unannounced intrusions. What is important here is to consider inequalities in relation to access to IT and also skills in using it. Whilst this evaluation data is yet to emerge, where online and telephone consultation has been used more generally in primary care, evidence suggests it has been positively received by practitioners and service users.[42] Indeed, there is also evidence of positive uptake of other technology-enabled support, for example, in relation to breastfeeding advice.[42] What must be noted here, is that during the COVID-19 pandemic there is an increased need to safeguard children and families[43] and these activities may provide an important role in helping health visitors to establish and maintain relationships, supported by targeted face-to-face and clinic-based contacts where needed.

## THINKING SPACE

Take time to consider your experience of working as a health visitor. It may be useful to reflect on the following:
1. How is your service delivered?
2. How does this mode of delivery enable/inhibit therapeutic relationships?
3. What ideas do you have about developing your practice/service further to ensure therapeutic relationships with individuals, families and communities are central to your work?

## RELATIONSHIPS AND INCLUSIVE PRACTICE

Health visiting practice operates within a complex and dynamic social context. The remaining part of this chapter will consider how the service has responded to this with a particular focus on our role in developing therapeutic relationships with those who have experienced trauma and engaging with fathers, as well as the increasing need to decolonise health visiting practice.

## TRAUMA-INFORMED PRACTICE AND RELATIONSHIP-BUILDING

In Scotland there has been a recent drive for all services that support children and young people to be based on an understanding of human behaviour based upon possible trauma that may have been experienced in childhood.[44] Trauma-informed practice recognises that the behaviour of children or adults when engaging with care services such as health visitors could be a product of previously experienced traumas, therefore behaviours could appear aggressive, withdrawn or attention-seeking. Research into adverse childhood experience further considers the impact of stressful experience early in life can have on memory, learning and cognitive function.[45] Carl Rodgers recognised in his work that people react in very individualised ways to their illness or experiences with services and this is based upon their perceptions and life experience.[46] The strategy and practice of implementing trauma-informed practice and recognition of the effects of adverse childhood experience on later life is becoming well established in Wales and Scotland and Northern Ireland.[45,47,89] This work builds upon the evidence researched by Bowlby and Ainsworth[48] regarding attachment theories and how individuals develop their ability to feel safe and develop trustworthiness in others. Trauma-informed practice is not just about the way that practitioners understand and work with service users/clients who have experienced trauma but also how they focus on organisational practices and their ability to foster a safe physical environment.[23] Cultural awareness and choice are factors in trauma-informed practice, as well as power balances playing a part as it is essential for service users who have experienced trauma to have the ability to exert autonomy. Berger and Quiros[23] emphasise that consistency of service, location of service and predictability all play a significant part in establishing positive relationships with trauma-experienced people and, as well as strong working partnerships, the presence of emotional safety is critical. Therefore, the guidance in Scotland advises practitioners to develop relationships with service users/clients that are based on safety, choice, reliability, collaboration and trust.[89]

Trauma-based work may have particular relevance in our work with fathers. Men who have experienced trauma in their childhood, possibly partly as a result of being raised in a household with a severely depressed father, could therefore be at risk of repeating the experience for their children. Some research does indicate that infants have a greater chance of developing a disorganised attachment pattern which manifests in later life as having difficulties in establishing a trusting relationship with others and possible mental health problems, if raised by psychologically frightened and/or physically frightening parents. Many incarcerated men, a fair number[49] of whom will be fathers, are likely to have had some sort of trauma during their childhoods.[90] Their ability to exert autonomy whilst in prison is clearly severely compromised, so breaking that intergenerational cycle by offering the appropriate support and advice to fathers, as well as mothers, may go some way to prompting healthy attachments for the next generation.

## BUILDING RELATIONSHIPS WITH FATHERS

Baldwin et al,[50] in a systematic review of paternal mental health and well-being during the transition to fatherhood, found much relevance for health visiting practice. Their findings conclude that the role and lifestyle changes for men can result in feelings of stress, for which some fathers use denial or escape activities as a coping mechanism. Fathers appear to want more guidance and support, but barriers to this support include lack of tailored information resources and acknowledgement or engagement from health professionals.

Although the literature around paternal perinatal ill health appears to be in its infancy in comparison to maternal perinatal ill health,[51] the specialist community public health nursing (SCPHN) still should routinely be asking fathers about their experience of becoming a father at every contact.[52] Exploring fathers' thoughts, feelings and expectations may allow for a discussion around the transition to fatherhood, as well as an opportunity to screen for depression, which is thought to affect about 8% of new fathers and be more likely in the presence of maternal postnatal depression.[53] Postnatal depression may manifest later in men and is likely to be under-detected and under-reported. There is no definitive guidance about how and when to screen fathers, but what is essential is that it is considered, and that fathers as well as mothers are asked and given opportunities to talk about their mental health and well-being, fostering a family-centred approach.[53] Work with fathers can be compounded by an entrenched culture in health visiting that defines it as a mother and child service; it is here where all health visitors and health professionals must work together to challenge this perception, and ensure that work with fathers is not discretionary but a mandatory feature of our role.[54] Health visitors need to understand the gender-specific differences between parents (as much as they need an understanding on gender differences in children) for mental distress.

Many depressed men – unlike depressed women, who often present with feelings of sadness – can present as hostile, angry and more likely to be in conflict with others.[55] They may withdraw or engage in escape activities, such as working very long hours, or find themselves increasing their smoking, drinking or gambling habits.[50,56]

It is increasingly accepted that fathers' mental health and well-being is an important public health issue to which health visitors must respond to iHV.[107] Indeed, research Baldwin et al[57] indicates that men would welcome the opportunity to be asked about their health and well-being. However, there is also evidence that health visitors lack confidence in this area and are unprepared through their training to engage with and work with fathers.[58] Whilst there is an assumption that establishing effective relationships with fathers requires a different set of skills, this is not the case. Instead, Baldwin et al[57] suggests it is about reflecting on our assumptions and approaching work with fathers with an open mind, as well as using our existing skills to establish and maintain effective relationships. This also presents an opportunity for us to learn from fathers and work with them to shape the service into one that includes and values them. Arguably, what would enhance this process is increasing the diversity of the workforce and attracting more male nurses into the profession. However, with only 11% of the nursing workforce being made up of men[59] this is a challenge, particularly in Specialist Community Public Health Nursing. Here there are only 653 men out of a total of 28,996 practitioners, which equates to 2.25% of the workforce; moreover, these numbers are in steady decline.[60] Explanations for this include the challenge of changing the traditional profile of the professions, as well as a cyclical problem whereby a dearth of male role models leads to fewer men considering nursing as a potential career.[60] What is clear is that male health visitors add immense value to the service and can help shape it for supporting the changing nature of society and the erosion of stereotypical gender and professional roles.[60]

## THINKING SPACE

Take time to consider your experience of working with fathers. It may be useful to reflect on the following:

1. How does your service address the needs of fathers?
2. How does this mode of delivery enable/inhibit therapeutic relationships?
3. What ideas do you have about developing your practice/service to ensure therapeutic relationships with individuals, families and communities are central to your work?

### Case study 2

You visit Andy and Andreanna, with their new baby Alexandra, for the six-week contact. The family have been informed of your visit by a colleague as the new birth visit at 10 days. Your employer expects you to follow the Health Child Programme and to enquire after Andreanna's mental health at this contact. From the previous notes, you know both parents are usually in full-time work, Andy in local government and Andreanna as a nurse. When you visit the home, Andy is in the kitchen and appears to be working on his laptop. He makes you and Andreanna a drink, but then returns to his laptop, withdrawing from any further interaction.

Thought point: How would you promote Andy's engagement in this visit and offer equality of service provision to both parents?

## EQUALITY, DIVERSITY AND INCLUSION IN HEALTH VISITING

The call for increased diversity in the health visiting profession links to arguments calling for decolonisation of the service and wider social movements, not exclusively, but including, the Black Lives Matter movement, which reflects an increasing recognition that society needs to do more to promote equality, diversity and inclusion. Across the United Kingdom ethnicity, culture and language is recorded by the Census which identifies that in England and Wales 86% of the population are from white ethnic groups.[91] The Scotland census of 2011[92] identified Scotland as 92% white Scottish and British combined[61] and in Northern Ireland 98% of the population identify their ethnicity as white.[93] It is difficult to provide accurate data regarding how many health visitors in the United Kingdom are of black or minority ethnic origin, as the data often combines nurses, midwives and health visitors/SCPHN's. 2019 data indicates that around 64.4% of nurses (which may include SCPHN's) and 80.4% of midwives (which may also include SCPHN's) are of white ethnic origin.[62] It is also noted that as nursing grade increases, the number of staff from Black and Minority Ethnic (BME) backgrounds decreases further,[63] which is likely to be reflected in the numbers in the health visiting profession. This raises important questions about how as a profession we practise in an inclusive manner and contribute to decolonisation of the profession.

Colonisation is an intentional activity in which cultural domination is enabled through a belief in superiority and the promotion of one group of humans over another.[64] Asserts that decolonisation can be achieved by addressing power imbalances, specifically 'by sharing power, equalising privilege, and challenging the assumption of superiority and inferiority that sustain unbalanced power and privilege'. Therefore, the health visiting skills described earlier in this chapter, which focus on developing human valuing and strengths-based therapeutic relationships, should set health visitors in good stead to develop beneficial relationships. Valero-Garces[65] states that communication is a vital element of being human, and that a lack of effective communication impacts negatively on human health and well-being. Therefore, the communication skills inherent within our practice are essential in communicating effectively with those whose culture and language differ from our own.[65]

Whilst these features of our work are important, Emery-Whittington and Te Maro assert that decolonisation also requires a purposeful effort to recognise the advantage that white people have experienced, which shapes their beliefs and a 're-orientation' of the belief systems that white culture has built, and the way that white people think.[94] This imposition of our own beliefs and cultures reflects Peckover's[30] view that health visitors 'police' families with their own beliefs and values of maternal and paternal mental health, child development, parental behaviours, and parenting practice. Therefore, in order to develop helpful relationships with clients/families that have a culture or ethnicity different to our own, it is important that we not only employ effective relationship-building practice, but also consider how our own beliefs and possible sense of superiority over another human being may affect our clinical assessments and judgements.[95] This is not without notable challenges for health visitors and whilst this area of practice is not well researched, a study by Cuthill[66] indicates that, despite calls for cross-cultural competence, this is not clearly defined; furthermore, many professionals, including health visitors, feel uncertain and sometimes anxious about delivering culturally competent care. In response to this, the health visitors in this study were seen to adopt three responses. Firstly, some focused on 'fixing a culture' by finding out more about that culture in order to reduce uncertainty. Others adopted an approach that emphasised equality and sameness. The concern here is that, in doing this, important cultural differences might be negated and would therefore not lead to equity of experience. The third approach involved health visitors relying on 'research-based evidence' as a source of certain knowledge. This reflects earlier discussion whereby the voice of the cultural or ethnic minority is silenced in favour of the majority[30,94] and westernised discourses of research-based evidence are favoured, which do not adequately reflect or embrace cross-cultural knowledge or care.[66] What is needed here is for practitioners to recognise that some of the strategies they employ have the potential to negate culturally competent care, but also to perpetuate the very inequalities we aim to address.[66]

## THINKING SPACE

Take time to consider your experience of working as a health visitor. It may be useful to reflect on the following:

1. How does your service promote equality, diversity, and inclusivity?
2. How does this enable/inhibit therapeutic relationships?
3. What ideas do you have about developing your practice/service further to ensure that it meets the needs of a diverse population?

## CONCLUSION

This chapter has considered how the evolution of the health visiting service influences relationships with individuals, families and communities, as well as the response of the service to the changing nature of modern society. Whilst the content of the chapter is not exhaustive, it has included some important challenges for our profession with the intention of prompting critical reflection on both individual practice and service delivery.

### Summary of key learning points

- The health visiting service continues to be a highly regarded and fundamental source of support for parents with preschool children.
- Therapeutic relationships are an essential feature of health visiting practice and are established with individuals, families, populations and other community services.
- Building therapeutic relationships relies on partnership working, trust, authenticity and effective communication and motivational interviewing skills.
- The health visiting service needs to promote equality, diversity and inclusivity and to continue evolving to meet the changing needs of the communities we serve.

## REFERENCES

1. Institute of Health Visiting (2020). Developing you in practice. https://ihv.org.uk/for-health-visitors/developing-you-in-practice/. Accessed 30 June 2020.
2. Rodger, A. (2017). Newly qualified health visitor: therapeutic relationships. *Journal of Health Visiting*, 5(6), 270–272.
3. Brooke, J., & Salmon, D. (2015). A qualitative study exploring parental perspectives and involvement in health visiting services during the Health Visitor Implementation Plan in the South West of England. *Health and Social Care in the Community*, 25(2), 349–356.
4. Oxford Dictionary (2019). *Oxford dictionary*. https://www.lexico.com/en/definition/reciprocity. Accessed 31 January 2020.
5. National Institute for Health and Care Excellence (2009). Solihull approach to parenting group. https://www.nice.org.uk/sharedlearning/solihull-approach-parenting-group. Accessed 31 January 2020.
6. Scottish Government. (2019). Family Nurse Partnership: Revaluation report. https://www.gov.scot/publications/revaluation-family-nurse-partnership-scotland/. Accessed 31 January 2020.
7. Cowley, S., Whittaker, K., Malone, M., Donetto, S., Grigulis, A., & Maben, J. (2015). Why health visiting? Examining the potential public health benefits from health visiting practice within a universal service: A narrative review of the literature. *International Journal of Nursing Studies*, 52. doi: 10.1016/j.jnurstu.2014.07.013.
8. Cowley, S., Whittaker, K., Malone, M., Donetto, S., Grigulis, A., & Maben, J. (2018). What makes health visiting successful – or not? 1. Universality. *Journal of Health Visiting*, 6(7), 352–360.
9. Scottish Government. (2015). Universal health visiting pathway in Scotland: Pre-birth to pre-school. https://www.gov.scot/publications/universal-health-visiting-pathway-scotland-pre-birth-pre-school/. Accessed 31 January 2020.
10. Department of Health. (2011). Health Visitor Implementation Plan 2011–2015. https://assets.publishing.service.gov.uk/government/uploads/system/uploads/attachment_data/file/213759/dh_124208.pdf. Accessed 31 January 2020.
11. Turnell, A., & Edwards, E. (1997). Aspiring to partnership. The signs of safety approach to child protection. *Child Abuse Review*, 6(3), 179–190.
12. Sanders, J., Channon, S., Gobat, N., et al. (2019). Implementation of the Family Nurse Partnership programme in England: Experiences of key health professionals explored through trial parallel process evaluation. *BMC Nursing*, 18(13). https://bmcnurs.biomedcentral.com/articles/10.1186/s12912-019-0338-y. Accessed 31 January 2020.
13. Miller, W. R., & Rose, G. S. (2009). Towards a theory of motivational interviewing. *American Psychologist*, 64(6), 527–537.
14. Public Health England (2015). The new paradigm of medicine and health: What's in it for nurses. Let's explore coaching. https://publichealthmatters.blog.gov.uk/2015/07/07/lets-explore-nurse-coaching/. Accessed 31 January 2020.
15. Shumacher, J. A., & Madson, M. B. (2015). *Fundamentals of Motivational Interviewing: Tips and Strategies for Addressing Common Clinical Challenges*. Oxford: Oxford University Press.
16. Roberts, Y.H., Caslor, M., Turnell, A., Pearson, K., Pecora, P.J. (2019). An international effort to develop a fidelity measure for signs of safety. *Research on Social Work Practice*, 29(5), 562–571.
17. Koloroutis, M., & Trout, M. (2013). *See Me As a Person: Creating Therapeutic Relationships with Patients and Their Families*. Minneapolis: Creative Health Care Management.
18. Hinojosa, A. S., Davis, K., McCauley, B., Randolph, S., & Gardner, W. (2014). Leader and follower attachment styles: Implications for authentic leader-follower relationships. *The Leadership Quarterly*, 25(3), 595–610.
19. Freeman, M., & Jana, T. (2016). *Overcoming Bias*. London: Penguin Random House.
20. The Institute of Health Visiting (2021). Who are health visitors? https://cypf.berkshirehealthcare.nhs.uk/media/109513867/who-are-hvs-ihv-october-2021.pdf. Accessed 15 November 2021
21. Williams, Lippincott, & Wilkins (2015). *Fundamentals of Nursing Made Incredibly Easy!* London: Wolters Kluwer.
22. Bidmead, C., Cowley, S., & Grocott, P. (2017). Measuring the parent/health visitor relationship: Piloting the questionnaires. *Journal of Health Visiting*, 5(2), 72–80.
23. Berger, R., & Quiros, L. (2014). Supervision for trauma informed practice. *Traumatology*, 20(4), 296–301.
24. Dobson, A. (2017). Newly qualified health visitor: Starting out in safeguarding. *Journal of Health Visiting*, 5(5), 219.
25. House of Commons Health and Social Care Committee. (2019). First 1000 days of life. Thirteenth Report of Session 2017–2019. https://publications.parliament.uk/pa/cm201719/cmselect/cmhealth/1496/1496.pdf. Accessed 31 January 2020.
26. Cowley, S., & Houston, A. M. (2003). A structured health needs assessment tool: acceptability and effectiveness for health visiting. *Journal of Advanced Nursing*, 43(1), 82–92.

27. Nursing and Midwifery Council. (2004). Standards of proficiency for specialist community public health nurses. https://www.nmc.org.uk/globalassets/sitedocuments/standards/nmc-standards-of-proficiency-for-specialist-community-public-health-nurses.pdf. Accessed 31 January 2020.

28. Doi, L., Jespon, R., & Hardie, S. (2017). Realist evaluation of an enhanced health visiting programme. *PLoS One*, *12*(7). doi 10.1371/journal.pone.0180569.

29. The Times (2018). Delay sparks new call to abandon Scotland's named person scheme. Also known as 'state snoopers charter'. https://www.thetimes.co.uk/article/delay-sparks-new-call-to-abandon-scotland-s-named-person-scheme-also-known-as-state-snoopers-charter-msqrkkmp0. Accessed 31 January 2020.

30. Peckover, S. (2002). Supporting and policing mothers: an analysis of the disciplinary practices of health visiting. *Journal of advanced nursing, 38* (4): 369–377.

31. Institute of Health Visiting. (2019). History of Health Visiting. https://ihv.org.uk/about-us/history-of-health-visiting/. Accessed 31 January 2020.

32. Cowley, S. A., & Frost, M. (2006). *The principles of health visiting: Opening the door to public health practice in the 21st century*. London: Community Practitioner and Health Visitors Association.

33. James, J., & Rosan, C. (2019). Remodelling baby clinics: Opportunities to support parent-baby relationships. *Journal of Health Visiting, 7*(8), 400–404.

34. Abdu, L., & Cooper, K. (2016). The implications of mobile working for health visiting practice. *Journal of Health Visiting*. https://www.magonlinelibrary.com/doi/full/10.12968/johv.2016.4.7.360. Accessed 15 January 2020.

35. Bryar, R. M., Cowley, S. A., Adams, C. M., Kendall, S., & Mathers, N. (2017). Health visiting in primary care in England: A crisis waiting to happen? *British Journal of General Practice, 67,* 656.

36. Whittaker, K., & Carter, B. (2013). Modernising health visiting practice whilst keeping compassion in care. https://journals.sagepub.com/doi/10.1177/1367493513492902. Accessed 31 January 2020.

37. World Health Organisation. (2020). Coronavirus disease (COVID-19) pandemic. https://www.who.int/emergencies/diseases/novel-coronavirus-2019. Accessed 29 June 2020.

38. Institute of Health Visiting. (2020). Parenting through Coronavirus (COVID-19). https://ihv.org.uk/families/parenting-through-coronavirus-covid-19/. Accessed 29 June 2020.

39. NHS Education for Scotland. (2020). Remote consultation and recruitment. https://learn.nes.nhs.scot/28943/coronavirus-covid-19/remote-consulting-and-recruitment. Accessed 29 June 2020.

40. Technology Enabled Care. (2020). COVID-19 and near me. https://tec.scot/. Accessed 29 June 2020.

41. van Gurp, J., van Selm, M., Vissers, K., can Leuwen, E & Hasselaar, J., (2015). How outpatient palliative care teleconsultation facilitates empathic patient-professional relationships: A qualitative study. *Public Library of Science, 10*(4), 1–13.

42. NHS England. (2020). Using online consultations in primary care. https://www.england.nhs.uk/wp-content/uploads/2020/01/online-consultations-implementation-toolkit-v1.1-updated.pdf. Accessed 1 July 2020.

43. Social Care Institute for Excellence. (2020). Safeguarding children and families during the Covid-19 crisis. https://www.scie.org.uk/care-providers/coronavirus-covid-19/safeguarding/children. Accessed 1 July 2020.

44. Couper, S., & Mackie, P. (2016). Polishing the Diamonds: Addressing adverse childhood experiences in Scotland. https://www.scotphn.net/projects/adverse-childhood-experiences/introduction/. Accessed 31 January 2020.

45. Bunting, L., Montgomery, L., Mooney, S., MacDonald, M., Coulter, S., Hayes, D., Davidson, G. & Forbes, T. (2018). Evidence review: Developing trauma-informed practice in Northern Ireland. https://www.safeguardingni.org/sites/default/files/sites/default/files/imce/ACEs%20Report%20A4%20Feb%202019%20Developing%20a%20Trauma%20Informed%20Approach%20-%20Full%20Evidence%20Review.pdf. Accessed January 31, 2020.

46. Rodgers, C. (1951). Client-centered therapy. *Journal of Clinical Psychology, 7*(3), 294–295.

47. Public Health Wales. (2017). The Welsh Adverse Childhood Experience National Survey. https://www.google.co.uk/url?sa=t&rct=j&q=&esrc=s&source=web&cd=6&cad=rja&uact=8&ved=2ahUKEwjoi9GFrLHnAhUxQUEAHbBGAQwQFjAFegQIBBAB&url=https%3A%2F%2Fphw.nhs.wales%2Fnews%2Fnew-survey-shows-both-good-welsh-public-sector-awareness-of-adverse-childhood-experiences-aces-and-opportunities-for-improvement%2Fknowledge-and-awareness-of-adverse-childhood-experiences-in-the-public-service-workforce-in-wales%2F&usg=AOvVaw3UH3vqaaE1mboFd93vd5wB. Accessed 31 January 2020.

48. Ainsworth, M., & Salter, M. D. (1978). The Bowlby-Ainsworth attachment theory. *Behavioural and Brain Sciences, 1*(3), 436–438.

49. Barlow, J., & Underdown, A. (2008). Attachment and infant development. In: *Child and Adolescent Mental Health Today: A Handbook*. Brighton: Pavilion Publishing/Mental Health Foundation.

50. Baldwin, S., Malone, M., Sandall, J., & Bick, D. (2018). Mental health and well-being during the transition to fatherhood: a systematic review of first time fathers' experiences. *JBI Database of Systematic Reviews and Implementation Reports, 16*(11), 2118.

51. Paulson, J. F., & Bazemore, S. D. (2010). Prenatal and postpartum depression in fathers and its association with maternal depression: A meta-analysis. *JAMA, 303*(19), 1961–1969. doi: 10.1001/jama.2010.605.

52. Davies, J. (2015). Fatherhood Institute: supporting fathers to play their part. *Community Practitioner, 88*(1), 13.

53. Ramluggun, P., Kamara, A., & Anjoyeb, M. (2020). Postnatal depression in fathers: A quiet struggle. *British Journal of Mental Health Nursing, 9*(4), doi:10.12968/bjmh.2019.0042.

54. Family Included. (2016). Why do UK Health Visitors not Engage with Fathers? https://familyincluded.com/uk-health-visitors/.

55. National Institute of Mental Health. (2020). Men and Depression. https://www.nimh.nih.gov/health/publications/men-and-depression/index.shtml.

56. Veskrna, L. (2010). Peripartum depression: Does it occur in fathers and does it matter? *Journal of Men's Health, 7*(4), 420–430.

57. Baldwin, S., Malone, M., Sandall, J., & Bick, D. (2019). A qualitative exploratory study of UK first-time fathers' experiences, mental health and well-being needs during their transition to fatherhood. *BMJ Open, 9*, e030792. doi: 10.1136/bmjopen-2019-030792. https://bmjopen.bmj.com/content/9/9/e030792.info.

58. Oldfield, V., & Carr, H. (2017). Postnatal depression: Student health visitors' perceptions of their role in supporting fathers. *Journal of Health Visiting, 5*(3), 143–149.

59. Nursing & Midwifery Council. (2018). The NMC register. https://www.nmc.org.uk/globalassets/sitedocuments/other-publications/the-nmc-register-2018.pdf. Accessed 1 July 2020.

60. Harris, P. (2018). A few good men. https://www.communitypractitioner.co.uk/sites/default/files/media/document/2018/cp_feb2018.pdf. Accessed 1, 2020.

61. Scottish Government. (2020). National Performance Framework. https://nationalperformance.gov.scot/. Accessed 31 January 2020.

62. Nursing & Midwifery Council. (2019). Diversity data 2018–2019. https://www.nmc.org.uk/globalassets/sitedocuments/annual_reports_and_accounts/edi/edi-2018-19-data-tables.pdf. Accessed 2 July 2020.

63. NHS England. (2019). Workforce Race equality standard. An overview of workforce data for nurses, midwives and health visitors in the NHS. https://www.england.nhs.uk/wp-content/uploads/2019/03/wres-nursing-strategy.pdf. Accessed 2 July 2020.

64. Fay, J. (2018). Decolonising mental health services one prejudice at a time: Psychological, sociological, ecological, and cultural considerations. *Settler Colonial Studies, 8*(1), 47–59.

65. Valero-Garces, C. (2014). *Health, communication and multicultural communities: Topics on intercultural communication for healthcare professionals.* Cambridge: Cambridge Scholars Publishing.

66. Cuthill, F. (2014). Understanding the ways in which health visitors manage anxiety in cross-cultural work: A qualitative study. *Primary Health Care Research Development, 15*(4), 375–385.

67. Burns, S.H. (2012). Kilbrandon's Vision. Healthier Lives: Bette futures. The Tenth Kilbrandon Lecture, Sir Harry Burns, Chief Medical Officer for Scotland. The Scottish Government. https://www.strath.ac.uk/media/1newwebsite/departmentsubject/facultyofhumanitiesandsocialsciences/documents/10th_Lecture_-_Harry_Burns.pdf.

68. Mittelmark, M.B. et al. (2016). The Handbook of Salutogenesis. Cham: Springer.

69. Parenting across Scotland 2021. Scotland: the best place in the world to bring up children? 1st ed. [ebook] Edinburgh: Parenting across Scotland, pp.9–10. https://www.parentingacrossscotland.org/media/1162/pas-the-best-place.pdf. Accessed 12 November 2021.

70. Department of Health 2011. Educating Health Visitors for a transformed service. 1st ed. [ebook] London. https://www.gov.uk/government/publications/educating-health-visitors-for-a-transformed service. Accessed 12 November 2021.

71. Quinn, E. (2011). Working in Partnership: The Family Partnership Model - By Hilton Davis and Crispin Day, Support for Learning, 26(3), pp. 137–138. doi:10.1111/j.1467-9604.2011.01493_2.x.

72. Olds, D., Henderson, C., Tatelbaum, R., & Chamberlin, R. (1986). Improving the Delivery of Prenatal Care and Outcomes of Pregnancy: A Randomized Trial of Nurse Home Visitation. Pediatrics. 77. 16–28.

73. Olds, D. (2003). Reducing program attrition in home visiting: what do we need to know?, Child abuse & neglect, 27(4), pp. 359–361. doi:10.1016/S0145-2134(03)00022-X.

74. Cross, B. & Cheyne, H. (2018). Strength-based approaches: a realist evaluation of implementation in maternity services in Scotland, Journal of public health, 26(4), pp. 425–436. doi:10.1007/s10389-017-0882-4.

75. Miller, W. R., & Rollnick, S. (2013). L'entretien motivationnel. Aider la personne à engager le changement, 2.

76. Rollnick, S., Miller, W. R., & Butler, C. (2008). Motivational interviewing in health care: helping patients change behavior. Guilford Press.

77. Madson, M. B., Mohn, R. S., Schumacher, J. A., & Landry, A. S. (2015). Measuring client experiences of motivational interviewing during a lifestyle intervention. Measurement and Evaluation in Counseling and Development, 48(2), 140–151.

78. Rogers, C. R. (1959). A theory of therapy, personality, and interpersonal relationships: As developed in the client-centered framework (Vol. 3, pp. 184–256). New York: McGraw-Hill.

79. Teal, C.R. et al. (2012). Helping medical learners recognise and manage unconscious bias toward certain patient groups, Medical education. Received 15 February 2011; editorial comments to authors 26 April 2011; accepted for publication 19 July 2011, 46(1), pp. 80–88. doi:10.1111/j.1365-2923.2011.04101.x.

80. Low, C.M. et al. (2018) Measuring reflective supervision within home visiting: changes in supervisors self-perception over time, Infant mental health journal, 39(5), pp. 608–617. doi:10.1002/imhj.21736.

81. Johnston, M. (1999) On becoming non-judgmental: some difficulties for an ethics of counselling, Journal of medical ethics, 25(6), pp. 487–490. doi:10.1136/jme.25.6.487.

82. Parker-Radford, D. (2014) The impact of specialist health visitors for homeless and vulnerable families, Journal of health visiting, 2(11), pp. 592–596. doi:10.12968/johv.2014.2.11.592.

83. Bowlby, J. (1979). The bowlby-ainsworth attachment theory. Behavioral and Brain Sciences, 2(4), 637-638.

84. Miller, W.R. and Rollnick, Stephen (2012) Motivational interviewing : helping people change. 3rd ed. New York, NY: Guilford Press.

85. Day, C. & Harris, L. (2013). The Family Partnership Model: Evidence-based effective partnerships, Journal of health visiting, 1(1), pp. 54–59. doi:10.12968/johv.2013.1.1.54.

86. Jourard, S. M. (1971). The transparent self. Van Nostrand Reinhold Company.

87. Sanders, J. et al. (2019). Implementation of the Family Nurse Partnership programme in England: experiences of key health professionals explored through trial parallel process evaluation, BMC nursing, 18(1), pp. 13–13. doi:10.1186/s12912-019-0338-y.

88. Stetler, K. et al. (2017). Lessons Learned: Implementation of Pilot Universal Postpartum Nurse Home Visiting Program, Massachusetts 2013 -2016, Maternal and child health journal, 22(1), pp. 11–16. doi:10.1007/s10995-017-2385-x.

89. Scottish Government (2018). Adverse childhood experiences (ACES). https://www.gov.scot/ publications/adverse-childhood-experiences/. Accessed 1 January 2020.

90. Schimmenti, A., Passanisi, A., Pace, U., Manzella, S., Di Carlo, G. & Caretti, V., (2014). The relationship between attachment and psychopathy: A study with a sample of violent offenders. Current Psychology, 33(3), pp. 256–270.

91. Office of National Statistics (2019). Ethnicity. https://www.ons.gov.uk/peoplepopulationandcommunity/culturalidentity/ethnicity. Accessed 15 November 2021.

92. Scotland's Census (2021). Ethnicity. https://www.scotlandscensus.gov.uk/census-results/at-a-glance/ethnicity/. Accessed 15 November 2021.

93. Northern Ireland assembly (2013). Census 2011: Detailed Characteristics of Ethnicity and Country of Birth at the Northern Ireland level. http://www.niassembly.gov.uk/globalassets/documents/raise/publications/2013/general/13813.pdf. Accessed 15 November 2021.

94. Emery-Whittington, I., & Te Maro, B. (2018). Decolonising occupation: Causing social change to help our ancestors rest and our descendants thrive. New Zealand Journal of Occupational Therapy, 65(1), 12–19.

95. FitzGerald, C. & Hurst, S. (2017). Implicit bias in healthcare professionals: a systematic review, BMC medical ethics, 18(1), pp. 19–19. doi:10.1186/s12910-017-0179-8.

96. Luker K. & Chalmers K. (1989) The referral process in healthvisiting. International Journal of Nursing Studies 26(2), 173–185.

97. Condon, J. T., Boyce, P., & Corkindale, C. J. (2004). The first-time fathers study: A prospective study of the mental health and well-being of men during the transition to parenthood. Australian and New Zealand Journal of Psychiatry, 38(1–2), 56–64.

98. Channon, et al. (2016). Motivational interviewing competencies among UK family nurse partnership nurses: a process evaluation component of the building blocks trial. BMC Nursing, 15(1).

99. https://ihv.org.uk/wp-content/uploads/2019/11/7.11.19-Health-Visiting-in-England-Vision-FINAL-VERSION.pdf. Accessed 11 February 2021.

100. Scottish Government. (2018). Getting it right for every child (GIRFEC). https://www.gov.scot/policies/girfec/. Accessed 31 January 2020.

101. Scottish Government. (2018). Adverse childhood experiences (ACES). https://www.gov.scot/publications/adverse-childhood-experiences/. Accessed 31 January 2020.

102. Scottish Government. (2019). Children and Young People (Information Sharing) Bill. https://www.gov.scot/news/children-and-young-people-information-sharing-bill/. Accessed 31 January 2020.

103. European Court of Human Rights (2019). European Convention on Human Rights. European Convention on Human Rights (coe.int). Accessed December 26, 2021.

104. John Boothman (2018). Delay sparks new call to abandon Scotland's named person schem, also known as 'state snoopers charter'. The Sunday Times. 22nd July 2018. Accessible on-line from: Delay sparks new call to abandon Scotland's named person scheme, also known as 'state snoopers charter' | Scotland | The Sunday Times (thetimes.co.uk).

105. Donetto, S. and Maben, J. (2015) 'These places are like a godsend': a qualitative analysis of parents' experiences of health visiting outside the home and of children's centres services. Health Expectations 18(6), 2559–2569.

106. Bennett (2015). https://vivbennett.blog.gov.uk/2015/02/02/health-visiting-listening-to-parents-transforming-services-viv-bennett/.

107. Institute of Health Visiting. 2020. Parent Tips (PT) - Emotional Health and Wellbeing – Fathers. Accessible on-line from: https://ihv.org.uk/for-health-visitors/resources-for-members/resource/ihv-tips-for-parents/mental-health/emotional-health-and-wellbeing-fathers/.

# 6

# ASSESSMENT

FELICITY JONES

## CHAPTER CONTENTS

INTRODUCTION

CLINICAL DECISION-MAKING

THE USE OF ASSESSMENT TOOLS

BARRIERS TO USING ASSESSMENT TOOLS

ASSESSMENT AND SCREENING TOOLS FREQUENTLY USED IN PRACTICE

WORKING IN PARTNERSHIP WITH PARENTS

WORKING WITH THE FAMILY

STRENGTH-BASED APPROACH AND MATCHING AGENDAS

VIRTUAL ASSESSMENTS AND THE IMPACT OF THE COVID-19 PANDEMIC

CONCLUSION

## LEARNING OUTCOMES

*At the end of the chapter the reader will be able:*

- To demonstrate an awareness of the assessment process in the health visiting service.
- To explore the skills that health visitors use when undertaking assessments.
- To develop an understanding of the supporting factors and barriers to the assessment process.

## INTRODUCTION

The Nursing and Midwifery Council have identified that assessment is a core component of health visiting practice.[1] As part of the universal HV programme,[2] health visitors offer a holistic assessment of children and families considering physical, psychological and environment impact.[3] These assessments are ongoing processes that start from initial contact with the family and are revisited and reviewed as circumstances change,[4] requiring the health visitor to have complex assessment skills as needs may not always be visible or readily disclosed.[5] The ability to assess requires a high level of professional knowledge and judgement and is central for empowering and supporting families.[6] Assessment should be family-centred; gaining a comprehensive understanding of the family, its strengths as well as any risks that impact on its health. In addition to needing professional judgement and knowledge of evidence base, one of the most important aspects of undertaking in-depth assessments is the ability to build a relationship with the family.[4,7] It has been suggested that building relationships is the main component of a health visiting service, central to empowering parents to develop confidence and knowledge of parenting within the context of local community services and amenities.[7]

This chapter will explore the assessment process, the clinical skills required to undertake assessments and some of the barriers to the assessment process. It will also explore some of the more frequently used assessment and screening tools in the health visiting service. In concluding, it will consider the COVID-19 pandemic of 2020 and the impact this has had on the rapidly developing use of virtual assessments, not only in the health visiting service but across the NHS.

## THINKING SPACE

As health visitors we undertake complex and dynamic holistic assessments that aim to empower parents and families. These use a partnership, strength-based approach.

What skills do you need as a health visitor to undertake these assessments?

## CLINICAL DECISION-MAKING

To gain an understanding of the assessment process, it is important to reflect on how clinical decision-making is undertaken and what key factors influence it. Clinical decision-making in nursing is seen as 'a complex process involving observation, information processing, critical thinking, evaluating evidence, applying relevant knowledge, problem solving skills, reflection and clinical judgement to select the best course of action which optimizes a patient's health and minimizes any potential harm'.[8:7] It has been argued that the assessment process is more complex in community nursing than hospital nursing – the health visitor having to balance actual with potential problems and also consider possibly conflicting views of needs from different family members.[9]

A pivotal case study of 15 health visitors analysed the health visiting assessment process and the skills that underpin identifying and assessing family health needs.[4] This study found that assessment is a complex and interactive process that had seven key components:

- Interpersonal skills
- Knowledge in use
- Processing knowledge to aid assessment
- Facilitating factors
- Strategies adopted to aid assessment
- Assessment as an intervention
- Inhibitory factors

These factors will be explored during this chapter.

'Knowledge of use' recognises the evidence base and guidelines that support the assessment process. As part of knowledge processing, health visitors need to reflect on their knowledge of the family: for example, re-assess the family's health needs, the impact of the planned interventions on these needs and how they compared to the expected norm. The expected norm is evaluated against a research evidence base, policy and professional experience of working with other families or situations. Practitioners' previous experience and tacit knowledge are seen across research as a core aspect of decision-making in nursing.[8,10,11]

Alongside previous knowledge, intuition or gut feeling can assist the health visitor in the assessment process. Intuition can be defined as 'the process whereby the nurse knows something about the patient that cannot be verbalised without difficulty, or for which the source of knowledge cannot be determined'.[11:43] Intuition is often related to external cues and plays a key role in nursing assessment. Research has found that intuition is present in nearly all steps of the decision-making process and it is a component of nursing clinical care, being used in conjunction with cues and guidelines.[12] Practitioners rely on their evidence base to synthesise and analyse intuitive thoughts when planning care.[10] Their intuition was found to be affected by professional knowledge, experience, skill level, personal characteristics and relationships with the client.[11]

Research has identified that health visitors offer a flexible approach during assessment, often gauging when to say something, trying to recognise if a person is both ready to hear information and consider the best way to present that information. In Appleton and Cowley's study, it became more apparent that health visitors did this when they were trying to maintain access to families.[4] This research was published in 2008, prior to the contemporary discussion on the importance of partnership working, strength-based approaches and matching agendas with families. More recent research has highlighted that health visitors still, to a degree, gauge how to deliver information as they may be concerned of the emotional impact it may have on the parent.[13] What is evident is that support from the health visiting service provider organisation and managers can influence the assessment and decision-making process.[11,14] Guidelines for assessment appeared to have minimal impact on their undertaking.[4] This may be because as nurses gain experience they feel more confident to make client-based decisions rather than simply follow guidelines.[11] However, this may lead to criticism: being over-reliant on professional experience may not explicitly include the structured use of evidence, which may reduce the reliability and validity of the decisions made.[15] Health Visitors not adhering to guidelines may also be frustrating for managers, as their planned support for a family may be beyond those the HV service is commissioned to deliver.[14] As full-time equivalent health visiting numbers reduce,[5] resulting in service cutbacks and time constraints, this may also have an impact on decision-making processes and the services that can be offered.[9] To make complex, autonomous decisions, health visitors need to work in a supportive culture that trusts practitioners' experience and ability to make decisions.[14] This is a time when the health visiting service needs strong leadership that can consider innovative ways to develop practice in a way that supports autonomous decision-making.[16]

To be competent practitioners, health visitors need ongoing professional development to support their clinical decision-making skills. Research has found that the working environment, personal capacity and fear of missing serious conditions all impact on clinical decision-making.[10] Practitioners need to have the time and ability to reflect and learn; this can be in the form of initial training programmes, ongoing professional development, communities of practice and clinical supervision.[8] Clinical decision-making models, such as Cognitive Continuum Theory[17] or the Hypothetic-Deductive Model,[18] can offer theoretical frameworks and a common language which allow nurses to support and reflect on clinical decision-making. This could lead to greater understanding of the decision-making process, aiding communication and justification of decisions made.[19,20]

## THE USE OF ASSESSMENT TOOLS

Core to the assessment process is the assessment and screening tools used within the health visiting service. There is an abundance of tools used to support the assessment process. Many tools, such as family health needs assessment and risk assessment tools, have historically been developed by local provider services and lack an evidence base.[7,21] With the development of national healthy child programmes across the UK[2,21a,22] and the continuing accumulation of evidence, there is the ongoing adoption of evidence tools, such as the Ages and Stages Questionnaire.[23]

Assessment tools offer structure both to process of the assessment that supports analysis, as well as an opportunity for further clarity when recording the assessment. Alongside professional judgement, they support the holistic evaluation of family environments, identifying the need for specific interventions and assisting timely referral.[22]

Their structure has been found to be particularly useful in assisting inexperienced health visitors, offering support in the teaching and development of skills of assessment for students and newly qualified health visitors.[24,25] They can also offer structure that enables health visitors to justify the service that they offer providing a safety net to ensure holistic assessments are undertaken; this is particularly important when the profession is at a high level of scrutiny from commissioners.[15,24] The use of assessment tools may support health visitors to articulate their decision-making process and findings, while the frameworks may facilitate conversations to support parents.[13]

## BARRIERS TO USING ASSESSMENT TOOLS

Research has shown that there are barriers to practitioners using assessment and screening tools, including the need for organisations to offer training in the use of the tool, on-going support and supervision for staff.[25–30] Lack of ongoing training and support has been identified as a barrier to the use of the promotional guide and Health Visitor Observation and Assessment of Infant Tool.[25,26] It was found that the longer a practitioner had been trained in the use of the tool, the more confident they were to use it.[25] A lack of training in the use of screening tools seems to inhibit the use of the tools and less accuracy in their use.[27] In both the use of the Whooley questions (also referred to as depression identification questions) and the promotional guide, research has found that ongoing training and regular updates have been shown to enhance health visitors' knowledge of the tool and confidence in its use.[28,29] Although training may be a time-consuming process, particularly where services are already under pressure, organisations need to consider the value of the training time, both during implementation and for ongoing development of staff, as this could impact on the success

of their use in practice.[30] Resources such as aide-memoires may be useful to prompt, guide and standardise practice.[25]

With the number of FTE health visitors decreasing by 31.8% between October 2015 and June 2019, back to pre-Call for Action figures,[5] the implication of having enough time to undertake assessments needs to be considered as another barrier. Staffing levels and increasing caseload sizes will impact on the service that can be offered.[31] Organisations need to consider the cost-saving approaches they take in terms of assessment. The use of screening tools, such as the ASQ-3, as a tick box exercise rather than part of a holistic assessment may leave hidden needs of both children and families unidentified. This is particularly important as vulnerable families may often be less motivated to seek out the support of services. This could cause the widening of inequalities and increased long-term societal costs.[5]

Time constraints were noted as a barrier in relation to undertaking the promotional guide, with some areas only allocating 20 minutes for this assessment to be completed.[26,29] By contrast, health visitors reported that time constraint was not really considered a barrier in relation to using the Whooley questions.[28] If service guidelines put time limits on more complex assessments the ability to perform them as they were initially designed to be used may be hindered. This will also impact on the building of relationships with clients, which both parents and health visitors felt to be beneficial in improving the assessment process.[25] Where services are stretched there needs to be consideration of the time taken to record assessments; the implications of policies that lead to the duplication of record keeping may impact on concordance with these requirements and further affect the time that health visitors have to build relationships with clients.[25,32] While computer systems offer improved accessibility to records,[33] the complexity of some IT systems, availability of IT equipment and programmes that crash can make data inputting for assessments more time-consuming.[30]

## ASSESSMENT AND SCREENING TOOLS FREQUENTLY USED IN PRACTICE

### Family health needs assessment

The assessment of family health needs is central to health visiting practice, supporting health visitors to identify need, service provision and referral to other agencies and voluntary services. There have been many locally developed family health needs assessment tools but one of the main limitations of these 'formal' tools is the lack of a substantial evidence base to support their use.[34–36] The development of these tools often reflects the Framework of Assessment for Children in Need and Their Families.[37] This offers an ecological framework that allows a comprehensive assessment of a family, incorporating parenting capacity, family and environmental factors and the child's developmental needs.

In Scotland, 'Getting it Right for Every Child'[38] advocates the use of the 'My World Triangle'; this is used with SHANARRI well-being indicators and Resilience Matrix to analyse the history discussed. Where the needs raised are not complex the Resilience Framework may not always be used.[38] As with other family health needs assessments, its development has been informed from the knowledge of the application of the Framework of Assessment for Children in Need and Their Families.[37,39] The 'My World Triangle' offers a holistic and ecological assessment from the child's perspective. It is grounded in child development theory, identifying strengths and risks, analysing how these impact on the child's health and developing outcomes to increase well-being.[39,40] The assessment tool supports multi-agency working, underlining that services don't work in isolation and highlighting where more specialist information needs to be sought. It is reported that this tool has a strong evidence base,[40] with its emphasis on risk assessment offering an additional dimension not seen in the Assessment Framework Triangle.[41]

To support the delivery of the Healthy Child Wales Programme, the Family Resilience Assessment Instrument and Tool (FRAIT) has been developed by University of South Wales, in conjunction with health visitors, to assess key contacts with children under five years.[3] FRAIT consists of the Family Resilience Assessment Tool (FRAT) that Health Visitors use to assess the resilience of families and the Family Resilience Assessment Instrument (FRAI) that is used to assess/score family resilience as perceived by the HV. Like the My Word Triangle, this assessment tool is built around an ecological model of health considering the child in its wider context of social, economic and environmental factors.[22] It is used to identify protective factors as well as needs, including safeguarding concerns,[3] assisting health visitors in decision-making and care planning, as well as further interventions and resources. Through the use of FRAIT the aim is to have an all-Wales approach to identifying family needs; by late 2017, all HVs in Wales had been trained in its use.[42] On evaluation of the Family Resilience Assessment Instrument and Tool, some health visitors felt that the tool made the contact less personal. They stated that the tool lacked flexibility and the sensitive questions within it could raise needs that might not be met. It was also reported that use of the FRAIT revealed more about family background. The recommendations of the report included the need to revisit the tool, including the development of additional training to health visitors on the purpose and application of the tool.[43]

### Promotional guides

The Antenatal/Postnatal Promotional Guides were first developed by the European Early Promotion Project in 2000.[44] Their use in practice was recommended in the Healthy Child Programme,[2] and during the Health Visiting Call for Action over 4300 health visitors and students were trained in their use.[45] The guides are evidence-based, supporting a partnership approach to assessment which offers a structured but flexible process that promotes early child development and transition to parenthood. This semi-structured assessment enables identification of family health needs, including parental strengths and concerns in order to match agendas and develop effective care plans. The antenatal and promotional guide have 11 and 10 topic guides respectively. The topic guides are used as conversational prompts to facilitate a 'guided conversation' of each topic with the parents. The conversation is further supported by topic cards, with the health visitor asking the parent/s to pick out the topic cards they deem most relevant to them. This offers a parent-led, flexible approach to the conversation. The health visitor can then draw on the other cards as the conversation develops, thereby informing an assessment of family strengths and needs.[45] Although the antenatal cards can be used at any point, it is suggested that they are used in the second trimester as this is a good time to reflect on the pregnancy; later in the pregnancy parents may be concentrating more on the birth. The postnatal guide is designed to be used by eight weeks in order to enable early identification of potential needs.[46]

The guides offer a framework for the assessment process while still preventing it from becoming a box-ticking exercise.[45] Research has found that two years after the promotional interviewing approach was used in the early postnatal period, mothers were more responsive to their children.[47] It also found that Health Visitors more accurately identified family health needs and had increased job satisfaction.

To support health professionals to use the promotional guides, training is required and there needs to be an opportunity to reflect on the use of guides through such mechanisms as clinical supervision. This would help to enable health visitors in feeling more confident in this assessment approach, allowing the client to shape the agenda.[29] There also needs to be organisational support for the implementation of the guides, including allocation of sufficient time to use them in practice; the promotional interview takes approximately 60 minutes.[45] Barriers to the use of the promotional guides include inadequate time to use the assessment, lack of professional confidence post training, lack of client awareness of the purpose of the review which includes the role of the health visitor, client's awareness of a health need and health visitors feeling it is just adding an additional task to their workload.[26,29]

## Assessment for perinatal depression and anxiety

Perinatal mental health and assessment of mental well-being are core skills for health visiting and also a public health priority.[2,48] The impact of parental mental health during the transition to parenthood and beyond can impact on the whole family, including the child's mental health, physical health, attachment, social development and educational outcomes.[49] Documented rates of perinatal depression vary greatly, with estimates of 10% of women suffering from antenatal depression and 13% suffering from postnatal depression.[50,51] It is approximated that about half of the cases of perinatal depression and anxiety go undetected, although this is probably a conservative estimate[49] (see Chapter 13, Perinatal Mental Health for more in-depth discussion on this).

Assessment of antenatal and postnatal mental health is outlined in the NICE Antenatal and Postnatal Mental Health: Clinical Management and Service Guidance (CG 192).[52] The guidelines advise using the depression identification questions (Whooley questions) and the two-item

Generalized Anxiety Disorder scale (GAD-2) as part of a general discussion about a woman's mental health and well-being. These should be used at the woman's first contact with primary care or her booking visit, and during the early postnatal period. NICE suggests referring women to a secondary mental health service if they have a severe history of mental illness.[52] When asking the Whooley questions, if a woman responds positively to one of the questions or if there is a clinical concern then the practitioner should consider using either the Edinburgh Postnatal Depression Scale (EPDS) or the Patient Health Questionnaire (PHQ-9) for further assessment. In relation to the GAD-2 scale, if the score is three or more then the practitioners should consider doing a further assessment using the GAD-7 scale. Referral to a GP or, if a severe mental health problem is suspected, to a mental health professional should be considered as an outcome of this assessment.

The Whooley questions were first evaluated to be used as a screening tool for depression in 1997.[53] To use these questions, the health professional should be trained in asking them sensitively at a time when they can undertake a supportive, open discussion with the mother.[54] In a study of 47 health visitors, although they felt that they had time to ask the questions, without sufficient training they tended to lack the confidence to use them.[28] A meta-analysis on the diagnostic accuracy of the Whooley questions showed the high sensitivity and moderate specificity of the use of the questions across a range of settings and among different populations. They demonstrate the ability to rule out depression; few people who answer no to both questions are depressed.[55] Research has demonstrated the validity for use in the antenatal period, although they suggest further research is needed to look at their use by health visitors in the postnatal period.[54]

The Generalized Anxiety Disorder 2-item (GAD-2) is based on the GAD-7 questions and was devised in 2007.[56] There is little evidence to support their use in relation to perinatal depression.[57,58] There has been a recent debate on whether to use an EPDS subscale, with questions 3, 4 and 5 of the EPDS being anxiety-based questions.[59] It has been identified that item 3 showed moderate evidence of its psychometric value and items 4 and 5 demonstrated strong evidence of being psychometrically sound in assessing antenatal anxiety.[58]

The EPDS is noted for use in the 2020 updated NICE guidance;[52] evidence shows it has been accepted for use by women. The EDPS, which was devised in the 1980s, is a self-reported, 10-item scale that was designed specifically to screen for possible depression or depressive symptoms in perinatal populations.[60] It is probably the most widely used perinatal screening tool, having been translated into 57 languages, although only 40% of the translated versions are validated for the specific population and country.[61] Each item is scored 0–3, and when used in a community setting, it has a recommended cut off score of 12/13. As with all screening tools it should not be used as an assessment on its own, but it should be supported with a clinical interview and professional judgement.[61] Whether asking the Whooley questions or using the EPDS, the use of clinical interviews to explore women's views on their psychological well-being will increase identification of perinatal depression.[62] The EPDS has been shown to increase detection rates of perinatal depression by 57%.[63] It has also been found to be acceptable for use by women and health professionals. In a research study of 391 women, the EPDS was preferred to the Whooley questions even though they were comparable in their detection rates; EPDS questions were rated as more comfortable and easier to answer, mainly due to their wording.[64] Limitations of the EPDS have been noted: these include cultural sensitivity, different cut off scores, ambiguous questions, miscalculation of scores, false positives and transient depression.[65] To improve accuracy of use of the EPDS, research highlights the need for health professionals to be trained in its use.[61,66]

With rates of depression in men in the perinatal period being an average of 10%,[67] training also needs to include assessment and support for fathers. Recent research showed that health visitors lacked training and confidence in working with fathers with perinatal depression.[68] Training and on-going supervision will assist health visitors in developing communication skills to open up conversations about mental health and developing planning to support fathers.[66]

### Ages and stages questionnaire

The Ages and Stages Questionnaires are widely used across the world, having been found to be cost-effective and having a high rate of validity.[69] In 2014, the Department of Health stipulated that from April 2015 the ASQ-3 would be used by health visiting teams in England when undertaking the 2–2.5 Year Health Review as part of the Healthy Child Programme.[2,70] It is used as a population indicator to measure child development from 2–2.5 years in England as part of the Public Health Outcomes Framework.[71] Prior to this, the majority of areas were using local adaptions of screening tools when undertaking the 2–2.5-year review.[72]

The Ages and Stages Questionnaire was developed in the late 1980s by Jane Squires and Diane Bricker at the University of Oregon, the 3rd edition was published in 2009. Designed to identify development delay in children between one month and 5.5 years, the ASQ-3 has five domains: communication, gross motor, fine motor, problem-solving and personal and social development. The ASQ:SE-2 was published in 2015, focusing on social and emotional development, assessing seven areas: self-regulation, compliance, communication, adaptive functioning, autonomy, affect and interaction with people.[73] The questionnaires are screening tools completed by the parent, focusing on the parent's expert knowledge of their child when identifying strengths as well as concerns.[73] It can be completed by the parent/carer independently or with the support of a health professional and has the flexibility of being able to be used in a variety of settings.[69] The ASQ can offer health promotion opportunities, exploring with the parents ways to support their child's developmental which they may not have considered before.[74]

The use of the Ages and Stages Questionnaires has generally been reported as acceptable by parents. Parents have expressed that it is easy to complete, and they enjoyed using it.[69,72,75] It gave the parents reassurance and enabled them, not only to identify aspects of their child's development that may be of concern, but also helped them to consider ways to play with their children in activities that supported their development.[72] However, some parents felt the ASQ-3 had the potential to cause anxiety, particularly if their child couldn't do something asked in the questionnaire, or over some of the safety items, for example, climbing on a chair. A limitation of the questionnaire is that it does not reassure users by stating that it was looking at a range of ability.[76] A further issue noted was its use in England and the Americanised language in the questionnaires; parents reported that some terms were unfamiliar to them and made the questionnaire awkward to use.[72,75,76]

In international studies, the ASQ-3 and ASQ:SE has been found to be effective across a variety of countries and cultures,[69,77] and it has been translated into various languages for use across the world.[69,72,73] To make the questionnaire more user-friendly in England, the ASQ-3 was adapted from US English to British English.[72,76] When undertaking developmental reviews it is important to consider the language and cultural sensitivity of the tool.[78,79] Cultural and contextual factors may impact on child development, for example extended families interactions may lead to higher social skill or parents being protective of their children may limit a child's ability to explore.[78,79]

The ASQ has also been reported to be acceptable to health professionals.[72,75] It gave a more standardised approach to the assessment and both professionals and parents stated that it led to more of a partnership approach.[72] In research, 91% of parents reported that they were provided with sufficient feedback from the health professional when the ASQ was used.[72] Where parents did not feel involved in the assessment process, communication of the score was noted as an issue. An aspect of this could be the family's lack of relationship with the health professional doing the assessment; many parents may not have met the health visitor before the developmental review.[72] Professionals may also use the screening tools in different ways; an example of this could be that the professional completed the ASQ rather than the parent.[76] The use of the ASQ could be impacted by the assessment venue and the amount of time given to do the assessment. There is a danger that the assessment can just become a box-ticking exercise with the paperwork taking priority. This could lead to the most disadvantaged children and families, who may have the greatest health and developmental needs, being put at risk as they may struggle to engage and ask for professional help.[5]

The ASQ-3 and ASQ: SE should act as a guide and should be used alongside professional judgement, to form a holistic assessment.[5] Consistent training of health professionals is needed to support them in incorporating the use of the ASQ-3 into the 2–2.5-year review and online training on E-LFH has been developed to support this.[76,80]

## WORKING IN PARTNERSHIP WITH PARENTS

To support partnership working with parents in the assessment process, services should seek to provide personalised care that includes continuity of practitioner.[5] Continuity is seen as contributing to successful, nurturing relationships and is valued by mothers.[5,6,32,81] It enables parents to feel known by a health visitor who has an understanding of the family situation, respects their views and can offer personalised care.[81] The practitioner's role is to act as a co-ordinator, understanding the service provision that enables families to build on their strengths and meet planned goals.[6] Repeated contact with the same practitioner is an important aspect of a parent feeling satisfied with the health visiting service;[81] without it parents are more likely to feel that the health visiting service they receive is not personalised and feels more like a 'tick box' exercise.[5]

As well as continuity of practitioner, parents have identified other characteristics in a health visitor that help build a relationship. Research has shown that parents also valued empathy, approachability, respect, genuineness and appearing calm, being caring and friendly as positive traits of a health visitor. Empathy was described as 'understanding' that made parents feel heard and aided them in being able to talk about their thoughts and feelings in the assessment process.[82] Parents also valued a practitioner's ability to listen and to respond to parents' circumstances in a sensitive way.[81] Parents stated that they valued a relationship with someone who was not a family member or friend, someone they could express their needs to and be brutally honest with.[82]

A recurring theme in research is parents' desire to be treated in a non-judgemental way.[6] It was important that the health visitors they met did not judge them or did not make them feel judged.[81] Where parents felt the practitioner was interested in their family's well-being and praised them, it made them feel respected, thus building their confidence and trust in the judgements they made as parents.[82] Mutual trust has been shown as an important element in the building of a good relationship between parents and the practitioner.[82]

In partnership working, both health visitors and parents bear a responsibility for how that relationship functions. However, practitioners need to be aware that some parents may struggle to be trusting so health visitors need to consider what skills they must use to build that relationship.[83]. Many parents may not understand the scope of the health visitor's role and the support available from the health visiting service.[84] In a study that explored 10 parents and 12 health visitors' experiences of health assessments, parents were often found to be anxious about assessments due to feelings of being tested and not being involved in the decision-making.[24] In a strength-based, partnership approach, parents' feeling of involvement is essential. Health visitors need to consider how they can facilitate partnership working. In the same study, some health visitors reported finding it difficult to explain the assessment process to parents, and others noted that they felt parents were not always interested as they were more preoccupied with their baby.[24] There is a need for health visitors to be open about the assessment process, otherwise some families may become suspicious or feel that the assessment process is merely intrusive.[29,40] Parents have also indicated that health visitor behaviour can impact on relationship building and can lead them to disengage with the health visiting service. These behaviours included the health visitor not being polite or punctual and not introducing themselves.[81,82]

The venue of the health visiting contact can also have an impact on relationship building between parents and health visitors. This is particularly significant in a time when health visiting numbers are reducing.[5] There is a variation in funding and service delivery between the different nations in the UK and also between local authorities in England.[85] Some areas have strengthened their health visiting services, whilst others have disinvested in them, looking to rationalise the five core contacts and how they are delivered. The home has been deemed the best environment for assessments to take place.[6] Parents stated that they felt home visits were beneficial, believing that health visitors gave them more attention which helped them to divulge issues in more detail.[86] Health visitors have reported similar beliefs, feeling parents were more receptive and responsive in their homes. Home contacts also enabled them to assess how a family lived, providing opportunities to observe and identify concerns that would not have been possible in a clinic setting.[32,86] This view is supported by the Institute of Health Visiting who feel that home visits offer health visitors a holistic perspective of the home environment that can facilitate early identification of need.[5] Parents have reported that contacts in a clinic may impact on them asking questions; this was due to the fact the clinic environment often felt too busy, or the parent didn't recognise a member of the health visiting team.[32]

Although home visits were seen to be of extreme value by both parents and health visitors, the ability to have contact by phone was regarded as important, particularly during relationship development when parents felt less confident.[82] Drop-in clinics not only gave parents the ability to access the health visiting service but were also valuable as they offered the opportunity for social networking.[86] When reviewing service delivery, a balance needs to be considered between service restrictions and the impact of the environment on relationship building and the assessment process.

## WORKING WITH THE FAMILY

The health visiting service is a whole family service, working with a diverse range of families across the UK.[87] The Healthy Child Programme has a strong emphasis on supporting families and 'ensuring that contact with the family routinely involves and supports fathers, including non-resident fathers'.[2:10] The service must engage fathers: when conducting a needs assessment, it's important to acknowledge their impact on the family and child. Although national guidance recognises the importance of fathers in family health, it highlights that services do not do enough to recognise this and support fathers.[2] This view has been reiterated by Public Health England who highlight the need to strengthen father-inclusive services.[88] Health visiting contacts are still predominantly with the mother.[13] This is despite the early intervention agenda highlighting the importance of both parents in child development and changes in national policy such as shared parental leave.[89] This means that health visitors are more likely to have contact with fathers, which allows them to help the fathers engage with the service.[90]

Research has highlighted some of the barriers that the health visiting service has in engaging with fathers; these include personal, organisational, strategic and societal factors.[90] The health visiting service is often perceived as a 'mother and child' service, leading to feelings of exclusion for dads.[70] Some underlying factors for this may include that the workforce is predominantly female, a lack of specialist training on fatherhood, workload capacity to adapt services when they are already struggling to meet the Healthy Child Programme and that some mothers may be reluctant to include their partner.[90] To increase the engagement of fathers, the health visiting service needs to look at arranging appointments and health promotion groups at times that will increase the chances of fathers attending.[2] Commissioning guidelines highlight that services should be available at times and locations that meet the needs of children and their families.[88] However, the health visiting service still mainly offers contacts with parents from Monday to Friday, 9 am to 5 pm. This often makes it difficult to engage with fathers who are in employment[81] and also has implications for mothers: recent figures show that just under 50% of parents with children under three years old are both in full-time employment.[91]

Communication with fathers is essential in raising awareness of the whole family approach of the health visiting service. The service needs to adapt to try and engage fathers; this can include simple measures such as addressing fathers during assessments and encouraging their input into the assessment process.[2] Improving communication on fathers' presence at contacts could increase the inclusion of fathers in assessment contacts; fathers have noted that their ability to be involved in visits was not always discussed by the health visitor.[81] Additional training for health visitors on fatherhood issues and how to support their health needs may improve the confidence of staff in engaging fathers.[70,90] Local policy change to involve fathers needs to be more consistently evident in practice.[81]

There is great diversity in family composition and other family members, such as grandparents and step-parents, may also influence decision-making that relates to a child's health and well-being. However, research would suggest that it is not common for health visitors to involve extended family members in assessment and the decision-making process.[13] Health visiting services should be working towards a whole family approach, making this clear from the initial contact.[87,90] Engaging the family members who have a significant impact on the child's life would enable a health visitor to have a better understanding of the family networks, improve decision-making and parental acceptance of interventions to support child well-being.[13] By individual health visitors, teams and service leads making even small changes it could lead to greater involvement of fathers in assessment and a whole family approach.[90]

## STRENGTH-BASED APPROACH AND MATCHING AGENDAS

Partnership working with families, using a strength-based approach, is fundamental to the assessment process. The Healthy Child Programme advocates a strength-based approach, acknowledging that parents want an assessment process that 'recognises their strengths, concerns and aspirations for their child,'[2:20] highlighting their resourcefulness and skill. This assessment approach underlines the strengths in the family as well as any difficulties that they may be experiencing, thereby engaging families in addressing their own issues. It employs partnership working to identify the most relevant, realistic goals and solutions to the family that are more likely to be met.[92] Through using strength-based approaches, families become active participants rather than passive consumers. Through empowerment and acknowledgement of the strengths, it can provide hope to address other issues that they previously may have felt they could not confront. This approach recognises that a professional is not a fixer who knows all the answers but is a co-facilitator of plans and goals.[93:13]

An important aspect of the strength-based approach is the ability to match agendas, discussing the priorities of the family in relation to those identified by the practitioner. The ability to match agendas is seen as important in all areas of health work as it supports joint decision-making in relation to behaviour change.[94] Central to this approach is the relationship between the parent and the health visitor, supported by a holistic assessment that enables parents to develop their confidence in parenting.[6] Health visitors need to develop sensitive assessment skills to facilitate individual and personalised support that will work in partnership with parents and empower them.[95] The language and tone of voice used by the health visitor can help to create equality in power; humour is also reported to be used.[13] The practitioner needs to be able to listen to the priorities and concerns of the family, while being able to express their professional concerns in ways that families can understand and appreciate. Professional knowledge can be used to promote understanding and responsiveness in relation to

a child's needs;[95] professional curiosity is also required when assessing needs and developing family-centred outcomes. From here, priorities can be set, goals can be negotiated, and plans can be devised.[96] Mothers have been reported as valuing this strength-based approach to assessment.[5] This approach is complex, even when priorities are agreed, there may not be a shared understanding between the health visitor and parent about the importance of the issue to the child's wellbeing. Due to the dynamic, changing nature of family life, parents' priorities may change between contacts.[13] If parents' strengths, concerns and choices are not respected then this may have an impact on both their relationship with the health visitor and whether the assessment can address issues that support family health.[81]

The development of strength-based and agenda-matching approaches has been supported by programmes such as FNP (Family Nurse Partnership), MESCH (Maternal Early Childhood Sustained Home-visiting) and the development of transformational models of health visiting such as Blackpool Better Start.[95] Within the healthy child programme, the use of agenda-matching assessment tools that use strength-based approaches, such as the promotional guide and motivational interviewing,[2] have helped balance what are important needs for the families and needs identified by professionals.

## VIRTUAL ASSESSMENTS AND THE IMPACT OF THE COVID-19 PANDEMIC

The NHS Long Term Plan[97] highlighted the move within the NHS for patients to have the ability to access care through alternative routes, such as online consultations. The onset of the COVID-19 pandemic moved this agenda forward in the NHS as there became an urgent need to assess patients in a way other than just face-to-face contacts.

The speed of change in Spring 2020 was dramatic, with NHS Digital stating that just 15% of 23 million primary care appointments took place by phone or online in December 2019; this had increased to 49% by April 2020.[98] Although there has been guidance on this move,[99,100] changes have been fast-paced, with fewer constraints from governance than compared to normal times in the NHS.[101]

Although many health visiting services were moving towards greater digital service offers, including the use of the text-messaging service ChatHealth,[102] the COVID-19 pandemic saw an increase in virtual contacts. At the height of the pandemic there was an adaption in the delivery of the healthy child programme, which was guided by COVID-19 prioritisation within Community Health Services.[103] As a further NHS response to the pandemic, many health visitors were redeployed. A survey of practitioners, evaluating the impact of COVID-19 on health visiting, reported that 60% of respondents stated that at least one member of their health visiting team was redeployed between March and June 2020. This meant that 38% of the respondents had experienced an increase in the number of children they were responsible for.[104]

To support service delivery, face-to-face contacts were limited to mainly vulnerable families or those with urgent needs,[104,105] health visiting services continued core contacts via an increase in virtual contacts by phone or online video link. For example, 94% of respondents to the UCL survey reported that they delivered antenatal contacts by phone and 45% by online video link.[104] However, as provider services made this move, there was variability in the availability and ability to use video technology in some areas.[105]

The Institute of Health Visiting supported service adaption, developing advice for practitioners on how to carry out contacts virtually.[100] This helped service providers to consider the skills and service requirements needed for virtual contacts, including physical set-up of virtual systems, training, ongoing support when working remotely, and additional resource requirements. It considered aspects such as the increase of stress for health visitors due to remote, lone working, thus highlighting the importance of having the ability to 'check-in' each day. During the initial stage of the pandemic, health visitors reported concerns about the rapid change in service to virtual contacts and how this may leave vulnerable children and families at increased risk due to their needs being overlooked.[105] The access to virtual contacts for vulnerable people, including those suffering domestic abuse, has also been highlighted as a concern by the Kings Fund.[106]

Reflecting on this rapid move to virtual contacts, previous research has shown that technology, such as ChatHealth, has been viewed positively by parents and professionals; it offers timely messaging and increased access to service which has provided reassurance to parents.[107] Video consultations, in general practice, have been deemed more beneficial than phone consultations as both patients and practitioners feel that the video consultations were more formal, and the video gave the ability to pick up verbal cues. Patients state that an existing relationship with the health professional was beneficial to the video consultation. However, both patients and clinicians believed these consultations could be limited in their use, for example, it was felt that they were not in the place to deliver sensitive news. They also felt that there were issues with technology disruptions impact on consultations, such as screens freezing and poor audio.[108] The COVID-19 pandemic increased the speed of the move to online patient assessments and this necessitated urgent review in order to evaluate the successes and also limitations of virtual assessments.[104] This should include any inequalities of access to health care for vulnerable patients and families and the impact of virtual working on staff, including training needs.[106]

## THINKING SPACE

The NHS Long Term Plan establishes the move to greater use of digital technology in the NHS. As health visiting was starting to develop its digital offer, including ChatHealth, the COVID-19 pandemic saw a dramatic shift in the use of technology, particularly in relation to online assessments.

Consider what the impact may be of online assessments on:
- the assessment process
- the skills a health visitor requires to undertake assessments online
- the impact on children and families.

## CONCLUSION

Throughout this chapter the complexity of health visiting assessments has been examined. These dynamic assessments are holistic, considering the physical, psychological and environmental impact on families. They are constantly being reviewed as the child and family's health and well-being circumstances change.

There are multiple components to the assessment and decision-making process. Assessment tools offer structure and help to articulate the decisions made both to families and commissioners. When undertaking an assessment, it is underpinned by professional experience, a high level of interpersonal skills, knowledge of evidence base and of the assessment tool that is being used. Historically, assessment tools used within the health visiting service have been locally designed and have not been research-based. As part of the Healthy Child Programme,[2,21a,22] there has been a move to the national adoption of evidence-based assessment tools such as the ASQ and promotional interview guide. As these have become embedded into practice, research has demonstrated that, if they are to be used by a health visitor in the way they were designed, then the provider

organisations must ensure that they include time for training programmes and on-going support for practitioners, including the opportunity for supervision and reflection. To develop a supportive culture that enables health visitors to make autonomous clinical decisions, there also needs to be guidelines that allow assessments to be an interactive process with parents, with sufficient time to undertake them at a venue that is conducive to this process. If a provider organisation does not support health visitors in this way, findings suggest that practitioners will be less likely to have confidence in the use of the assessment tool, be less motivated to use them, may use them inaccurately and may not be able to communicate their use to parents. This will impact on children and families as the outcomes of the assessment may not empower families and meet their needs.

The health visiting assessment process should be a partnership with parents: strength-based, supportive and empowering of families. The cornerstone of the assessment process is reported to be the relationship between the family and the health visitor. This relationship is a two-way process, but health visitors need the interpersonal skills to support the construction of that relationship. As discussed in this chapter, parents have reported that health visitors can have positive and negative traits that may impact on a relationship and the assessment process. Where there is poor communication and an inadequate relationship, parents have reported that they lack awareness of the purpose of the assessment, including the role of the health visitor. Continuity of a named professional is seen as contributing to successful, nurturing relationships and is valued by mothers. It enables parents to feel known by a health visitor who understands their family situation, respects their views in a non-judgemental manner and can offer personalised care. It is also important for health visitors to ensure that assessments are inclusive of family members who have a significant impact on the child's life; historically, they have been more from the mother's view point. These will all support a partnership approach to assessment, recognising the strengths in the family as well as any difficulties that they may be experiencing, thereby engaging families in addressing their own needs.

As health visiting continues to further adopt digital health care, including virtual assessments, it must be made sure that these services are introduced for the benefit of the families they work with and not just due to financial constraints. The COVID-19 pandemic has seen a rapid increase in the use of virtual contacts and some of these changes will be adopted into standard health visiting practice. The pandemic had a considerable impact on the UK's financial deficit – government-approved spending increased by nearly £190 billion in the first three months of the pandemic to enable the introduction of measures in support of public services, businesses and individuals.[109] This budget deficit will need to be recouped and is likely to include a cut in public spending, which will consequently impact on the health visiting service at a time when staffing levels have been decreasing since 2015. Additionally, because of the pandemic unemployment has risen; this is likely to result in a rise in child poverty rates. As services look at innovative ways to increase the use of digital technology in health visiting, it is therefore more important than ever that it is used to add value to the service and does not have a negative impact on the most vulnerable families. As a service, health visiting must audit and research these changes in practice to ensure that they do not lead to a widening of inequalities and increased impact on the long-term outcomes of children therefore increased societal costs.

## KEY LEARNING POINTS

In summary, the key points of learning from this chapter are:

■ For health visitors to undertake assessment they require professional knowledge, intuition, knowledge of the assessment tools, support of organisational guidelines and flexibility to work within their professional accountability. Assessment is core to the role of the health visitor and requires professional knowledge, intuition, knowledge of the assessment tool and support of organisational guidelines.

■ Organisational support, including practice time to undertake assessments, adequate training and ongoing supervision, is required to support health visitors to use assessment tools accurately.

■ Partnership working with families, using a strength-based approach, is fundamental to the assessment process.

■ The COVID-19 pandemic has increased the use of online patient assessments; this requires urgent review in order to evaluate the successes, and also limitations, of virtual assessments.

## REFERENCES

1. Nursing and Midwifery Council. Standards of proficiency for specialist community public health nurses. https://www.nmc.org.uk/globalassets/sitedocuments/standards/nmc-standards-of-proficiency-for-specialist-community-public-health-nurses.pdf. Accessed 2 September 2020.
2. Department of Health. Healthy child programme: Pregnancy and the first 5 years of life. https://www.gov.uk/government/publications/healthy-child-programme-pregnancy-and-the-first-5-years-of-life. Accessed 2 September 2020.
3. Burton, A. (2019). Recommended universal components by age across the UK. In A. Emond (Ed.), *Health for all Children* (5th ed., pp. 355–365). Oxford: Oxford University Press.
4. Appleton, J. V., & Cowley, S. (2008). Health visiting assessment processes under scrutiny: A case study of knowledge use during family health needs assessments. *International Journal of Nursing Studies, 45*(5), 682–696.
5. Institute of Health Visiting. Health Visiting in England: A vision for the future. https://ihv.org.uk/wp-content/uploads/2019/11/7.11.19-Health-Visiting-in-England-Vision-FINAL-VERSION.pdf. Accessed 23 February 2020.
6. Cowley, S., Malone, M., Whittaker, K., Donetto, S., Grigulis, A., & Maben, J. (2018). What makes health visiting

successful – or not? 2. The service journey. *Journal of Health Visiting*, 6(8), 404–412.

7. Cowley, S., Whittaker, K., Malone, M., Donetto, S., Grigulis, A, & Maben, J. (2015). Why health visiting? Examining the potential public health benefits from health visiting practice within a universal service: A narrative review of the literature. *International Journal of Nursing Studies*, 52(1), 465–480. doi: 10.1016/j.ijnurstu.2014.07.013.

8. Standing, M. (2010). *Clinical Judgement and Decision-Making: Nursing and Interprofessional Healthcare*. Maidenhead: McGraw-Hill Education.

9. Luker, K. A., & McHugh, G. A. (2016). Evaluating Practice. In K. A. Luker, G. A. McHugh, & R. M. Bryar (Eds.), *Health Visiting: Preparation for Practice* (pp. 252–287). Chichester: John Wiley & Sons Ltd.

10. Johansen, M. L., & O'Brien, J. L. (2015). Decision making in nursing practice: A concept analysis. *Nursing Forum*, 51(1), 40–48.

11. Nibblebank, C. W., & Brewer, B. B. (2018). Decision-making in nursing practice: An integrative literature review. *Journal of Clinical Nursing*, 27, 917–928.

12. Melin-Johansson, C., Palmqvist, R., & Ronnberg, L. (2017). Clinical intuition in the nursing process and decision-making – A mixed-studies review. *Journal of Clinical Nursing*, 26, 3936–3949.

13. Astbury, R., Shepherd, A., & Cheyne, H. (2016). Working in partnership: the application of shared decision-making to health visitor practice. *Journal of Clinical Nursing*, 26, 215–224. doi: 10.1111/jocn.13480.

14. Pound, R. (2013). Influences on relationship-based health visiting, part 2: Discovering the need for balance through a new epistemology. *Journal of Health Visiting*, 1(9), 522–528.

15. King, C. (2016). 'Sticking to carpets' – Assessment and judgement in health visiting practice in an era of risk: a qualitative study. *Journal of Clinical Nursing*, 25, 1901–1911.

16. Harlow, J., & Smith, M. (2016). Safeguarding Children: Debates and Dilemmas for Health Visitors. In K. A. Luker, G. A. McHugh, & R. M. Bryar (Eds.), *Health Visiting: Preparation for Practice* (pp. 170–217). Chichester: John Wiley & Sons Ltd.

17. Standing, M. (2008). Clinical judgement and decision-making in nursing – Nine modes of practice in a revised cognitive continuum. *Journal of Advanced Nursing*, 62(1), 124–134.

18. Thompson, C., & Dowding, D. (2002). *Clinical Decision-Making and Judgement in Nursing*. Edinburgh: Churchill Livingstone.

19. Cader, R., Campbell, S., & Watson, D. (2005). Cognitive continuum theory in nursing decision-making. *Journal of Advanced Nursing*, 49(4), 397–405.

20. Parker-Tomlin, M., Boschen, M., Morrissey, S., & Glendon, I. (2017). Cognitive continuum theory in interprofessional healthcare: A critical analysis. *Journal of Interprofessional Care*, 31(4), 446–454.

21. Appleton, J. V., & Cowley, S. (2004). The guideline contradiction: Health visitors' use of formal guidelines for identifying and assessing families in need. *International Journal of Nursing Studies*, 41(7), 785–797.

21a. The Scottish Government. Universal Health visiting pathway in Scotland: Pre-Birth to pre-school. https://www.gov.scot/binaries/content/documents/govscot/publications/advice-and-guidance/2015/10/universal-health-visiting-pathway-scotland-pre-birth-pre-school/documents/00487884-pdf/00487884-pdf/govscot%3Adocument/00487884.pdf?forceDownload=true. Accessed 25 October.

22. Welsh Government. *Healthy Child Wales Programme*. http://gov.wales/topics/health/publications/health/reports/healthy-child/? Accessed 2 September 2020.

23. Squires, J., Bricker, D., & Twombly, E. (2015). *Ages & Stages Questionnaires®: Social-emotional, second edition (ASQ®:SE-2): A parent-completed child monitoring system for social-emotional behaviors*. Baltimore: Paul H. Brookes Publishing Co.

24. Hogg, R., Kennedy, C., Gray, C., & Hanley, J. (2013). Supporting the case for 'progressive universalism' in health visiting: Scottish mothers and health visitors' perspectives on targeting and rationing health visiting services, with a focus on the Lothian Child Concern Model. *Journal of Clinical Nursing*, 22, 240–250.

25. Holland, A. (2019). Development of an all-Wales Health Visitor Observation and Assessment of the Infant tool. *Journal of Health Visiting*, 7(11), 542–551.

26. Barlow, J., & Coe, C. (2013). New ways of working: promotional interviewing in health visiting practice. *Journal of Health Visiting*, 1(1), 44–50.

27. Svanberg, P. O., & Barlow, J. (2013). The effectiveness of training in the Parent-Infant Interaction Observation Scale for health visitors. *Journal of Health Visiting*, 1(3), 162–166.

28. Beauchamp, H. (2014). What factors influence the use of the Whooley questions by health visitors? *Journal of Health Visiting*, 2(7), 378–387. doi: 10.12968/johv.2014.2.7.378.

29. Morton, A. (2014). Beyond 'train and hope': Identifying factors that affect implementation of the Promotional Guide in practice. *Journal of Health Visiting*, 2(12), 670–680.

30. Rankin, J., & MacInnes, S. (2014). Training and development needs of health visitors: 27–30-month child health review. *Journal of Health Visiting*, 2(8), 442–448.

31. Institute of Health Visiting. Health Visitors in England fear for some children's futures as their numbers are reduced: Results from a Survey of English Health Visitors December 2017. https://ihv.org.uk/wp-content/uploads/2017/12/171204-Institute-of-Health-Visiting-survey-results-safeguarding-children-2-12-17.pdf. Accessed 2 September 2020.

32. Binmead, C., Cowley, S., & Grocott, P. (2016). The role of organisations in supporting the parent/health visitor relationship. *Journal of Health Visiting, 4*(7), 366–374.

33. McMillan, B., Eastham, R., Brown, B., Fitton, R., & Dickinson, D. (2018). Primary care patient records in the United Kingdom: Past, present, and future research priorities. *Journal Medical Internet Research, 20*(12), e11293.

34. Cowley, S., & Houston, A. (2003). A structured health needs assessment tool: Acceptability and effectiveness for health visiting. *Journal of Advanced Nursing, 43*(1), 82–92.

35. Houston, A. M., & Cowley, S. (2002). An empowerment approach to needs assessment in health visiting practice. *Journal of Clinical Nursing, 11*(5), 640–650.

36. Mitcheson, J., & Cowley, S. (2003). Empowerment or control? An analysis of the extent to which client participation is enabled during health visitor/client interactions using a structured health needs assessment tool. *International Journal of Nursing Studies, 40*, 413–426.

37. Department of Health. Framework for the assessment of children in need and their families. http://www.dh.gov.uk/en/Publicationsandstatistics/Publications/PublicationsPolicyAndGuidance/DH_4003256. Accessed 2 September 2020.

38. Scottish Government. A guide to getting it right for every child. https://www.gov.scot/policies/girfec/. Accessed 2 September 2020.

39. Coles, E., Cheyne, H., Rankin, J., & Daniel, B. (2016). Getting it right for every child: A national policy framework to promote children's well-being in Scotland, United Kingdom. *The Milbank Quarterly, 94*(2), 334–365.

40. Aldgate, J. & Rose, W. Assessing and managing risk in getting it right for every child. https://lx.iriss.org.uk/sites/default/files/resources/0069411.pdf. Accessed 2 September 2020.

41. Stafford, A., Parton, N., Vincent, S., & Smith, C. (2012). *Child protection systems in the United Kingdom: A comparative analysis.* London: Kingsley.

42. University of South Wales. Family Resilience Assessment Instrument and Tool (FRAIT) Guidance v.17/05/17. http://www.primecentre.wales/resources/FRAIT%20Guidance.pdf. Accessed 2 September 2020.

43. Welsh Government. Evaluation of the Healthy Child Wales Programme: Interim report. https://gov.wales/sites/default/files/statistics-and-research/2019-01/evaluation-of-the-healthy-child-wales-programme-interim-report.pdf. Accessed 2 September 2020.

44. Roberts, R., Loxton, R., Campbell, J., Frame, M., Kirkum, M., Lake, M., et al. (2002). The European Early Promotion Project: Transition into parenting. *Community Practitioner, 75*, 464–468.

45. Day, C., Morton, A., Ibbeson, A., Maddison, S., Pease, R., & Smith, K. (2014). Antenatal/postnatal promotional guide: Evidence-based intervention. *Journal of Health Visiting, 2*(12), 658–669.

46. Day C. Promoting early infant development. https://www.nursinginpractice.com/clinical/womens-health/promoting-early-infant-development/. Accessed 2 September 2020.

47. Purra, K., & Davis, H. (2005). The outcome of the European early promotion project: Mother child interaction. *International Journal of Mental Health Nursing, 7*(1), 82–94.

48. Public Health England. Healthy Child Programme: The 4-5-6 approach for health visiting and school nursing. https://vivbennett.blog.gov.uk/wp-content/uploads/sites/90/2016/10/2905781-PHE-4-5-6-School-nursing-infographic_FINAL.pdf. Accessed 2 September 2020.

49. Department of Health and Social Care. Early years high impact area 2: Maternal mental health. Health visitors leading the Healthy Child Programme. https://assets.publishing.service.gov.uk/government/uploads/system/uploads/attachment_data/file/754790/early_years_high_impact_area_2.pdf. Accessed 2 September 2020.

50. Miles, S. (2011). Winning the battle: A review of postnatal depression. *British Journal of Midwifery, 19*(4), 221–227.

51. World Health Organization. (2015). *Maternal mental health.* Geneva: WHO.

52. National Institute of Clinical Excellence. Antenatal & postnatal mental health: Clinical management and service guidance. https://www.nice.org.uk/guidance/cg192. Accessed 2 September 2020.

53. Whooley, W. A., Alvins, A. L., Miranda, J., & Browner, W. S. (1997). Case Finding instrument for depression: Two are as good as many. *Journal of General Internal Medicine, 12*, 439–445.

54. Howard, L. M., Ryan, E. G., Trevillion, K., Anderson, F., Bick, D., Bye, A., et al. (2018). Accuracy of the Whooley questions and the Edinburgh Postnatal Depression Scale in identifying depression and other mental disorders in early pregnancy. *The British Journal of Psychiatry, 212*, 50–56.

55. Bosanquet, K., Bailey, D., Gilbody, S., Harden, M., Manea, L., Nutbrown, S., & McMillan, D. (2015). Diagnostic accuracy of the Whooley questions for the identification

of depression: A diagnostic meta-analysis. *BMJ Open, 5.* doi: 10.1136/bmjopen-2015-008913.

56. Kroenke, K., Spitzer, R. L., Williams, J. B., Monahan, P. O., & Löwe, B. (2007). Anxiety disorders in primary care: Prevalence, impairment, comorbidity, and detection. *Annals of Internal Medicine, 146,* 317–325.

57. Fairbrother, N., Corbyn, B., Thordarson, D. S., Ma, A., & Surm, D. (2019). Screening for perinatal anxiety disorders: Room to grow. *Journal of Affective Disorders, 250,* 363–370. doi: 10.1016/j.jad.2019.03.052.

58. Sinesi, A., Maxwell, M., O'Carroll, R., & Cheyne, H. (2019). Anxiety scales used in pregnancy: Systematic review. *British Journal Psychiatry Open, 5*(e5), 1–13. doi: 10.1192/bjo.2018.75.

59. Cattanach, J., & Taylor, J. (2019). The effects of antenatal anxiety assessment by health visitors on outcomes for mothers and babies. *Journal of Health Visiting, 7*(3), 120–131.

60. Cox, J., Holden, J., & Sagovsky, R. (1987). Detection of postnatal depression. Development of the 10-item Edinburgh Postnatal Depression Scale. *British Journal of Psychiatry, 150,* 782–786. doi: 10.1192/bjp.150.6.782.

61. Cox, J., Holden, J., & Henshaw, C. (2014). In *Perinatal mental health: The Edinburgh Postnatal Depression Scale (EPDS) manual* (2nd ed.). London: RCPsych publications.

62. Fellmetha, G., Opondoa, C., Hendersona, J., Redshawa, M., Mcneillb, J., Lynnb, F., & Alderdicea, F. (2019). Identifying postnatal depression: Comparison of a self-reported depression item with Edinburgh Postnatal Depression Scale scores at three months postpartum. *Journal of Affective Disorders, 251,* 8–14.

63. Hearn, G., Iliff, A., Jones, I., Kirby, A., Ormiston, P., Parr, P., Rout, J., & Wardman, L. (1998). Postnatal depression in the community. *British Journal of General Practice, 48*(428), 1064–1066.

64. Littlewood, E., Ali, S., Dyson, L., Keding, A., Ansell, P., Bailey, D., et al. (2018). Identifying perinatal depression with case-finding instruments: A mixed-methods study (BaBYPaNDA – Born and Bred in Yorkshire PeriNatal Depression Diagnostic Accuracy). http://eprints.whiterose.ac.uk/134342/1/3012281.pdf. Accessed 2 September 2020.

65. Matthey, S., & Agostini, F. (2017). Using the Edinburgh Postnatal Depression Scale for women and men – Some cautionary thoughts. *Archive of Women's Mental Health, 20,* 345–354.

66. Marks L. Overview of challenges to implementation of good practice in perinatal mental health promotion and management, in universal primary care and community services. https://compasswellbeing.co.uk/media/155067/lucy-marks.pdf. Accessed 2 September 2020.

67. Paulson, J. F., & Bazemore, S. D. (2010). Prenatal and postpartum depression in fathers and its association with maternal depression: A meta-analysis. *Journal of American Medical Association, 303,* 1961–1969.

68. Whitelock, A. (2016). Why do health visitors screen mothers and not fathers for depression in the postnatal period. *Journal of Health Visiting, 4*(6), 312–321.

69. Singh, A., Jung Yeh, C., & Boone Blanchard, S. (2017). Ages and Stages Questionnaire: A global screening scale. *Boletin Medico del Hospital Infantil de Mexico, 74*(1), 5–12.

70. Bennett V. Ages and Stages Questionnaires: 3rd edition (ASQ-3TM) and parents' contribution to the 2 year health review. https://vivbennett.blog.gov.uk/2014/11/21/ages-stages-questionnaires-penny-crouzet/. Accessed 2 September 2020.

71. Department of Health. Public health outcomes framework 2016–2019. https://assets.publishing.service.gov.uk/government/uploads/system/uploads/attachment_data/file/520457/At_a_glance.pdf. Accessed 2 September 2020.

72. Kendall, S., Nash, A., Braun, A., Bastug, G., Rougeaux, E., & Bedford, H. Evaluating the use of a population measure of child development in the Healthy Child Programme Two Year Review. https://discovery.ucl.ac.uk/id/eprint/1493007/1/Kendall%20et%20al%20Evaluating%20child%20development%202014.pdf. Accessed 2 September 2020.

73. Agesandstages.com. ND 4 decades of development. https://agesandstages.com/about-asq/asq-development/. Accessed 2 September 2020.

74. Marks, K. P., Sjö, N. M., & Wilson, P. (2018). Comparative use of the Ages and Stages Questionnaires in the USA and Scandinavia: A systematic review. *Developmental Medicine and Child Neurology, 61*(4), 419–430.

75. McKnight, S. (2014). Implementing the Ages and Stages questionnaire in health visiting practice. *Community Pract, 87*(11), 28–32.

76. Kendall, S., Nash, A., Braun, A., Bastug, G., Rougeaux, E., & Bedford, H. (2019). Acceptability and understanding of the Ages & Stages Questionnaires®, Third Edition, as part of the Healthy Child Programme 2-year health and development review in England: Parent and professional perspectives. *Child: care, health and development, 45*(2), 251–256. doi: 10.1111/cch.12639.

77. Kvestad, I., Taneja, S., Kumar, T., Bhandari, N., Strand, T., & Hysing, M. (2013). The assessment of developmental status using the Ages and Stages Questionnaire-3 in nutritional research in north Indian young children. *Nutrition Journal, 12*(50). doi:10.1186/1475-2891-12-50.

78. Velikonja, T., Edbrooke-Childs, J., Calderdon, A., Sleed, M., Brown, A., & Deighton, J. (2017). The psychometric

properties of the Ages & Stages Questionnaires for ages 2-2.5: A systematic review: ASQ-3 TM and ASQ:SE systematic review. *Child: Care Health and Development, 43*(1), 1–17. doi: 10.1111/cch.12397.

79. Charafeddine, L., Dani, A., Badr L. K., Sinno, D., Tamim, H., Khoury, J. et al. (2019). The psychometric properties of the Ages and Stages Questionnaires-3 in Arabic: Cross-sectional observational study. *Early Human Development, 136*, 33–38.

80. E-Learning for Health. Ages and Stages Questionnaires. https://www.e-lfh.org.uk/programmes/ages-and-stages-questionnaires/. Accessed 2 September 2020.

81. Donetto, S., Malone, M., Hughes, J., Morrow, E., Cowley, S., & Maben, J. Health visiting: The voice of service users Learning from service users' experiences to inform the development of UK health visiting practice and services (Department of Health Policy Research Programme, ref. 016 0058). https://www.kcl.ac.uk/nmpc/research/nnru/publications/reports/voice-of-service-user-report-july-2013-final.pdf. Accessed 2 September 2020.

82. Binmead, C., Cowley, S., & Grocott, P. (2016). The health visitor contribution to the parent/health visitor relationship. *Journal of Health Visiting, 4*(4), 212–220.

83. Binmead, C., Cowley, S., & Grocott, P. (2016). The parental contribution to the parent/health visitor relationship. *Journal of Health Visiting, 4*(10), 48–55.

84. Bennett V. Health Visiting: You said – We Did – We Will. https://vivbennett.blog.gov.uk/2015/03/10/health-visiting-you-said-we-did-we-will/. Accessed 2 September 2020.

85. Institute of Health Visiting. Health Visiting in England: State of Health Visiting in England. https://ihv.org.uk/wp-content/uploads/2020/02/State-of-Health-Visiting-survey-FINAL-VERSION-18.2.20.pdf. Accessed 2 September 2020.

86. Doi, L., Jepson, R., & Hardie, S. (2017). Realist evaluation of an enhanced health visiting programme. *PLoS One, 12*(7). doi: 10.1371/journal.pone.0180569.

87. Boddy, B. (2019). Newly qualified health visitor: Assessment and support for fathers' mental health. *Journal of Health Visiting, 7*(11), 515–517.

88. Public Health England. Best start in life and beyond: Improving public health outcomes for children, young people and families Guidance to support the commissioning of the Healthy Child Programme 0–19: Health visiting and school nursing services. https://assets.publishing.service.gov.uk/government/uploads/system/uploads/attachment_data/file/716028/best_start_in_life_and_beyond_commissioning_guidance_2.pdf. Accessed 2 September 2020.

89. Gov.uk. Shared parental leave. https://www.gov.uk/shared-parental-leave-and-pay. Accessed 2 September 2020.

90. Bateson, K., Darwin, Z., Galdas, P., & Rosan, C. (2017). Engaging fathers: Acknowledging the barriers. *Journal of Health Visiting, 5*(3), 26–32.

91. Office of National Statistics. Families and the labour market, UK: 2019. https://www.ons.gov.uk/employmentandlabourmarket/peopleinwork/employmentandemployeetypes/articles/familiesandthelabourmarketengland/2019. Accessed 2 September 2020.

92. Bailey, B. (2014). Solution – Focused work in practice. *Journal of Health Visiting, 2*(2), 110.

93. The Institute for Research and Innovation in Social Services (IRISS). Insights: Strength-based approaches for working with individuals. https://www.iriss.org.uk/resources/insights/strengths-based-approaches-working-individuals. Accessed 2 September 2020.

94. Coulter A, Collins A. Making shared decision-making a reality: No decision about me, without me. https://www.kingsfund.org.uk/sites/default/files/Making-shared-decision-making-a-reality-paper-Angela-Coulter-Alf-Collins-July-2011_0.pdf. Accessed 2 September 2020.

95. McGregor, D. (2018). Better start: The Blackpool universal health visiting service. *Journal of Health Visiting, 6*(7), 334–338.

96. E-Learning for Health. Healthy Child Programme. www.e-lfh.org.uk/. Accessed 2 September 2020.

97. NHS. The NHS long-term plan. https://www.longtermplan.nhs.uk/. Accessed 2 September 2020.

98. NHS Digital. Appointments in general practice – April 2020. https://digital.nhs.uk/data-and-information/publications/statistical/appointments-in-general-practice/april-2020. Accessed 2 September 2020.

99. NHS. Principles for supporting high quality consultations by video in general practice during Covid-19. https://www.england.nhs.uk/coronavirus/wp-content/uploads/sites/52/2020/03/C0479-principles-of-safe-video-consulting-in-general-practice-updated-29-may.pdf. Accessed 2 September 2020.

100. Institute of Health Visiting. Professional advice to support best practice: Virtual Contacts by Health Visitors. https://ihv.org.uk/wp-content/uploads/2020/03/Virtual-Contacts-FINAL-VERSION-27.3.20.pdf. Accessed 2 September 2020.

101. Collins, B. What is Covid-19 revealing about innovation in the NHS? https://www.kingsfund.org.uk/blog/2020/08/covid-19-innovation-nhs. Accessed 2 September 2020.

102. NHS Innovation Accelerator. Health Visitors go digital for millennial parents with the support of ChatHealth. https://nhsaccelerator.com/health-visitors-go-digital-millennial-parents-support-chathealth/. Accessed 2 September 2020.

103. NHS England. Covid-19 prioritisation within Community Health Services. https://www.england.nhs.uk/coronavirus/publication/next-steps-on-nhs-response-to-covid-19-letter-from-simon-stevens-and-amanda-pritchard. Accessed 2 September 2020.

104. Conti, G., & Dow, A. The impacts of Covid-19 on Health Visiting in England First Results. https://discovery.ucl.ac.uk/id/eprint/10106430/1/Conti_Dow_The%20impacts%20of%20Covid-19%20on%20Health%20Visiting%20in%20the%20UK-POSTED.pdf. Accessed 2 September 2020.

105. Institute of Health Visiting. Health visiting during Covid-19: An iHV report. https://ihv.org.uk/our-work/publications-reports/health-visiting-during-covid-19-an-ihv-report/. Accessed 2 September 2020.

106. Collins, B. Technology and innovation for long-term health conditions. https://www.kingsfund.org.uk/sites/default/files/2020-07/Technology%20and%20innovation%20for%20long-term%20health%20conditions%20August%202020.pdf. Accessed 2 September 2020.

107. Palmer, C. Use of a text messaging service for communication with parents and carers. https://journals.rcni.com/primary-health-care/evidence-and-practice/use-of-a-text-messaging-service-for-communication-with-parents-and-carers-phc.2019.e1472/pdf. Accessed 2 September 2020.

108. Donaghy, E., Atherton, H., Hammersley, V., McNeilly, H., Bikker, A., Robbins, L. et al. (2019). Acceptability, benefits, and challenges of video consulting: A qualitative study in primary care. *British Journal of General Practice*, *69*(686), e586–e594.

109. BBC. Coronavirus: How much will it cost the UK? https://www.bbc.co.uk/news/business-52663523. Accessed 2 September 2020.

# 7

# EVIDENCE-BASED PRACTICE AND EARLY INTERVENTION TO SUPPORT CHILDREN AND FAMILIES

CLARE MCGUIRE ■ CLAIR GRAHAM ■ DIANE ALLCOCK ■ JANINE STEWART

## CHAPTER CONTENTS

INTRODUCTION

EARLY YEARS POLICY AND PRACTICE

WHAT IS EVIDENCE-BASED PRACTICE?

HIERARCHY OF EVIDENCE

LIMITATIONS OF THE HIERARCHY

RESEARCH AND EVIDENCE IN HEALTH VISITING

EVIDENCE-BASED PRACTICE: MORE THAN EVIDENCE

SHARED DECISION-MAKING

QUALITY IMPROVEMENT

QUALITY

QUALITY MONITORING AND REVIEW

CARE ASSURANCE

EARLY INTERVENTION

EARLY INTERVENTION AND INVESTMENT IN THE EARLY YEARS

TARGETED HOME VISITING

HUMAN ECOLOGY THEORY

EARLY INTERVENTION AND CHILD DEVELOPMENT

RISK

MANAGING RISK

RISK ASSESSMENT

CONCLUSION

## LEARNING OUTCOMES

*To:*

■ develop a critical understanding of evidence-based practice and the application of evidence to support child-centred decision-making.

■ critically evaluate the context of holistic assessments for children and families.

■ assess the systematic influence and coordinated approach to quality improvement across organisations/services to improve outcomes for children and families.

■ reflect an increased understanding of risk assessment and the management of risk through early intervention practices.

## INTRODUCTION

The early years are a critical period for every child to establish, protect and promote their health and well-being in childhood and throughout their lives. Early years are also an opportunity for you as a heath visitor to identify need and intervene early to improve outcomes, reduce inequalities, and to support parents and carers to optimise health and well-being outcomes in the short- and long-term. Through knowledge, skill and assessment, health visitors understand factors impacting child health and well-being and the ways in which the quality of the parent-infant relationship influences development. This understanding extends to preventative and early interventions to address additional and unmet need. Children in the UK experience poorer outcomes in comparison to other countries – with rises in infant mortality, comparably low breastfeeding rates and increasing development concerns cited as contributing factors.[1] Your unique and universal role utilises evidence-based practice to identify and respond to health and well-being needs for children and to understand the world around a child and its impact. Health visitors establish and maintain therapeutic relationships and are often the key professional responsive to factors actually or potentially impacting a child's health and well-being. This relationship is considered central to health visiting practice.

## EARLY YEARS POLICY AND PRACTICE

Political devolution gives powers from the UK Parliament to the other countries in determining some of their own national policy. Subsequently, early years policy and practice varies across the UK; however, wherever you work, a universal provision of health visiting services is evident in each of the four UK countries, with a consistent aim to reduce health inequalities and improve outcomes for children throughout their childhood and beyond. Early intervention, incorporating play into the education curriculum and parenting are examples of similarities reported. In England, minimum service delivery is stipulated, and additional targeted services provided dependent on need. There are further considerations when short-term need arises requiring additional support and for more complex need when multi-professional or multi-agency work is required. This is defined through four levels of intervention: Community; Universal; Universal Plus; and Universal Partnership Plus – delivered through the 'Healthy Child Programme 0-19' and the 4-5-6 approach.[2]

In Scotland 'Getting it Right for Every Child' (GIRFEC) is a universal approach across children and young people's services, based on evidence and practitioner experience and delivered through a transitional implementation model. A realist evaluation was part of a range of evidence to inform the development of an enhanced health visiting service in Scotland.[3] This three-phase evaluation concluded the benefits in creating more opportunities to identify health and well-being issues early. The GIRFEC approach is focused on the child, recognises the potential impact of wider influences on health, well-being and development and the need for everyone to work in partnership.

The 'Healthy Child Wales Programme' and 'Healthy Child, Healthy Future' programmes in Northern Ireland are like Scotland in their approach to universal provision. Differences are noted in England and Northern Ireland who incorporate integrated reviews of child development between health and education.

Universality in health visiting has been explored by considering a range of research and illuminating the history and core practice in primary prevention and early intervention.[4] Child well-being sets the foundations of early years policy and practice in the UK and internationally, and understanding factors impacting well-being is reflected in the literature, particularly through the assessment and measurement of a child's well-being. Whilst there are varying definitions of well-being, reaching a consensus to define indicators of well-being is multi-dimensional and complex. The concept of children's well-being is underpinned by 'Salutogenesis', introduced by Aaron Antonvosky in the late 1970s.[5] Holistically health creating and assets-based, salutogenesis has a close connection and application with health visiting practice through understanding wellness, well-being and the promotion of health. Adopting a salutogenic approach in working with families proactively enables and promotes relationships with parents and carers to identify and address issues which may impact on their health and well-being and their children's health and well-being.

This chapter will explore evidence-based practice in the context of health visiting and discuss its relationship with early intervention to support children and families.

## WHAT IS EVIDENCE-BASED PRACTICE?

This section will provide the opportunity to revise your knowledge on evidence-based practice, recognising your current and previous professional and academic experience.

The term 'evidence-based practice', in relation to health care, was shared from a medical perspective in the early 1970s and termed 'evidence-based medicine'. A commonly referred definition suggests evidence-based practice is '…the conscientious, explicit and judicious use of current best evidence in making decisions about the care of individual patients'.[6] This definition emphasises the correlation between evidence and practice with decision-making within everyday practice, with our decisions clearly stated and well supported. Evidence-based practice should therefore be supported through a clear, coherent, contemporary rationale which considers the client's preferences and utilises the professional's clinical judgement.

Whilst its inception is often cited in the medical profession, Florence Nightingale's influence on using the best available evidence to improve patient outcomes in the 1800s is also recognised, particularly on the environmental impact on health.[7] Gathering data to understand comparisons, for example; mortality rates and preventable mortality, informed Florence Nightingale's practice but she had a much broader desire that evidence be used to inform public policy and decision-making. Nightingale was at this early point using evidence gained through experimentation and critical examination and is recognised

as a pioneer of evidence-based practice within the discipline of nursing.

It was during the 1970s that medicine focused on the value of research evidence, efficacy and the incorporation of evidence to clinical practice. Before this point, health care professionals practiced through more traditional means, doing what they had been taught and trained to do, with little or no reference to research findings incorporated into their clinical practice.

Recognising the differentiation between process and outcome, Dawes et al[8] suggest that evidence-based practice '…requires that decisions about health care are based on the best available, current, valid and relevant evidence. These decisions should

---

**BOX 7.1**

### A CONTEMPORARY HISTORY OF EVIDENCE-BASED PRACTICE

- The impact of the economic crisis during the early 1970s propelled the examination of treatment efficacy and value for money to be cogitated.
- Professor Archie Cochrane led early evidence-based medicine movement, by incorporating higher-level critical thinking and suggesting the integration of patient values to implement research findings.
- The publication of his definitive monograph on evaluation led to the establishment of the Cochrane collaborations in 1972.
- Before this, most medical decisions were based on individual physician's assessment and preference and did not incorporate a patient-centred focus.
- Despite this recognition of the principles of evidence-based medicine in the early 1970s, it wasn't until two decades later in 1992 that the phrase evidence-based practice was coined.
- Although Cochrane's early work contended that Randomised Controlled Trials (RCTs) provided the most reliable form of evidence, it took two decades of the promotion of the use of RCTs to support foundational decision-making in medicine, and for these principles to be duly recognised and adopted.

be made by those receiving care, informed by the tacit and explicit knowledge of those providing care, within the context of available resources'. This is relevant in your role by working in partnership with those receiving care: children; young people; parents; carers and families. Shared decision-making will be discussed later in the chapter.

Evidence-based practice underpins health visiting education and is used to bridge the gap between theory and practice and is firmly rooted in the premise that patient care should be informed by sound evidence which practitioners utilise and synthesise in care delivery. Evidence-based practice is now widely applied within the professional roles of nursing, midwifery and health visiting, and therefore, essential as these professions account for almost 50% of the global health care workforce.[9] Evidence-based practice is vital within health visiting practice, given the fundamental principle to identify need, evaluate and apply the best available evidence to support early intervention and improved outcomes. A range of evidence underpins practice, but to adopt an evidence-based practice approach requires good evidence which will enhance and support our decision-making.

The Nursing and Midwifery Council[10] stipulates the requirement to always practise in line with the best available evidence. Evidence-based practice enhances critical thinking and decision-making and helps to promote consistency in practice; however adopting a child and person-centred approach enables you to apply this to individual needs. It may appear arduous to determine 'best evidence', given the wide array of evidence available. Therefore, consideration of the types of evidence that are utilised to inform practice and their value within this process and the associated outcomes are important.

Whilst scientific research, for example through RCTs, is regarded as the most reliable source of evidence in terms of treatment, not all areas of health care have this depth or type of research evidence or use this level of evidence in everyday

clinical practice. So, how do we apply evidence in practice? There is some agreement that the best available evidence combined with expert opinion and a holistic approach to the views and values of those receiving care is the most effective combination, although much wider influence through knowledge also informs practice knowledge gained from practice and experience.[11]

In UK health care, clinical and practice guidelines inform practice and support decision-making. An example of this is the National Institute for Health and Care Excellence (NICE) who provide evidence-based pathways, guidance, standards and recommendations in England. The Scottish Intercollegiate Guidelines Network (SIGN) has a similar role in Scotland utilising scientific evidence to enable translation to practice. With a shared goal to improve care quality, NICE and SIGN often collaborate to influence and benefit health care delivery and avoid duplication.

## HIERARCHY OF EVIDENCE

A valuable skill is understanding the origins of evidence and its quality. Evidence is often systematically considered in terms of its hierarchy, with a common illustration being a seven-level evidence pyramid.[12] Not all evidence is comparable in method, applicability and validity which is a concept represented through the pyramid. Whilst the evidence pyramid may be ranked in order of importance, there are some forms of research considered to be stronger in aspects than others.[13] The top of the hierarchy represents the most reliable evidence with those less reliable and at higher risk of bias at the bottom. Evidence pyramids are intended to be a guide and useful in considering the quality of evidence, therefore research evidence must always be interpreted and never just accepted.

In relation to systematic reviews, their strength is undisputed in summarising all available literature on a topic by reviewing the literature systematically and rigorously and putting it into context. One of the most recognisable and accessible publications of systematic reviews are Cochrane Reviews, which we mentioned earlier. RCTs are placed next in the hierarchy and may prove more challenging in their use and applicability in health visiting, due to health and social complexities and the variables and discrete influences impacting families and communities.[14]

Qualitative studies and expert opinion are presented at a low level within the hierarchy of evidence although their contribution to decision-making in health visiting is valued.[15] Best practice guidelines are often used within health visiting practice to make the principles of evidence-based practice more accessible for practitioners to incorporate into clinical practice and decision-making. Best practice guidelines are based on the most rigorous research evidence available but do also include expert opinion within an area of practice, for example infant feeding and childhood obesity.

## LIMITATIONS OF THE HIERARCHY

There are limitations with the hierarchy of evidence, and you should consider the evidence in relation to what you are looking at. For example, is it evidence to determine the effectiveness of an intervention or treatment? Or is it required to determine the patient experience or concordance with an intervention to improve outcomes? Whilst the hierarchy helps identify the available research sources, there are also many more sources available which integrate research evidence, for example, government policy reports; guidelines; standards; protocols; and reports from international and national organisations. It is therefore important to determine your own unique hierarchy of evidence to address your problem or situation within practice.

Conducting research and developing knowledge of methods and methodology are evident in health visiting curricula and academic pathways. Promoting and supporting health visitors as researchers is invaluable to contribute and enhance

evidence, particularly on contemporary issues. As already indicated, critical thinking is an essential skill to support your evidence-based practice, the foundations of which are evident in undergraduate curricula and further enhanced through specialist knowledge and practice in postgraduate study.[16] Thinking critically and reflectively requires knowledge to base reasoning and decisions, principally as decision-making is multifaceted in health care. You will have a developed understanding of critical and reflective practice and it will be useful to consider and develop this further in the context of health visiting practice.

## RESEARCH AND EVIDENCE IN HEALTH VISITING

In preschool-aged children, evidence-based health visiting practice focuses on promotion and improvement of health to support better outcomes. Research and evidence (what is known) in health visiting has developed over the past 20 years, with prevention and early intervention a priority across UK early years policy. Knowledge translation (what is done) is an evolving concept relating to the sharing, application and implementation of research in practice the 'practice' in evidence-based practice. Knowledge acquisition is more complex and multi-factorial, as mentioned previously, from research, clinical guidelines (e.g., NICE, SIGN) and models of care, all of which contribute to health care improvements.

THINKING SPACE

- Identify a clinical guideline that relates to your professional practice, one which you may not have become so familiar with.
- Consider any recommendations, their supporting evidence and how this guideline is applied in your current practice.
- Take time to discuss and share with a colleague.

## EVIDENCE-BASED PRACTICE: MORE THAN EVIDENCE

Understanding the hierarchy of evidence is useful to support the application of evidence-based intervention, but you should recognise that evidence-based practice is more than evidence alone and requires the application of clinical/professional judgement, a vital dimension to support an evidence-based approach to care.[17]

There will be times when there is a lack of evidence or the evidence will not be directly applicable, and you will be required to make informed judgements based on the available evidence, giving consideration of both the context and complexity of the situation. Strategies to support your decision-making process could, for example, be through supervision, reflection and reflexivity. You should seek opportunities to learn more about the fundamentals of clinical supervision. A good source may be the NHS education provider in the UK country you are working, for example, NHS Education for Scotland and Northern Ireland Practice and Education Council for Nursing and Midwifery.

---

### BOX 7.2
### EVIDENCE-BASED PRACTICE AND PROFESSIONAL JUDGEMENT

■ Clinical/professional judgement in health visiting practice is understood as the interpretation made about a situation or child and/or family's needs, concerns or health problems.

■ It is a product of theoretical, experiential and often intuitive learning, used to determine whether (and which) evidence should be applied.

■ Intuition is acknowledged for its close relationship with experience and is grounded in both knowledge and experience – integral to making sound professional judgements.

■ Whilst evidence-based practice can and is used to inform your decision-making, it cannot replace professional expertise and judgement.

---

Evidence-based practice within health visiting requires the mutually dependent dimensions of evidence and professional judgement; as evidence without the application of professional judgement (although recognising you may currently be in a supervised learning role) could lead to rigid care practices, whilst professional judgement without evidence would lead to out of date practice. However, an important additional dimension is undoubtedly the child and parent/carer's preference. These preferences must be acknowledged to enable effective partnership working and to gain their consent before the undertaking interventions.

## SHARED DECISION-MAKING

Establishing effective ways to discuss evidence with parents and carers, to promote informed choice, can be challenging. With a rise in consumerism, expectations relating to health care have notably risen. Knowledge of health and where this is accessed from has significantly changed in recent years with the exponential growth of social media. This contrasts to a time when health professionals in the 20th century were often the main source of health advice and patients less actively involved in decisions affecting their health.

To support effective shared decision-making, facilitative discussions with parents/carers are conducted which enable informed choice and in turn promote a person-centred approach. Technological advances and knowledge acquisition from a range of sources, for example online, can also present challenges and are discussed further in Chapter 9. The skills to navigate evidence and confidence to engage in discussions are therefore essential to support and empower parents and carers to reach an informed decision. Parents can also be considered experts in relations to their child's health needs, for example, where there are continuing and complex needs.

Health visitors have a responsibility to establish and maintain an effective, trusting and therapeutic relationship with parents and carers to promote child and family health and well-being. Utilising shared language is essential to this development from a human rights perspective, to allow the parent/carer equal access and shared decision-making, which is set in the foundations of health literacy. Health literacy, sometimes referred to as health information literacy, is the capacity of individuals to obtain, process, and understand basic health information and available service provision needed to make appropriate health decisions.[18] As a health visitor, you are uniquely placed to achieve this through universal service provision. This relationship can be enhanced by consistent evidence-based advice, important to promote engagement and connect with families and communities. Relationship-centred, trauma-informed, and responsive care can help identify personal outcomes for families, recognising their hopes and aspirations.

### Case study: part 1

Our case study introduces you to a woman 34 weeks pregnant with her first child and their partner, who meets the health visitor in their home antenatally. Some information shared by the midwife before your contact are noted below:

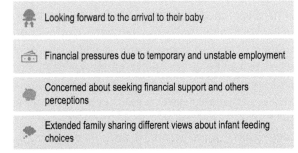

Looking forward to the arrival to their baby

Financial pressures due to temporary and unstable employment

Concerned about seeking financial support and others perceptions

Extended family sharing different views about infant feeding choices

Take time to explore and consider the antenatal contact and your role as a health visitor given the information provided; we have noted some

key points in Box 7.3, and you may wish to add to these. Keep a note of your initial considerations and we will revisit the family in Part 2 of the case study later in the chapter.

An antenatal contact establishes a relationship between the health visitor and parent(s) which may also influence and enhance future engagement with health visiting services. Consider a time where you have met a parent(s) for the first time and the opportunities and/or challenges this presented in establishing and sustaining your relationship. Did the situation you are reflecting on influence your future practice and if so in what ways?

Health visiting practice builds on the firm foundations of good, open communication skills and practice, which utilises transactional analysis to work in partnership with parents, carers and families. Transactional analysis is founded on the philosophical assumptions that people are equal and have the capacity to think and make decisions, which is facilitated through open communication to achieve the goal of change.[19] The guiding principles of transactional analysis rely on the process

---

**BOX 7.3**
**KEY CONSIDERATIONS IN THE ANTENATAL CONTACT**

- Partnership working with midwifery.
- Holistic assessment.
- Explore parental preparedness and support parenthood transition.
- Understand the relationship with the unborn baby.
- Promote health and well-being.
- Share local information and resources.
- Identify additional need which may require multi-agency or multi-professional support antenatally and in the postnatal period.
- Infant feeding choices through a meaningful conversation.
- Financial inclusion routine enquiry and referral pathways.
- Explore parental mental health.

of communication, as well as its content. That is, it is essential not only that you pay close attention to what people say but also to how they say it and their non-verbal communication. These are referred to as the social level and the psychological level, respectively. These aspects should complement your exploration of Chapter 5.

Health visitors and parents/carers working together to improve the well-being of their child is enabled through building a relationship.[20] Parents having an active role in decision-making, agreement on well-being need, health visitors having meaningful conversations and building trusting relationships were some factors highlighted which could strengthen or negatively impact a shared decision-making approach. Collaborative communication is a vital skill for you as a health visitor and foundational to higher level critical appraisal and a key outcome of your professional development. The validation of information to and from other services, and the views of parents/carers, promotes a common understanding to mitigate potentially negative impacts on your relationships.

## QUALITY IMPROVEMENT

Evidence-based practice and early intervention are key factors in a universal service striving for optimum health outcomes for children and their families. Access to health care, on its own, is not enough and requires monitoring of quality through a co-ordinated systematic approach. A country's health care system requires commitment through policy and strategies to enable continuous quality improvement. Demonstrating effectiveness through service contribution and outcomes in health visiting practice is evident across the UK; however, there are varying approaches when defining key indicators and measurement of performance which we will explore further in this section. Quality improvement and evidence-based practice are complementary in

terms of the evidence used to inform everyday practice in health care, essential to improve care delivery and promote consistency and now explicitly represented in UK nursing and midwifery curricula.

## QUALITY

There are a range of definitions as to what 'quality' means across internationally diverse health care settings. Following a review by Lord Darzi, quality was defined as requiring three dimensions: clinical effectiveness; patient safety; and patient experience, which led to developments in health policy and subsequently safeguarded through legislation.[21] The World Health Organisation[22] focus on six indicators in relation to quality of care: safe; effective; timely; efficient; equitable; and person-centred. Promoting and embedding these quality indicators have been at the forefront across UK health settings since the 1990s, with quality improvement and quality assurance evolving in parallel. Safety and effectiveness predominate health care quality monitoring whilst equity and efficiency are the most infrequently measured.

Quality improvement (also referred to as improvement science) can be viewed as both a philosophy to help organisations function and change processes, and a range of tools to promote consistency in care delivery. Strategic approaches to measurement and improvement are often represented through overarching mechanisms and legislation, which is evident globally, nationally and locally. Globally, the United Nations established sustainable development goals to address poverty and inequalities through three key dimensions: economic, social and environmental. Within the UK examples of this strategic alignment are seen within legislation, for example, prioritising the well-being of children and young people in Northern Ireland[23] and Scotland.[24] Locally, you may have been involved in or are aware of 'quality improvement collaboratives', which have gained momentum in recent years to enable multi-professional groups to work together and be supported to achieve improvement on an agreed aim and increasing capacity and capability for improvement.

Legislative and strategic developments in times of economic austerity can increase pressure on health care budgets and service provision. Evolving public health priorities and demographic changes can also have a detrimental impact, for example, the global coronavirus pandemic and its subsequent effect on health and the economy in the short and longer term. Internationally, the best functioning health care organisations intertwine improving value and efficiency with improving quality and reducing waste and many health care systems model themselves on quality of care, health of the population; and value and sustainability.

A clearly defined aim for improvement initiatives is enabled by adopting a SMART (Specific, Measurable, Achievable, Realistic, Timely) approach, to promote success and help identify outcome measures. There are a wide range of tools to provide focus and structure to improvement projects, some of which you may already be familiar with. You will find more information on quality improvement with examples and templates online from the Institute for Healthcare Improvement.

Improving health outcomes through evidence-based processes are often the primary focus of evidence-based practice as one type of quality improvement; however, not all quality improvement is based on scientific evidence and may instead be driven by local processes and data.[25]

Methods for quality improvement provide a framework and consideration should be given to the most suitable for the specific purpose. For example, Lean/Six Sigma is useful when waste in the health care system can be removed to make better use of resource and therefore improve

efficiency. You may already be familiar with the 'Plan, Do, Study, Act' (PDSA) cycle,[26] which is often used to test change in small scale projects. This cyclical four step approach can inform learning at each stage and guide further change cycles, although change does not necessarily lead to improvement.[27] Regardless of the methods and tools applied, a systematic and continuous approach is vital to drive any improvement project. The visual infographic (Figure 7.1) provides more information. Within the PDSA model, it is also recommended you consider three key questions: What are we trying to accomplish?; How will we know that a change is an improvement?; and, What changes can we make that will result in an improvement?

PDSA provides learning opportunities where test cycles can be adjusted for subsequent cycles therefore establishing where improvement occurs. The stages enable feasibility of each change idea which can inform larger scale implementation. The practice of upscale and spread of small-scale testing may be complex and challenging for organisations, for example, the context in which the small test of change was effective in may not be transferrable or directly applicable on a larger scale. Contemporary health visiting has benefited from a focus on improvement; an example from Scotland is the testing of an enhanced programme and pathway in health visiting which has been incrementally implemented across the country.[28]

You should take time to explore opportunities to share quality improvement activities you are leading or contributing to as this can help build evidence on specific areas of practice. Across the UK and globally, there are repositories which promote and support the improvement agenda in health and social care, and we recommend you also explore sharing evidence through conference presentations, journal publication, blogs and vlogs, and other technology enabled platforms.

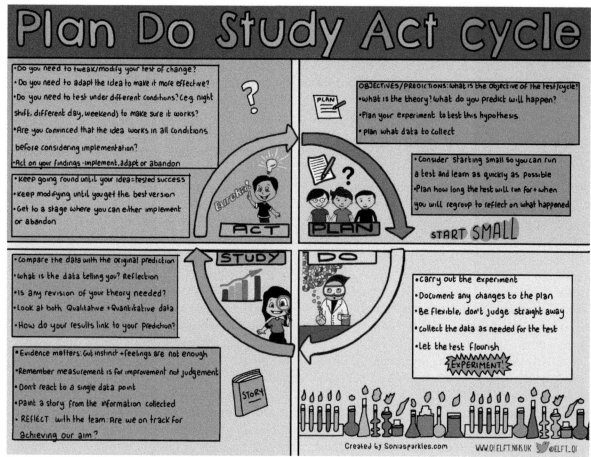

Figure 7.1 ■ PDSA Infographic. (With kind permission from Quality Improvement department at East London NHS Foundation Trust, who have developed this visual with Sonia Nosheen.)

## QUALITY MONITORING AND REVIEW

Governance in health care was introduced by the World Health Organisation[29] in their health report in 2000, with effectiveness and accountability considered key components in its 'stewardship'. A systematic review[30] revealed a lack of 'good practice' examples although commonalities in frameworks nationally and globally, such as risk management; clinical audit; evidence-based care and effectiveness; and patient/client/carer experience and involvement were evident.

Establishing and sustaining quality standards can help measure and demonstrate care quality; however it can be complex. A lack of clarity and understanding of measurement and practitioner competence in data collection can impact on reliability of results in ever-changing health care systems and population needs. Reported in 1966 by a pioneer in health research, the Donabedian model is widely adopted as an enabler to assess, monitor and benchmark measures.[31] Designed as a framework of 'structure, process and outcome', it helps evaluate quality and identify areas

---

**BOX 7.4**

**DONABEDIAN MODEL: EXAMPLES IN HEALTH VISITING PRACTICE**

- Structural measures–electronic record systems or the number or health visitors employed.
- Process measures–percentage of children who had developmental screening undertaken by the health visitor.
- Outcome measures–percentage of children who have a healthy weight. With outcome measures frequently viewed as the gold standard in measuring quality; many factors can impact on these and balancing measures may need to be included to provide a clearer picture such as the characteristics of a population.

---

requiring improvement. The three aspects, which may now seem overly simplistic and reductionist from its inception, are deeply rooted in health service research.

Data are collected and analysed at individual and population level in relation to child health and well-being and the UK government align outcome measures with the World Health Organisation and UNICEF. Infant mortality, breastfeeding, and immunisations uptake are some examples of information collected and recorded by all four UK countries. Other sources such as the Royal College of Paediatrics and Child Health (RCPCH) provide health monitor outcomes and make recommendations to improve child health and well-being with data sets including life expectancy at birth, poverty, education and employment. Internationally, The Organisation for Economic Co-operation and Development (OECD) data portal provides insight on monitoring the health and safety of children, children's home and family life, education, activities and life satisfaction offering global comparisons.

Key performance indicators, which although will vary across the UK, can illuminate population health data and provide some comparisons globally, nationally and locally (e.g., breastfeeding, immunisations and infant mortality). In England, key indicators are accessible within a public health dashboard system making comparable data across the country visually accessible. Cowley et al[32] discussed a lack of evaluative evidence for health visiting's contribution to public health outcomes and reducing inequalities, however, they identified the benefits of a salutogenic approach through prevention and early intervention.

Strategic monitoring, inspection and regulation of standards for safety and quality in health and social care is undertaken by national regulators in the UK. This is evident in multi-professional health and social care inspections undertaken across the UK incorporating scrutiny on systems and processes alongside individual child pathways to ensure care quality and safety. As a health visitor, you are likely to or may have already been involved in care inspections, which can include review of clinical documentation and may be accompanied by in-depth interviews to provide a more holistic context. Outcomes of these processes are reported and highlight areas of good practice and recommendations for improvement requiring formal action plans.

In recent years public inquiries into care quality in the NHS revealed poor standards of care and significant concern on patient safety. Of significance is the Report of the Mid Staffordshire NHS Foundation Trust Public Inquiry (often referred to as the Francis Report), which made 290 recommendations incorporating: professional regulatory governance; stakeholder engagement; education; and leadership. In response, the UK regulator for nursing and midwifery, the Nursing and Midwifery Council (NMC), made changes to its regulatory standards and procedures to promote high quality of care and public safeguarding and instil public confidence in the profession.[33]

## CARE ASSURANCE

Opportunity to influence governance at a practitioner level is evident through care assurance and accreditation programmes, resulting in quality standards which have influenced improvement work across the NHS.[34] Initially developed in acute hospitals, programmes have been adapted to community care settings to navigate the process of change for improvement. It is recognised that frontline practitioners have the knowledge and expertise and are therefore best placed to identify areas for change to improve services, outcomes and experience. The programmes also promote engagement of change by providing a clear route to the aim, providing structure and make the collection of data meaningful. Measurement of quality of care is evidenced through a set of care standards devised by the practitioners in partnership with other stakeholders.

An example in health visiting practice is a care assurance system developed and implemented by a Tri-Board collaborative in Scotland as part of 'Excellence in Care'. This system provides a structured measurement of dimensions and priorities aligned with the Healthcare Quality Strategy for NHS Scotland.[35] Consistency and sustainability of quality standards are promoted through practitioners and stakeholder's working together and towards the standards. Data gathered are visually represented within an electronic dashboard system, which is an approach used in NHS areas across the UK.

## EARLY INTERVENTION

Building on what we have already explored in relation to evidence-based practice and quality improvement, promoting and improving health and well-being to support better outcomes are a key focus in preschool-aged children. Research and evidence in health visiting practice have significantly developed over the past 20 years, with prevention and early intervention a policy priority across the UK.

Knowledge translation is an evolving concept relating to the sharing, application and implementation of research to practice. However, the growth in new knowledge developments for health visiting practice has notably largely stemmed from the neurosciences and developmental psychology fields, as opposed to from health visiting practice itself. These developments underpin the premise that early intervention in every child's life, starting from conception, can optimise brain development and is the key to strategies to improve carer attachment; educational attainment; criminality and behavioural challenges; reducing obesity; and improving overall health outcomes. Early intervention in effect means identifying and providing effective and timely support before health and well-being is negatively impacted. One example of early intervention relates to maternal mental health and the use of the two Whooley questions as recommended within National Institute for Health and Care Excellence (NICE) guidance[36] during the antenatal and postnatal period to support maternal mental health.

Maternal mental health and stress are associated with poor birth outcomes, which includes

---

**BOX 7.5**

### EXAMPLE OF EARLY INTERVENTION–MATERNAL MENTAL HEALTH

- Two-item Generalised Anxiety Disorder Scale (GAD-2) is both quick and easy to administer and used to support an early discussion of both ante- and post-natal anxiety and depression.
- Depending on responses from the questions, further application of the Edinburgh Postnatal Depression Scale (EPDS) or Patient Health Questionnaire (PHQ-9) can be made to assess the individual more fully.
- Additional recommendations are available within the NICE guidance to support assessment and decision-making in practice.

preterm birth, higher infant mortality rates, and low birth weight. This is in addition to the negative impact of stress on raised maternal cortisol, norepinephrine and inflammatory levels on the fetal environment and implications for fetal health, as well as the potential negative impact on the formation of mother-child attachment. You can continue your learning on perinatal mental health in Chapter 13.

Early intervention matters and has a crucial role in identifying and offering children and their parents/carers and families support to reach their potential. As a health visitor it is important to recognise that early intervention is not a panacea and will not solve every risk to a child's development but is vital to minimise the negative impacts in childhood and into adulthood. Having knowledge of human ecology theory, which we'll discuss more later, helps us to understand how a child's development is inseparable from their environment and how this can impact across the life course.

Interventions in health visiting practice are underpinned by effective and continual needs assessment. Recognising a child's need, and in the context of their family structure, enhances a child centred approach to maintaining and improving their health and well-being. The core principles of health visiting practice inform universalism for the preschool population and early identification of need provides more individualised and targeted support when required. Early intervention is at the forefront of public policy in the UK and influenced by multiple levels of research on areas such as neurodevelopment; attachment; parenting; and longer-term impacts. It is also helpful to consider 'primary prevention' as part of the discussion here, in terms of the opportunities to promote health and development and subsequently prevent or avoid issues arising which may negatively impact.

Early intervention is often conveyed as the stage after primary prevention, for example, early in a child's life or early in the scope of complexity or crisis – where timely intervention can help prevent further escalation or deterioration. However, primary prevention and early intervention are also terms which are used interchangeably and whilst they may be linked (for example, both related to proactive action in preventing occurrence or responding early enough to reduce impact) there are differences.

Promoting responsive and positive parent-infant relationships is an example of both primary prevention (in the antenatal period) and early intervention in health visiting, and requires knowledge and skill incorporating a range of theory and practice. Whilst included in health visiting curricula, continuing professional development can further enhance the transition of theory to practice in this area. Knowledge in neurodevelopment can support health visitors to work in partnership with parents and carers to promote their understanding of interactions and relationships with their child(ren). The Solihull approach is an example of an evidence-based programme which considers these factors. Solihull was devised collaboratively between health visitors and child psychologists in the late 1990s. The approach focuses on containment, reciprocity and behaviour management and continues to demonstrate the positive impact on parent-child relationships and the resulting societal and population benefits.[37]

Trauma informed approaches are represented in policies and professional practice guidance. For health visitors, this is two-fold in understanding, identifying and reducing the risk and impact of adverse childhood experiences (ACEs) for children; and recognising any previous trauma and its impact in adulthood (i.e., for parents/carers). Research on ACEs was initially explored in the USA in the 1990s[38] and has relevance in our discussion here in terms of prevention and early intervention. Routine enquiry, increasing knowledge on trauma informed practice and skill in effectively responding; and partnership working are some key factors for health visitors to consider. Childhood adversity and trauma is explored in more detail in Chapter 11.

## EARLY INTERVENTION AND INVESTMENT IN THE EARLY YEARS

The assessment of a child's well-being benefits from being underpinned by the United Nations Convention on the Rights of the Child (UNCRC). The convention is unique in terms of its consideration of all aspects of a child's life, and their rights (social, civil and political), through 54 articles. The UK signed the convention to confirm their commitment to children's rights in 1991 with the UNCRC being the most widely adopted global treaty. Children's rights and well-being are interconnected, and they work in partnership; for example, if a child's rights are fully considered this is more likely to have a positive influence on their well-being.

### THINKING SPACE

- Consider how you capture children's views, irrespective of age – discuss with colleagues.
- What informs your approach?
- Are the views of young children always considered and reflected within multi-agency discussions and assessments?
- In what way(s) do you include children's views in your assessment and clinical documentation?

The value of early years investment to improve life chances for children, particularly children who are disadvantaged, is recognised. Home visiting and promoting the home learning environment through parental support are essential to enhancing positive outcomes, although evidence

is lacking on the effectiveness of interventions. Early years policy in the UK and internationally is informed by the work of James Heckman. As economists, Heckman and colleagues explored the longer-term benefits of investing in early childhood, concluding prevention provided better return on investment than cure and visually represented in Figure 7.2.[39] This work has influenced international programmes, for example, the 'first thousand days' in the USA in 2010, a concept since adopted within the UK as 'The 1001 Critical Days'. There is wide recognition of early influences and opportunities these early days present, for example on: child development; parent-infant relationship; children at risk; and nutrition. Policy and practice focus commitment to early years in Scotland has been maintained since 2008 through quality improvement approaches and workforce development, with the primary object to improve outcomes for children.

### Case study: part 2

We're now going to revisit the family introduced earlier during the new birth contact. Consider the following information by taking account of the chapter content so far in relation to: salutogenic approach; evidence-based practice; shared decision-making; and relationship-building.

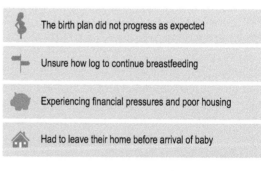

The birth plan did not progress as expected

Unsure how log to continue breastfeeding

Experiencing financial pressures and poor housing

Had to leave their home before arrival of baby

- Within the context of early intervention, what are some of the aspects you are considering for the family and specifically your role in promoting and supporting health and well-being?

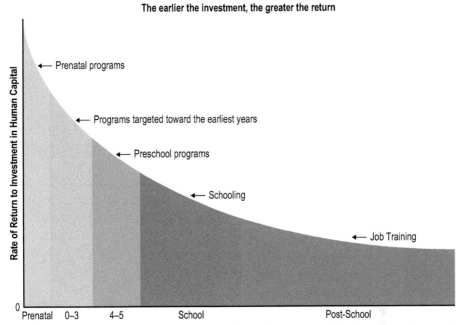

Figure 7.2 ■ The Heckman Curve. (Adapted with permission from: https://heckmanequation.org/resource/the-heckman-curve/.)

- What tools and approaches could help you understand, assess and analyse the context of the baby's life at this time?
- In what ways will you explore the parent's perspective, for example, what is or may impact health and well-being?
- How will you work collaboratively with the parents to support early intervention?
- What help might you need from others to address identified health and well-being needs?
- What evidence will support you to engage in a meaningful conversation about breastfeeding and infant feeding choices?
- On reflection, is there anything you would you change in terms of your approach or decisions noted at the first part of the case study?

## TARGETED HOME VISITING

Targeted home visiting has received international research interest to address inequalities and improve health outcomes, particularly when there are social complexities affecting health and well-being. Promoting health through enablement is an important factor in reducing inequalities with parents and carers feeling informed to reach decisions about theirs and their child's health. As previously highlighted, establishing and building effective relationships, through parental engagement and shared decision-making, are critical skills for health visitors.

In their systematic review, Duncan, MacGillivary and Renfrew[40] explored the costs and savings of targeted parenting interventions in relation to promoting parent-child interactions in comparison to the universal health visiting service. The review identified evidence of savings in the longer term, for example in relation to criminal justice, and challenged policy makers to consider long term benefits and not solely rely on short-term priorities. One example of a targeted programme which has reported longer term cost-benefit is the Family Nurse Partnership (FNP) programme (also known internationally as the Nurse-Family

Partnership). FNP focuses on young first-time mothers to address and improve outcomes, whilst also recognising the modifiable risks, for example, in relation to abuse or neglect.[41] One of the theoretical foundations of FNP is human ecology theory, which we will explore further now.

## HUMAN ECOLOGY THEORY

Human ecology theory helps to explain how the intrinsic individualities of children and their surroundings interrelate to influence growth and development. Bronfenbrenner's ecological theory[42] recognises complexity around a child and the impact this may have on how they grow and develop, which is based on the understanding that the child is at the centre. As a child-centred approach this theory is reflected in models of health visiting practice in the UK and explicitly in Scotland through Getting it Right for Every Child (GIRFEC). According to Bronfenbrenner's ecological systems theory, children are typically involved in a variety of ecosystems, from those close at home to larger systems in schools and wider society.

Each of the ecological systems identified within Figure 7.3 inevitably interacts with and influences

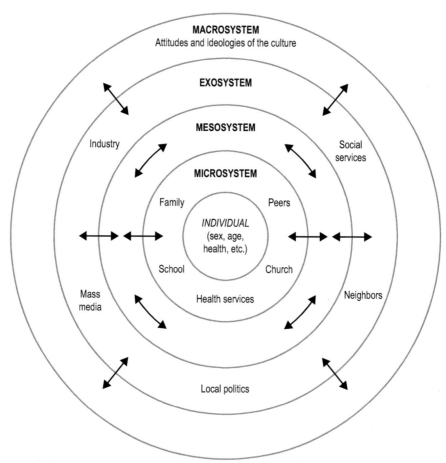

**Figure 7.3** ■ Bronfenbrenner's ecological theory of development. (From https://commons.wikimedia.org/wiki/File:Bronfenbrenner%27s_Ecological_Theory_of_Development_(English).jpg and https://en.wikipedia.org/wiki/GNU_Free_Documentation_License.)

the others in all aspects of the child's life. However, the model organises contexts of development into five specific levels of external influence. These levels are categorised from the individual level to the broadest.

The model identifies how human development is inseparable from our environments across the life course and through mapping the settings where most social interactions occur; this micro-level analysis makes it possible to explore how we all shape and influence the people around us, whilst acknowledging that we are also simultaneously shaped through these interactions. Through illuminating the multiple interrelated and connected influences surrounding us, Bronfenbrenner's theory helps to decipher how the complexities in these ring environments progress and contain our development. A significant realisation from this theory relates to siblings in the same ecological system having different experiences.

Early intervention is recognised as working towards reducing risk factors and increasing the protective factors in a child's life. Health visitors have a crucial role in understanding risk factors that can impact children's development. Risk factors can impact across the life course, increasing the chance of physical and mental health issues; criminality; addiction to substances; and maltreatment in later life. Human ecology theory recognises these factors interact in complex ways and at different levels. Acknowledging a child's development is inseparable from their environment, health visitors can have a positive influence on outcomes across the life course.

## EARLY INTERVENTION AND CHILD DEVELOPMENT

Increasing protective factors and reducing risk factors for children can be achieved through early intervention. Mitigating risks from an individual, family, community and societal perspective, in order to improve health and well-being, are the characteristics considered to be protective factors. Often both risk and protective factors can be separate parts of the same situation.

Whilst for many families universal services such as GPs, health visiting and early years education services will be enough, others will require more targeted interventions. Early intervention can be most effective when it targets children and families/carers on a selective or indicated basis.

- **Targeted selective** interventions informed by demography, for example, financial challenges and poverty, one parent or young parent families. Whilst there may not be specific issues presented by children, interventions are based on risk factors and have the potential to address health and well-being needs and improve outcomes, for example, as mentioned earlier in relation to Family Nurse Partnership.
- **Targeted indicated** interventions are offered based on identified need and the additional support that may be required to address need(s). Early interventions in these situations can reduce or reverse impact in the short and longer term, for example, a child living with parent(s) who have a substance misuse issue.

Early intervention approaches often focus on supporting the four key aspects of child development: physical, cognitive, behavioural, and social and emotional development.[43] These areas are considered to have the potential to make significant impact and improvements across the child's life course.

- **Physical development**: relating to all aspects of physical health. Examples of outcomes impacted by early interventions are decreasing infectious disease incidence, maintaining healthy weight and obesity reduction.[44]

Immunisation practice is a widely recognised early intervention.

- **Cognitive development**: examples relate to speech, language and communication development, literacy and numeracy, problem solving abilities. As achievement of these skills are correlated to educational attainment, outcomes and their interventions are reading, testing, educational achievement and longer-term outcomes in future academic studies and employability. An example of a recognised successful early intervention are projects promoting literacy and the connection between parents/carers and their child from the earliest opportunity.

- **Behavioural development**: a child being able to monitor and regulate behaviour is an important aspect of behavioural development. The skills to self-regulate contribute to establishing good relationships and school achievement. Examples of early intervention include the Solihull approach and early years education services support. Solihull was devised collaboratively between health visitors and child psychologists in the late 1990s, with the approach focusing on containment, reciprocity and behaviour management.

- **Social and emotional development**: this relates to emotional intelligence and managing negativity. As with behavioural development, establishing good relationships, which have a positive impact, can promote mental health and reduce the risk of poor mental health outcomes. Early interventions are often in the promotion of socialisation, relationships and self-confidence.[45] This is supported in infancy through nurturing and supporting positive parent-child relationships beginning in the antenatal period.

The examples discussed will be familiar to you in relation to early intervention and the four child developmental domains; it is therefore also important to discuss three key 'risk' areas which are strongly associated with adverse outcomes during childhood and beyond; child abuse, substance misuse and risky sexual behaviour.

## RISK

Whilst risk is understood as the likelihood or probability of a particular outcome given the presence of factors in a child's life, it is also not just about considerations of concern or harm but also about the inherent aspect of all human development. Risk is a multi-dimensional and dynamic concept; it is not static but fluid, and characterised by a range of events and movements in the context and environment where it occurs. Health visitors need to gain an adequate understanding of the child's environment and circumstances, signs of safety, unmet needs and reasoning, and how risk conditions may have emerged. Through utilising these understandings, health visitors and other professionals, through a safeguarding lens, assess actual and potential harm. Early intervention is therefore essential in protection from harm and reduces the need for child protection interventions. The projection of probable risk or harm also means there is a potential for error in terms of what is considered that may or may not occur. Chapter 12 provides the opportunity to explore safeguarding further.

Trauma-informed practice is identified within policies and professional practice guidance. For health visitors, this is two-fold in understanding, identifying and reducing the risk and impact of adverse childhood experiences (ACEs) for children and in recognising any previous trauma and its impact in adulthood (i.e., for parents).[46] Research on ACEs was initially explored in the USA in the 1990s and has relevance in our discussion here in terms of prevention, early intervention and understanding and managing risk. You will find Chapter 11 helpful for more depth to these discussions. Routine enquiry practices within health visiting increases knowledge on trauma-informed practice and promotes skill in effectively responding through partnership working.

## MANAGING RISK

The key principle for you as a health visitor in managing risk should be partnership working and collaboration. All relevant professionals and agencies, in partnership with parents and carers, should collaborate on a comprehensive assessment and analysis. Maintaining the child at the centre of risk assessment is essential and requires explicit agreement with partner agencies as to how the views of the child/children and parents/carers are inclusive. Assessment is a continuous process which places the child's needs, welfare and wishes and feelings at the centre and are open and transparent with parents/carers to encourage and support their understanding of early intervention and garner their engagement.[47]

Through effective partnership working, you consider strengths, protective factors and resilience proportionately with complexities and protection from harm. Managing risk requires that all interventions with children and their families/carers should incorporate evidence-based practice principles and child ecology. Gathering relevant and comprehensive information about what is happening to a child, and applying knowledge from theory, research and experience to achieve an informed understanding of a child and their family/carer's experiences. A core component of managing risk effectively is understanding the risk, resilience and resistance.

## RISK ASSESSMENT

Identifying risk should be a consideration at every opportunity within health visiting practice whether this is through face-to-face, telephone, virtual contacts or through information received from other agencies; all contacts and all mediums

should be considered concerning risk to the child. The use of recognised assessment processes and frameworks help to guide consideration of risk factors, and whilst there may be discrete differences in the presentation of these factors within a framework and processes, the risk indicator similarities are apparent. For example, the 'assessment triangle' from the UK Assessment Framework[48] provides a visual aid for the risk assessment process, representing the risk indicators as the three sides of a triangle and the interactions between these: parenting capacity, social and environmental factors and risk indicators for child development (Figure 7.4).

In Scotland, this tool is visually represented as the 'My world triangle' as part of the GIRFEC approach and the risk is again evident as risk indicators for the child, for the child's wider world and the parent/carer.

Risk assessment is a complex task which should be driven by a supportive and investigative approach. It needs to be comprehensive and methodical to examine risks, past, present and future. In addition, recognising that whilst it is important to be alert and focused to the factors of adversity or complexity in a child's life, so too is it essential that you as a health visitor focus on strengths and resilience. These factors are often strengthened by positive and effective relationships and meaningful conversations.

## CONCLUSION

Evidence-based practice and early intervention contribute to holistic child-centred assessments to address health and well-being needs and improve outcomes for children and families. Through systematic and co-ordinated approaches to quality improvement, short- and longer-term outcomes can be engaged and achieved for families, communities and the wider population. Early intervention is a key policy priority across each of the four UK countries, cognisant of its importance in reducing

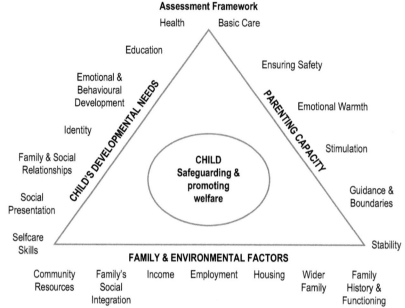

Figure 7.4 ■ Assessment framework. (From: http://www.nationalarchives.gov.uk/doc/open-government-licence/version/3/.)

health inequalities and improving outcomes and the impact of the world around a child. This chapter has explored a range of influencing factors which contribute to the effectiveness of the health visitor's role in applying evidence-based practice and early interventions, which are firmly established through building trusting relationships.

- Building an effective, trusting and therapeutic relationship with parents and carers promotes child and family health and well-being.
- Evidence-based practice and early intervention are key factors in a universal service striving to achieve optimum health outcomes for children and their families.
- A systematic approach is vital to drive any improvement project.
- Early intervention means identifying and providing effective and timely support before health and well-being is negatively impacted.
- Maintaining a child-centred approach to risk assessment is essential.

## FURTHER RESOURCES (PRINT AND ONLINE)

- Institute for Healthcare Improvement www.ihi.org
- Healthcare Improvement Scotland: https://ihub.scot/about-us/
- NHS Improvement: https://improvement.nhs.uk/home/
- Improving Quality Together NHS Wales: https://iqt.wales.nhs.uk/
- Sir Harry Burns TEDx Glasgow: What causes wellness? https://www.youtube.com/watch?v=yEh3JG74C6s
- Unicef: The Baby Friendly Initiative: https://www.unicef.org.uk/babyfriendly/

# REFERENCES

1. Royal College of Paediatrics and Child Health (2019). RCPCH Prevention Vision for Child Health. https://www.rcpch.ac.uk/resources/rcpch-prevention-vision-child-health. Accessed June 19, 2020.
2. Public Health England (2018). Best start in life and beyond: improving public health outcomes for children, young people and families. Guidance to support the commissioning of the Healthy Child Programme 0–19: Health visiting and school nursing services. https://assets.publishing.service.gov.uk/government/uploads/system/uploads/attachment_data/file/716028/best_start_in_life_and_beyond_commissioning_guidance_2.pdf. Accessed June 19, 2020.
3. Doi, L., Jepson, R., Hardie, S. (2017). Realist evaluation of an enhanced health visiting programme. https://journals.plos.org/plosone/article?id=10.1371/journal.pone.0180569. Accessed June 19, 2020.
4. Cowley, S., Whittaker, K., Malone, M., Donetto, S., Grigulis, A., & Maben, J. (2018). What makes health visiting successful – or not? 1. Universality. *Journal of Health Visiting*, *6*(7), 352–360.
5. Mittelmark, M. B., Sagy, S., Erikkson, M., Bauer, G. F., Pelikan, J. M., Lindstrom, B., & Espnes, G. A. *The handbook of salutogenesis*. Springer Open Access.
6. Sackett, D. L., Rosenberg, W. M., & Muir Gray, J. A. (1996). Evidence-based medicine: What it is and what it isn't. *British Medical Journal*, *312*(7023), 71–72.
7. Mackey, A., & Bassendowski S., (2017). The history of evidence-based practice in nursing education and practice. *Journal of Professional Nursing*, *33*(1), 51–55.
8. Dawes, M., Summerskill, W., Glasziou, P., Cartabellotta, A., Martin, J., Hopayian, K., et al. (2005). Sicily statement on evidence-based practice. *BMC Medical Education*, *5*(1), 1–7.
9. World Health Organization. (2016). Global strategic direction for strengthening nursing and midwifery 2016–2020. https://www.who.int/hrh/nursing_midwifery/global-strategy-midwifery-2016-2020/en/. Accessed September 18, 2020.
10. Nursing and Midwifery Council. (2018). The Code: professional standards of practice and behaviour for nurses, midwives and nursing associates. https://www.nmc.org.uk/standards/code/. Accessed June 19, 2020.
11. Geanellos, R. (2004). Nursing-based evidence: Moving beyond evidence-based practice in mental health nursing. *Journal of Evaluation in Clinical Practice*, *10*(2), 177–186.
12. Aveyard, H., & Sharp, P. (2013). *A beginners guide to evidence based practice in health and social care* (2nd ed.). Maidenhead: McGraw Hill Education: Open University Press.
13. Burns, P. B., Rohrich, R. J., & Chung, K. C. (2011). The levels of evidence and their role in evidence-based medicine. *Plastic and Reconstructive Surgery*, *128*(1), 305–310.
14. Ball, E., & Regan, P. (2019). Interpreting research to inform practice: The hierarchy of evidence framework. *Journal of Health Visiting*, *7*(11), 32–38.
15. Rolfe, D. E., Ramsden, V. R., Banner, D., & Graham, I. D. (2018). Using qualitative health research methods to improve patient and public involvement and engagement in research. *Research Involvement and Engagement*, *4*, 49. https://doi.org/10.1186/s40900-018-0129-8.
16. Aveyard, H. (2017). *A beginner's guide to evidence-based practice in health and social care* (3rd ed.). London: Open University Press.
17. van Bekkum, J. E., & Hilton, S. (2013). The challenges of communicating research evidence in practice: Perspectives from UK health visitors and practice nurses. *BMC Nursing*, *12*(17), 1–9.
18. Scottish Government (2017). Making it easier: A health literacy action plan 2017–2025. https://www.gov.scot/publications/making-easier-health-literacy-action-plan-scotland-2017-2025/. Accessed September 18, 2020.
19. Webb, L. (2011). *Nursing communication skills in practice*. Oxford: Oxford University Press.
20. Astbury, R., Shepherd, A., & Cheyne, H. (2016). Working in partnership: The application of shared decision-making to health visiting practice. *Journal of Clinical Nursing*, *26*(1–2), 215–224.
21. Health and Social Care Act 2012. (2012). http://www.legislation.gov.uk/ukpga/2012/7/contents/enacted. Accessed June 28, 2020.
22. World Health Organisation. (2020). What is quality of care and why is it important? https://www.who.int/maternal_child_adolescent/topics/quality-of-care/definition/en/. Accessed June 28, 2020.
23. Children's Services Co-Operation Act (Northern Ireland) 2015O. (2015). http://www.legislation.gov.uk/nia/2015/10/pdfs/nia_20150010_en.pdf. Accessed June 28, 2020.
24. Children and Young People (Scotland) Act 2014. (2014). http://www.legislation.gov.uk/asp/2014/8/contents/enacted. Accessed June 28, 2020.
25. LoBiondo-Wood, G., Haber, J., & Titler, M. G. (2019). *Evidence-based practice for nursing and healthcare quality improvement*. Missouri: Elsevier.
26. Langley, G. J., Moen, R. D., Nolan, K. M., Nolan, T. W., Norman, C. L., & Provost, L. P. (2009). *The improvement guide: A practice approach to enhancing organizational performance* (2nd ed.). San Francisco: Josey-Bass.

27. Taylor, M. J., McNicholas, C., Nicolay, C., Darzi, A., Bell, D., & Reed, J. E. (2014). Systematic review of the application of the plan-do-study-act method to improve quality in healthcare. *BMJ Quality & Safety, 23*(4), 290–298.

28. Doi, L., Jepson, R., & Hardie, S. (2017). Realist evaluation of an enhanced health visiting programme. https://journals.plos.org/plosone/article?id=10.1371/journal.pone.0180569. Accessed June 19, 2020.

29. World Health Organization. (2000). The World Health Report 2000 – health systems: improving performance. https://www.who.int/whr/2000/en/. Accessed June 28, 2020.

30. Pyone, T., Smith, H., & van de Broek, N. (2017). Frameworks to assess health systems governance: A systematic review. *Health Policy and Planning, 32*(5), 710–722.

31. Donabedian, A. (2005). Evaluating the quality of medical care. *Millbank Memorial Fund Q, 83*(4), 691–729. Reprinted from Millbank Memorial Fund Quarterly, 1966, 44(3), 166–203.

32. Cowley, S., Whittaker, K., Malone, M., Donetto, S., Grigulis, A., & Maben, J. (2015). Why health visiting? Examining the potential public health benefits from health visiting practice within a universal service: a narrative review of the literature. *International Journal of Nursing Studies, 52*(1), 465–480. doi 10.1016/j.ijnurstu.2014.07.013.

33. Nursing and Midwifery Council. (2015). Francis Report: our position. https://www.nmc.org.uk/about-us/policy/position-statements/francis-report/. Accessed June 29, 2020.

34. NHS Improvement. (2019). Guide to developing and implementing ward and unit accreditation programmes. https://improvement.nhs.uk/resources/guide-developing-and-implementing-ward-and-unit-accreditation-programmes/. Accesssed June 29, 2020.

35. Scottish Government. (2010). Healthcare quality strategy for NHS Scotland. https://www.gov.scot/publications/healthcare-quality-strategy-nhsscotland/. Accessed June 29, 2020.

36. National Institute of Health and Care Excellence. (2014). Antenatal and postnatal mental health: Clinical management and service guidance. https://www.nice.org.uk/guidance/cg192. Accessed June 29, 2020.

37. Douglas, H., & Johnson, R. (2019). The Solihull approach 10-week programme: A randomised controlled trial. *Community Practitioner, 92*(7), 45–47.

38. Felitti, V. J., Anda, R. F., Nordenberg, D., Williamson, D. F., Spitz, A. M., Edwards, V., et al. (1998). Relationship of childhood abuse and household dysfunction to many of the leading causes of death in adults. The Adverse Childhood Experiences (ACE) Study. *American Journal of Preventative Medicine, 14*(4), 245–258. doi 10.1016/s0749-3797(98)00017-8.

39. Heckman: the economics of human potential. The Heckman Curve. (2020). https://heckmanequation.org/resource/the-heckman-curve/. Accessed June 29, 2020.

40. Duncan, K. M., MacGillivary, S., & Renfrew, M. J. (2017). Costs and savings of parenting interventions: Results of a systematic review. *Child: Care, Health and Development, 43*(6), 797–811.

41. Olds, D. (2006). The Nurse-Family Partnership: An evidence-based preventative intervention. *Infant Mental Health Journal, 27*(1), 5–25.

42. Bronfenbrenner, U. (1979). *The ecology of human development: Experiments by nature and design.* Cambridge, MA: Harvard University Press.

43. Early Intervention Foundation. (2020). What is early intervention? https://www.eif.org.uk/why-it-matters/what-is-early-intervention. Accessed December 22, 2020.

44. Woodman, K. (2016). *Evidence briefing in support of the universal health visiting pathway.* Edinburgh: NHS Health Scotland.

45. Peckover, S. (2019). Brain-based discourses and early intervention: A critical debate for health visiting. *Journal of Health Visiting, 7*(7), 342–350.

46. Feletti, V. J. (2002). The relation between adverse childhood experiences and adult health: Turning gold into lead. *The Permanente Journal, 6*(1), 44.

47. Scottish Government (2008). *Getting it right for every child.* Edinburgh: Scottish Government.

48. HM Government. (2018). Working Together to Safeguard Children: A guide to inter-agency working to safeguard and promote the welfare of children. https://www.gov.uk/government/publications/working-together-to-safeguard-children--2. Accessed June 29, 2020.

# 8

# LEADERSHIP SKILLS FOR LEADING HEALTH VISITING PRACTICE

KAREN STANSFIELD ▪ VICKY GILROY

## CHAPTER CONTENTS

INTRODUCTION

NATIONAL CONTEXT

OVERVIEW OF LEADERSHIP THEORY

A MODEL OF LEADERSHIP DEVELOPMENT FOR HEALTH VISITING

SELF-AWARENESS – SEEING YOURSELF AS A LEADER/LEADERSHIP IDENTITY

DEVELOPING LEADERSHIP CAPABILITY

CONCLUSION

## LEARNING OUTCOMES

*To:*

- understand the importance of effective leadership in health visiting
- critically explore leadership theories that align to health visiting practice
- consider a model for leadership within health visiting
- reflect on personal leadership skills and consider areas for future development

## INTRODUCTION

This chapter will introduce the concept of leadership, exploring why and how leadership skills, capability and capacity can support health visiting practice to deliver best outcomes for children and families. One of the proficiencies for practice is 'strategic leadership for health and wellbeing',[16]

and Public Health England (PHE)[1] highlighting the important role of health visitors as leaders of the Healthy Child Programme, as such health visitors are expected to lead and be leaders. The reality of achieving this will be explored with consideration of the complex and diverse systems in which health visiting operates.

The last decade has seen a plethora of leadership theories in an attempt to find the solution to effective leadership to support excellent care in the NHS. The Kings Fund have written extensively on the type of approaches that may or may not facilitate the development of effective leaders and leadership within both health and social care settings. Despite this, there remains a gap in the direct application of leadership theories that support and enhance health visiting practice. This chapter will explore some of the key contemporary theories and consider their relevance to health visiting.

The ability to lead requires health visitors to be equipped with the leadership skills, the authority to act and the self-belief that they are leaders. Research by Stansfield[2] found that, when asked if they identified themselves as leaders, health visitors were not confident to make this claim; however, after further analysis of their self-reported skills and attributes, many of these aligned to the skills and capabilities of leaders as defined by the NHS Leadership Competency Framework.[3] This highlights the need to consider how to support health visitors to identify and recognise their personal leadership capacity. Stansfield[4] proposes a model of leadership for health visiting which aims to support the application of leadership to the context of health visiting (the model will be introduced later in this chapter).

The NHS Leadership Academy (NHSLA) and Health Education England (HEE) highlight that personal leadership development is not a static process; it is important that health visitors are encouraged and supported to consider opportunities for self-development. Following their introduction to leadership as part of pre-registration nurse education, health visitors need to consider their Continuing Professional Development (CPD) needs. Consideration will be given to potential opportunities for health visitors to develop their personal leadership potential and identity as part of a lifelong process.

## NATIONAL CONTEXT

NHS Policy acknowledges the need for effective leadership at all levels, with a focus on the delivery of high quality, effective and compassionate care through ensuring the NHS 'has the right staff, in the right numbers with the right skills' Department of Health (DH).[5] Across the UK the development of quality leaders at every level has been advocated as crucial to the modernisation agenda.[5–9]

HEE[10,11] highlighted the need for the development of leadership skills to be embodied in pre-registration standards for all healthcare students, with the aim of preparing the future workforce to lead effectively at all levels. This laid the path for a revised set of standards for pre-registration where leadership is explicitly stated in Platform 5, Leading and managing nursing care and working in teams, standards of proficiency for registered nurses.[12] The revised NMC Code of Conduct states that all nurses should '*Provide leadership to make sure people's wellbeing is protected and to improve their experiences of the health and care system*'.[12:22] In their paper 'Everyone's a leader' the RCN[13] highlight the tension for nurses experience working in the increasingly complex environment of health care; specifically acute shortages of a skilled workforce mean greater expectations of the new registrant to demonstrate leadership capacity and skills. With a significant period of austerity health visitors' numbers have been seen to drop over the last five years, leading to wide variance in service delivery across England (Institute of Health Visiting (iHV)).[14] Anandaciva et al[15] highlight the impossible task of delivering leadership in the NHS, due to a lack of attention to the context of the leader's environment and the complexity surrounding this.

Whilst currently under review, leadership continues to form a core part of the standards for health visiting practice within the Specialist Community Public Health Nursing (SCPHN) standards;[16] building on the pre-registration standards, it is expected that leadership capacity will remain central to the role of health visitors. The Recommended National Curriculum for SCPHN[17] delineates the need for practitioners to have leadership knowledge through education and skills and through application to the context of practice. This is important to consider as whilst programmes can impart knowledge to the learner it is only through the art and practice of leadership that individuals can identify themselves as leaders – a view supported by Stansfield[4] and Curtis et al,[34] who highlight the need for health visitors and nurses to be given the opportunity to reflect and apply their knowledge and skills in practice to consolidate their learning.

There is a growing body of evidence that organisations with 'good leadership' report better outcomes for patients. Development of leaders and leadership skills has been perceived as a means of constantly improving high quality, safe and compassionate healthcare in complex organisations.[18–20] Applying this principal to health visiting, The Healthy Child Programme (HCP)[21] acknowledges the importance of the health visitor as the lead professional in the community for child and family health delivering a programme of preventative and early intervention activities with families. However, specific literature on health visiting and leadership is limited and tends to refer to leadership within 'community nursing' or 'nursing' which does not readily translate to the public health context of health visiting.[22]

## OVERVIEW OF LEADERSHIP THEORY

### What is leadership?

#### Reflection point

Before reading on, consider the following points:
- What do you think leadership is?
- Do you consider yourself to be a leader?
- What skills and attributes do you think you will need to lead in your professional practice?

It is important to consider what the term 'leadership' means to health visitors in practice. The Chartered Institute of Professional Development (CIPD) defines it as the *'ability and capacity to lead and influence others, by means of personal attributes and/or behaviours, to achieve a common goal'.*[23] The NHS long-term plan[24] advocates the need for visible 'clinical leadership' at all levels, however, clinical leadership can mean different things in different contexts. These meanings are often conflated, which can make participating in senior organisational management more difficult for people with clinical backgrounds, alongside those with clinical roles not valuing their own leadership capabilities with the families and colleagues they support.

Leadership has been described as a process whereby an individual influences a group of individuals to achieve a common goal.[25–27]

Furthermore, Northouse[27] defines leadership as complex with a range of components: leadership is a process; leadership involves influence; leadership occurs in a group context; leadership involves goal attainment. The importance of the multi-faceted nature of leadership should not be underestimated and can at times act as a barrier to healthcare staff who do not identify themselves as leaders within clinical practice.[4]

One of the most cited definitions of leadership is from John Kotter who delineates between management processes that are concerned with planning, budgeting, organising, staffing, controlling and problem-solving and leadership processes that involve establishing direction, aligning people, motivating and inspiring.[28] According to Marquis and Hudson,[29] there is still some confusion about the relationship between leadership and management within nursing. Some view leadership as one of a number of functions of managers, while others argue that the skills required for leadership are more complex than those needed for management. As a health visitor, it is likely that you will have situations where you will be both leading and managing in tandem. The NHS Leadership Framework[53] acknowledges that to lead requires a range of capabilities including those traditionally focused on management tasks.

There is extensive literature on leadership theory spanning a number of decades; however one of the biggest challenges remains: how to produce effective leaders that have an impact on client/patient wellbeing. To enable us to understand how leadership can be applied to the practice of health visitors it is important that practitioners are able to consider which theory or approach may be most relevant to them. The next section will provide a short summary of some of the seminal leadership theories. It is important to consider that a theory is a view of a situation that can help us to explain or make sense of the context (Oxford Dictionary). Some theories are validated by evidence through structured research. However, the diverse environments that the health visiting workforce operates in adds a level of complexity that current theoretical models do not always accommodate with a general lack of direct research relating to the application and understanding of leadership within health visiting. The Leadership Development Model,[2] developed through empirical research, attempts to address this gap and provide a model of leadership that can be applied to health visiting practice.

## Historical development of leadership theory

Marquis and Hudson[29] suggest that historically leadership theories can be classified into the following main categories: trait or great man, behavioural, contingency/situational, transactional and transformational approaches. A common feature of all these theories is that they focus on the individual leader and how they behave or act. Arguably in all these views the leader needs followers who will be influenced or served by the leader. More recent contemporary theories of the 1990s and 2000s onwards focus more on the role of multiple leaders interacting together as a collective where leadership can be shared or distributed amongst a number of people. These collective leaders need to be compassionate and authentic with emotional intelligence.

The trait theories of the early 1900s considered that a leader was born with a set of attributes which allowed them to lead effectively. From this perspective you either had the skills or you didn't. Applying this to health visiting simplistically, you could argue that some health visitors can be leaders and some can't based on predisposed qualities they may or may not hold. This, however, does not take into account what the leader does and theorists of the 1930's and 1970's started to consider the behaviours of the leader.

The behavioural theorists concentrate on how the leader behaves in different situations.[30] In the 1930s, Kurt Lewin developed a framework based on a leader's behaviour. He argued that there are three types of leaders. Autocratic leaders who he proposed tend to make decisions in isolation from their teams and mainly in situations that require a rapid response. Democratic leaders allow the team to provide input before making a decision. This style is more participative and can be used when there needs to be a consideration of the wider teams' opinions and to ensure that everyone's voice is considered. Laissez-faire leaders are described as those who don't interfere. They allow people within the team to make decisions and act without direction.

### Reflection point

Consider the situations in health visiting that would require:
1. An autocratic approach
2. A democratic approach
3. A laissez-faire approach

Behavioural theories continued to evolve and considered a wide range of models and styles of behaviour which are beyond the scope of this chapter.[31] What is important is that these approaches are still evident within contemporary leadership models and offer a different perspective to situations that leaders may encounter. This marks the fundamental difference between the older trait theories and behavioural theories, as the behavioural theorists propose that you can train individuals to change their behaviour and learn leadership; therefore anyone can be a leader if given the training. This is evidenced in the wide range of contemporary leadership programmes aimed at supporting staff development of leadership attributes and behaviours (NHSLA, 2013).[19]

It is worth spending a few moments to consider servant leadership which was developed by Greenleaf in the 1970s and has been considered to be strongly aligned to the behavioural approaches to leading. This theory considered that the leader actively chooses to 'serve' those they are working with and leading. Greenleaf proposes that the leader aims to service those around them, and this is their primary purpose; importantly, this could include individuals and or organisations. The leader in this instance can use a range of behaviours to support them; however the Greenleaf Organisation (www.greenleaf.org) suggests that their approach is most strongly aligned to democratic behaviours. Interestingly, this approach remains a prominent theory, being supported by leading authors such as Stephen Covey,[32] the author of *7 Habits of Highly Effective People* (2004), and in recent nursing papers where it has been argued that this perspective still resonates with nursing where nurses 'serve' to meet the patients' needs and should be considered as a key theory to underpin nursing care.[32] However, arguably within health visiting, one of the key purposes is to promote health and wellbeing and independence[16] through health creating (salutogenic behaviour) which in essence doesn't resonate with a servant approach to providing support.

This leads us to consider the importance of the context of the leader's position and the influence of external factors on the approach. Such theories have been categorised by some as contingency and situational theories.[30] Hershey and Blanchard's situational research (1969)[71] showed that it was the situation that the leader found themselves in that influenced their leadership capacity. The need to consider context and the impact on an individual's behaviour is important for health visitors and will be drawn upon later in this chapter when we consider a leadership model for health visiting.

The final two dominant theories highlighted by Marquis and Hudson[29] are transactional and transformational. Transactional leadership focuses on the exchange between the leader and others. The focus is on the need to control and command supporting organisational compliance and meeting performance targets.[26,33,34] Furthermore, transaction focuses on the 'action' of one person on another to support the achievement of goals for example targets, as oppose to outcomes for individuals. Relating this to health visiting achieving a number of contacts per a contract is a transaction; however it does not focus on the outcomes for the family or the health behaviour that might have been influenced. These theories of an individual holding the power and making the decisions have been challenged, with calls for the NHS to move away from the Heroic Style of leadership and to move towards shared and collective responsibility, recognising that one person alone cannot lead large organisations and leadership is required at every level (Ham, 2011).[18,27,31]

Leadership development in health care highlights that transformational leadership theory is the most influential theory guiding health care leadership research in nursing.[35,64] This theory was first introduced by Burns in the 1970s, Bass[25] then built upon Burns's work, focusing more in-depth on how the leader influences their followers and the ethical components of leading effectively. Bass[25] explored in detail how the leader was able to influence through the generation of trust and role-modelling. He considered four key roles of the transformational leader. These are sometimes referred to as the four 'I's of transformational leadership:

## BOX 8.1

**Inspirational Motivation** The leaders offers vision and encourages those around to feel like they are a part of something big and worthwhile. In doing so, the leader is energised and focused with a clear purpose and direction.

**Individualised Attention** The leader focuses on the people around them, embracing diversity and building relationships. The leader is known to the team and they feel they know the leader; there is a feeling of mutual respect and trust.

**Intellectual Stimulation** The leader is focused on developing the followers to support their learning and performance. They value imagination and aspiration and look for new solutions. They are agile thinkers who like to see things from new and different perspectives.

**Idealised Influence** The leader acts as a role model. The leader is loyal and trustworthy, offering ethical and sound advice to their followers.

Reflecting on the application of this approach to health visiting it can be argued that the four 'I's of transformational leadership are well aligned to practice, where health visitors are creating vision with their colleagues and families, embracing diversity and focused on developing the best potential. In some situations, the health visitor needs to role model to guide and support new parents, for example, demonstrating attunement. Gilmartin and D'Aunno[35] identify that transformational leadership is associated with positive impact in relation to work-life balance, staff well-being, positive nursing outcomes, patient safety, openness about errors, and patient and staff satisfaction.

Transformational leadership arguably has a clear place within today's health care systems. However, despite this, recent reports highlight the need to consider moving away from a focus on the leader-follower model, which still dominates the transformational approach, and consider leadership as a collective.[36] Recent reviews of leadership theories have focused on leadership as a relationship between the leader and others.[37] Taking this stance, it takes two or more to have a relationship when a leader is only one person with one set of skills or behaviours. This view that leadership is about collective, as opposed to individuals, is promoted in the report Developing Collective Leadership (West et al[36]), where they suggest that 'collective leadership, as opposed to command-and-control structures – provides the optimum basis for caring cultures' (p13). West et al.[36] argue that, if we want staff to treat patients with respect, care and compassion, all leaders and staff must treat their colleagues with respect, care and compassion, which are central ingredients of therapeutic relationships. Health visitors leading programmes of care require strong therapeutic relationships.[38]

Collective leadership is therefore important to consider within health visiting. The Kings Fund Patient Centred Leadership Report,[15] describes a leadership approach that entails distributing and allocating leadership responsibility to wherever expertise, capability and motivation sit within organisations.

## BOX 8.2

Key features of this approach include:

- a partnership approach between staff and management
- strong promotion of collective leadership through staff engagement
- communication of information on engagement levels and linked improvements in service delivery throughout the organisation
- quick action after listening events to bring about change
- timely feedback to staff about achievements through a 'you said – we did' approach

West, M., et al. (2014) *Developing collective leadership for healthcare*. https://www.kingsfund.org.uk/sites/default/files/field/field_publication_file/developing-collective-leadership-kingsfund-may14.pdf.

Collective leadership promotes that everyone takes responsibility for the success of the organisation as a whole, with a move from focusing on their own jobs or sphere of practice. Within a collective leadership approach, West et al[36] promote the need for collective capability and focusing on the skills and personal development of the whole rather than self-service of a few, as seen in previous leadership development models.

A central component of collective leadership is the need for compassion. Compassionate leaders have been defined as those who use a high level of self-awareness and emotional intelligence to truly listen to what people tell them and then respond with empathy and actions that make a positive difference.[72] Daniel Goleman (2002) wrote extensively on the need for leaders to be emotionally intelligent; in its simplest form this means the ability to recognise one's own and others' emotions.

A growing body of evidence suggests that compassionate leaders are aware and attentive to the 'here and now', which enables them to tap into feelings and concerns that may otherwise have not been explored. West et al. (2017) suggest the compassionate leader is concerned with four key areas: attending, understanding, empathising and helping. For the leader to be effective, West et al. (2017) suggest that a collective approach is required where 'leadership is for all and by all' (p9). Compassionate leadership is an approach that would appear to support the work of Donetto et al.[38] where it is highlighted that the non-directive partnership based approaches to health visiting were seen as helpful in supporting mothers' self-confidence, whilst space for listening, reflective dialogue and therapeutic touch contribute to the development of trusting relationships with health visitors. This view aligns well to the complex context of health visiting practice where the practitioner needs to be flexible and adaptive to the needs of the individual, family and community and the system that they operate within.

## THINKING SPACE

Read the quote below and consider the compassionate leadership demonstrated by this health visitor. Would you have previously thought of this as leadership?

Quote from Jane Fisher, parent expert by experience:

*What you [health visitor] offered me was more profound and complex than what could be summarised on a monitoring form. Because what you offered me was hope. You offered me a safe space to share my mental pain and distress. You contained my distress and allowed me to feel heard and valued… you fought for me. When I had no strength to fight for my own care. You spoke up for me, for my needs. You were the voice for our family. Alone in this struggle, we would have no voice. We did not know what to say. But you did…. Thank you for believing that things would change.*

The iHV Vision for Health Visiting (iHV[39]) highlights that:

*Health visiting is part of a 'system' – we maximise the impact of the service by working collaboratively with partners. Clear leadership for children and families' public health is essential to ensure plans are in place which are co-ordinated across the area and across those responsible for the wider determinants of health. iHV (iHV[39] p45)*

This view is well aligned with the four nation's policy relating directly to health visiting and raises the need for health visitors to be effective leaders across systems; indeed, recent NHS policy has focused on the term 'systems leader'. A useful definition of systems leadership is '*Leadership across organisational and geopolitical boundaries, beyond individual professional disciplines, within a range of organisational and stakeholder cultures, often without direct managerial control'*. Comparing this definition to the role of health visitors as described in Cowley et al[40] report, health visiting is depicted through a set of values, skills and attitudes needed to deliver universal health visiting services across boundaries through salutogenesis (health creation), person-centredness (human valuing) and viewing the person in situation (human ecology). In this context key effective leadership in health visiting is the need to focus on the relationships and context of the practice.

The NHS Leadership Academy's Systems Leadership Development Framework[73] offers four domains:

- Innovation and improvement
- Relationships and connectivity
- Individual effectiveness
- Learning and capacity-building

As highlighted health visitors work within complex systems which are constantly evolving. Integrated care is a key feature of the NHS and health visitors need to be able to navigate and lead within this context. Applying the NHSLA's systems Leadership Development Framework (2020), health visitors need to develop capacity and capability in each domains of systems leadership.

Case study 8.1 considers how a health visitor might apply this framework to their practice.

### Case study 8.1

Judith is a health visitor who has a lead role in the promotion of Healthy Weight and Healthy Nutrition. She wants to influence her local area childhood obesity pathway using a systems leadership approach.

#### Innovation and improvement

- She needs to understand who she needs to talk to and who to take her pathway ideas to.
- She has a clear idea on how the pathway will support better and consistent access for her clients to additional support – she has reviewed the national obesity pathway and can evidence what good would look like.
- She knows that this needs to be about a service-wide approach but starts with a focus on her own area so she can build a strong case.

#### Relationships and connectivity

- She builds a strong relationship with the local authority lead for obesity and finds out when the strategy group meets, she gains her line managers support to attend.
- She connects with her Clinical Commissioning Group (in England) and establishes who in primary care has an interest in this area.
- She asks the families who have been identified as having overweight or obese children at their two-year review what would have been helpful from the service by holding a series of local engagement groups.

#### Individual effectiveness

- She talks to her colleagues and asks them their views showing her commitment and willingness to lead the change locally.
- She takes responsibility for leading this work within her service and ensuring that the key messages are shared.

#### Learning and capacity-building

- She considers what is working in her approach as part of a continuous learning – 'test, evaluate and adapt for continuous improvement'.
- She knows that it is not easy to influence change but keeps focus on the outcome for children and families.
- She seeks guidance from colleagues in other areas and links with her professional bodies for ideas to share learning attending National training on the topic.

This section of the chapter has explored a range of contemporary leadership theories. We will now consider a model for health visiting that builds on these recognising that there has been limited focus on leadership development within health visiting practice.

# A MODEL OF LEADERSHIP DEVELOPMENT FOR HEALTH VISITING

The leadership development model was developed from research undertaken as part of a Doctorate in Business Administration. The research focused on exploring how health visitors understand the social processes of leadership as a shared process that happens between individuals through relationships in an organisation, as opposed to looking at leadership as an individual activity only undertaken by formal leaders.[2]

The leadership model has been evaluated positively through two projects funded by The Burdett Nursing Trust in 2018 and 2019. These projects involved the leadership development model[2] being embedded in the leadership development training programme developed by the iHV. The leadership development model has subsequently been adopted by the iHV as the model of choice for their health visiting leadership development programme.

In addition, a leadership game has been developed to support the concepts embedded in the leadership development model to use as an interactive tool for learning about leadership. This was invented from research by Stansfield[41] and developed with the iHV and Focus Games. The leadership game has been used very successfully with a range of professionals (e.g. nurses, health visitors, school nurses, social workers etc.) and has been evaluated as a useful tool that relates to the leadership development model[4] to support the development of knowledge and understanding about leadership theories specifically shared, collective compassionate leadership.

## The leadership development model

The model is made up of four elements (see Figure 8.1).[4] The leadership development model asks health visitors to consider several questions

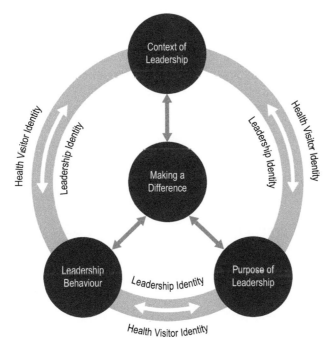

Figure 8.1 ▪ The Leadership Development Model.[4]

about the leadership activities they are undertaking. It starts by considering context: that is, **What** is it that you are leading? Followed by the purpose of leadership: that is, **Why** are you leading? Then leadership behaviour: **How** are you leading? Whilst considering professional and leadership identity: Are you clear on what your professional role is?; and, Do you see yourself as a leader?

The model works by explaining how a health visitor undertakes their leadership role and suggests that if you consciously recognise the what, why and how of your leadership, you will build your leadership identity. As we know, consciously seeing yourself as a leader and articulating your leadership role is essential for a leadership identity to develop.[42]

The four elements of the model are discussed in more detail below:

**Context of leadership – (What am I leading?)** – being able to understand the situation in which leadership exists, that is the social context, is central to many leadership definitions.[43] This is discussed throughout the chapter as the context frames the processes and consequences of leadership within organisations.[44] '*The social context of organisations is often intense, dynamic, multifaceted, ambiguous, information-rich and communication-dependent*'.[45:213] Therefore, how individuals in this case health visitors relate to each other within organisations can only be understood by being aware of the social contexts within which they work and lead.[4,42]

**Purpose of leadership – (Why am I leading?)** – this is often understood to mean the direction an organisation wants to go in as described by its vision and the strategies it needs to adopt to meet that vision.[31,42] This builds on the transformational leadership discussed above that clearly articulates the importance of having a vision. Being clear about purpose is important for health visitors, for it enables them to engage in shaping their own roles in the development and delivery of children and community services. If health visitors are to understand the strategic objectives of the multiple organisations that they work across and be able to take changes forward systematically, it is essential to be clear about why they are doing this.[2]

**Leadership behaviour – (How am I leading?)** – the behaviour of leaders in an organisation is seen as crucial to the culture that is created in the organisation. What leaders do is more important than what they say.[4,43] It is well recognised in the literature that 'action over words' in leadership is seen as a marker of authenticity[43] and the importance of making individuals understand the actions of the leadership through meaning and sense-making[27] is crucial to engaging colleagues in leadership. This is because seeing what can be accomplished through leadership action makes individuals feel inspired.[34,46]

**Making a difference** – the idea of 'making a difference to children and families' in health visiting was first articulated through the work of Whittaker et al.[47] They developed the concept whilst undertaking the study, 'Start and Stay: The Recruitment and Retention of Health Visitors'. In this study, they identified which, *beliefs and values influence professional identities and behaviour*, which form a distinctive *ideology of health visiting practice*, (p54). They summarised this in the phrase *making a difference to children and families*; they believe this single phrase best describes what health visitors see as the purpose of their role and what they are striving to achieve. It was their view that, '*fulfilment of making a difference was consistent with working to an acceptable professional health visiting ideology*' (p110), which builds on the notion of orientation to practice developed by Cowley et al.[40] in Why Health Visiting?

Making a difference demonstrates the outcome of the leadership activity undertaken by the health visitor that can be measured and seen in relation to improving children, families and community health.[4]

The leadership development model enables health visitors at all stages of their professional career to consider through understanding the **context** in which they lead; the **purpose** in why they are leading; and the **behaviours** they need to demonstrate to achieve the ultimate of making a difference. This will be different for all health visitors as they arrive in health visiting with different experiences, having accessed health visiting education through different routes: for example, nursing, child, adult, learning disability, mental health or through midwifery.[12,48] The leadership development model provides an opportunity for all health visitors and health-visiting students, regardless of the route by which they came into the profession, to reflect on where they are in their leadership journey.

## SELF-AWARENESS – SEEING YOURSELF AS A LEADER/ LEADERSHIP IDENTITY

### Identity

The fourth element of the model relates to being clear about your professional identity and creating a leadership identity.[2,4] The context of where you work can affect your identity; external factors, such as government policies, can impact on the identity of your role both as a health visitor and a leader. The leadership development model suggests that health visitor and leader identity is required for leadership to occur.

The literature suggests that identity gives leaders a sense of knowing who they are,[49] the goals and objectives they need to achieve, and what their own strengths and limitations are as a leader.[42] Research studies have supported the notion that to be a leader you have to see yourself as a leader first: that is you have to develop a leader's identity.[42,50] The reason is that if you think of yourself as a leader you are more likely to look for opportunities to undertake leadership and, therefore, build your leadership identity through experience and developing leadership skills.[42,50]

Health visitor identity is inextricably linked to their model of practise. Many health visitors (Band 6 in England) in the research study by Stansfield[2] recognised leadership as part of the health-visiting role. However, they did not always see themselves as leaders, especially in relation to the public health leadership role of the health visitor (Poulton, 2009).[51,52] Even though health visitors in the same study reported undertaking several well-recognised leadership activities[2,27,31,53] they still didn't see themselves as leaders, even though they understood the potential for health visitors to be both leaders and followers.[4]

### Case study 8.2

This case study illustrates how the leadership development model can be used in practice.

Julie, the mother of three-month-old baby Jack, has recently been diagnosed with post-natal depression and anxiety. Viola, the family's health visitor, will consider the **context (What is she leading?)** – the circumstances she is leading on in the work environment: that is family, team or organisational level. In this example the context of Viola's leadership is within the family and across professional/organisational boundaries; for example, working with GPs, the Perinatal Mental Health Team and voluntary/charity organisations. Perinatal illness may affect the bonding/attachment between Julie and Jack and her relationship with her partner. Given there are potentially several professionals/organisations working with the family, Viola will be required to liaise across organisational/professional boundaries and think about their leadership culture, as well as her own organisational culture, and how the different professionals/services work together or differently when addressing the needs of this family.

The **purpose (Why is she leading?)** — Viola will now think about what intervention she will make with the family and what her leadership role is: that is, What goal has Viola and the family agreed they are working towards? How will other organisations/professionals be involved in a co-ordinated way to achieve the goal? It is important at this step in the model for Viola to consider her model of practice and to be clear on what the goal of the intervention is to ensure that outcome measures can be considered at the same time. Viola will consider the needs of all members of the family and what is required to build their assets, whilst specifically supporting Julie through her post-natal depression and anxiety. Viola actively encourages the family members to express their feelings and be involved in all decisions about the family. Viola has agreed with the family and other services to co-ordinate the interventions across services to ensure the support received is seamless. Viola works with Julie and offers her therapeutic support visits; collectively, they agree on goals to support Julie's anxiety and depression. Viola takes a lead initially as Julie has low mood and energy, but as she begins to recover Viola is able to adapt her approach, and Julie initiates the contact and support. During these supportive contacts Viola is able to focus on both Julie and partner whilst considering the needs of Jack. Promotion of health to the whole family in this context is key.

Viola then considers her **leadership behaviours:** How will she behave as a leader? How will she demonstrate leadership through her actions with the family and other services? Role-modelling to the family and other services is very important because how she acts is more important than what she says. If the intervention is predicated on working together Viola

has to authentically demonstrate how working jointly with the family and other services will be undertaken and how the goals will be achieved. Because of Julie's post-natal depression and anxiety it's essential to role-model activities that promote attachment to Jack by Julie. In doing this, Viola demonstrates her expertise and understanding of effective strategies to support Julie and her family through her perinatal illness. Similarly, working together through a partnership approach with other professionals/organisations involved with the family enables Viola to demonstrate her leadership role by ensuring joint decision-making that has the family at the centre.

Viola will then consider if she has **made a difference** by reviewing the goals and outcomes related to the intervention agreed at the start. This is an important activity for Viola to undertake to demonstrate the value of the health visiting service and how she has worked with other services and what contribution this has made to the family.

From applying the model to her practice, Viola can clearly identify what her leadership intervention has been with the family to other professionals/organisations: the what, why and how of leadership. This enables Viola to consciously recognise her leadership role, which is important because the more Viola can identify her leadership activities, the more her leadership identity will grow. The model provides a framework for Viola to use in her personal development. By reflecting on such interventions, Viola can identify what further leadership opportunities would enable her to develop her leadership skills.

Finally, just to emphasise it is important to use the model to reflect on what went well and on what could have gone better, in terms of leadership development at a systems level as well as at an individual level. Health visiting can be complex and organisational challenges need to be captured as well as individual development when applying such models in practice.

# DEVELOPING LEADERSHIP CAPABILITY

## Developing leadership

There is little empirical evidence that directly links a specific leadership development programme with positive outcomes for patients.[18] So, there is no one best way to develop leaders or leadership. That is not to say that leadership/leader development programmes do not have benefits for the individual involved.[44] What is known to be valuable is leadership experience for individuals to be able to develop their leader/leadership skills that are supported through appropriate guidance in situ[18,42]; i.e. in the context/situation in which they work.[44]

Health visitors do not routinely access leadership development/training, even when commencing leadership roles. Professional practice appears to be what is valued and enables a health visitor to be a leader. This may provide one explanation as to why some health visitors don't identify themselves as leaders and may feel they lack leadership skills.[2] For health visitors it is seen as important to embed leadership within professional practice as it is understood through professional background and context. It is clear that health visitors are always practitioners first, and leadership is seen as part of being a professional.[4]

Historically, leadership modules in many health visitor education programmes have focussed on individual and team leadership skills and styles and have been related to the Healthcare Leadership Model specific to the country (e.g.[53] in England and Scottish Government, 2013).[54,74] Typically, leadership education has been delivered at the end of the health-visiting programme, although this is changing and more programmes are delivering leadership education throughout.[17] Stansfield[2] suggests what has been missing from leadership development, in both pre-qualifying and CPD programmes in health visiting, is a focus on developing a leadership identity.

The development of a leadership identity is important for health visitors as the literature highlights the importance of professional identity but also the importance of seeing oneself as a leader: identity has a significant impact on behaviour[42] and typically involves behaviours *in which individuals change their perceived identity as a leader.*[50:608] Therefore, it is essential that an introduction to role identity, that incorporates both being a health visitor and a leader, is included early in education programmes for health visitors and opportunities to reflect and apply in practice settings are available.

Health visitors don't view effective leadership training as a one-off course/module, but rather as a sequence of activities and support roles.[2] This approach to leadership development, that recognises the need for continuing support, is highlighted in the literature.[18,31]

How leadership programmes are designed, and the methods used to deliver them, dramatically alters the effectiveness of the training. What's needed is content that reflects the context and purpose of leadership for the professional group and the behaviours required in the leadership programme, together with methods of delivery that are inclusive and allow practitioners to try out new skills in a safe environment and practice them in the workplace. However, central to these developments is an understanding of the professional's identity and level of development required, as discussed by Lord and Hall[50] and Day and Harrison.[42]

Communities of Practice, mentorship, preceptorship and Action Learning Sets have been found to support the development of leadership[18,41] and are beneficial when embedding identity amongst practitioners.[18] These are activities that are available on some SCPHN and CPD programmes (e.g. iHV). Other activities that are known to support leadership development include being able to test out leadership situations in a safe environment. In addition, feedback is considered important and active learning through role-playing out leadership scenarios (e.g. courageous conversations in a safe environment) have been found to be beneficial.[41] It is equally important to learn about leadership in practice – continuously within a supportive environment with managers who involve health visitors in service design and delivery and provide shadowing opportunities (Whittaker et al, 2013).

Stansfield[2] suggests that the strongest influence for health visitors on leadership is role models. In addition, 'learning from doing', in line with social learning theory,[55] accumulating experiences that allow a person to test out decision-making skills and responsibility-taking are also extremely important.[18,49] This suggests that experience, combined with skills and knowledge in leadership with support and guidance, provides the best preparation for leadership. This is supported by Day and Harrison[42] who recognise the benefits of exposure to opportunities to develop leadership in practice.

## The importance of role-modelling to leadership development

A role model has been defined *as a cognitive construction based on the attributes of people in social roles an individual perceives to be similar to him or herself to some extent and desires to increase perceived similarity by emulating those attributes.*[56:136] 'Role-modelling is a traditional expectation' in nursing, whereby 'less experienced nurses' learn 'from more experienced nurses'. [57:101] In the leadership literature role-modelling is cited as a means of understanding and learning about leadership.[46,58]

Social learning theory[55] suggests that individuals learn what to do and how to behave by observing and emulating role models. This social learning begins when individuals focus their attention on modelled behaviours, meaning that they do not need to experience first-hand the activity to learn from it. This, it is suggested, is possible through observation of others rather than direct experience.[58] This almost certainly occurs 'even without conscious awareness on the part of the role model' (p 1470).[55,59]

Modelling is demonstrated most effectively through actions not words; this is similar to how leadership is role-modelled,[43,58] especially in ethical leadership approaches as these leaders are considered to have 'moral person attributes' (p 106).[60] In addition, it has been suggested that individuals can learn from both positive and negative role models.[58]

The reciprocity from being treated well by a supportive manager on how patients then experience healthcare positively has been well documented in the literature: staff satisfaction from good managers/leaders is directly linked to patient satisfaction.[26,64] In addition, we know that the way staff are treated has a reciprocal effect on how they behave towards clients/patients.[18]

The value and importance of role models to leadership can be understood through the attributes ascribed to role models. The important attributes for a leader are discussed widely in the literature.[31,43,61] These include being fair, knowledgeable, passionate, compassionate, credible, inspiring and motivating.[2,60,62]

In addition, how the leader makes you feel is recognised as being very important in leadership. Effective leaders provide a sense of value to the work that staff undertake and 'a sense of purpose, which inspires staff to be committed'.[63:108] Getting things done is important: i.e., action not just words is central to how effective leadership is recognised in leaders who are role models. In order for health visitors to be able to role-model leadership they need to see it and have the opportunity to build a relationship with leaders in order to know who to approach to influence.[4,52]

Looking up to others has been seen as a key component of the process of role-modelling.[58]

This view supports the earlier discussion that how health visitors learn leadership is by observing and copying leadership in clinical practice and by the experiences they acquire as a professional.[52,55] This experience of working with a role model also has the effect of verifying their own understanding of leadership by allowing health visitors to practise leading when they feel safe and confident.

It is abundantly clear that leadership programmes need to recognise the importance of role models, e.g. mentors/managers[58,59] and social learning theory. It also provides further understanding of how health visitors understand leadership as an unconscious activity that is undertaken through experience in their professional roles and suggests that bringing the activity of leadership more to the forefront, as part of understanding leadership within their role and as part of identity development, could be a beneficial aspect of leadership development.[4]

This resonates again with compassionate/authentic/inclusive leadership theories being espoused in the NHS[24] and discussed earlier in the chapter and in the nursing literature[64] as a way of delivering leadership in practice. Authentic leadership advocates the importance of the requirement for leaders to maintain consistency, in terms of how their expressed values are linked to their ethical conduct.[43]

## Leadership skills required by health visitors

Whilst there exists a range of competency frameworks espousing what leadership behaviour should be demonstrated by health professionals[18,53] there is no specific model that informs the development of leadership skills for every health professional.[50] The introduction of the HEE Leadership model is welcome as an attempt to provide a specific model of leadership development for undergraduate healthcare students.[11]

The undergraduate HEE framework in England identifies key skills that all healthcare professionals should have on registration. This model works on developing '*stage 1 – skills in self, stage 2 – working with others and stage 3 – improving healthcare services*'.[11:20–21]

In the study by Stansfield[2] it was discussed at length with participants the skills health visitors believed needed to be included in leadership training and was articulated as a developing tool kit that would help build confidence. These skills are identified in Table 8.1 and are the same leadership skills frequently identified in the Healthcare Leadership Model[20,53] and other nursing/health visiting leadership literature.[11,54]

The outcomes that health visitors feel would make training useful are increased self-esteem, building confidence to feel empowered to lead and the ability to be assertive.[2] These are similar to those identified in the literature (HEE, 2018).[11,34]

It has been identified that there is a need for leadership training for health visitors but also the need for support to develop those skills and use them. This includes the need to be aware of yourself as a leader and the need to be aware of personal feelings personal esteem. In addition, the need to build up the confidence of health visitors in their ability to lead is essential.

| TABLE 8.1 | |
|---|---|
| **Leadership skills identified that are required by health visitors[2]** | |
| **Communication** | **Prepare a business case** |
| Therapeutic interventions | Change management |
| Theory of leader/leadership styles/models of leadership | The best way to get a message across to people |
| Dealing with conflict | Visioning |
| Influencing policies | Developing the individual/self |
| Political astuteness | Motivation/Motivational interviewing |

Thus, a picture develops that leadership training; should support and provide opportunities to try out new things and experiences, as these are important to allow health visitors to develop as leaders. Recognise that you can't be a good leader unless you understand yourself.[2]

The need to be skilled in political astuteness reflects the changing nature of the role of the health visitor with the incessant change in government health policies[47] and the new skills and knowledge needed by health visitors.[48] Inevitably this is symptomatic of the changing nature of the environment that the health visitor works in and, yet again, the need to reformulate the identity of health visitors[65] as the context of their work environment changes. This reinforces the importance of health visitors consciously recognising the importance of context, the first element of the leadership model.

The ability to communicate with colleagues at different hierarchical levels and in different roles across a range of organisations and to carry the whole team along to achieve the goal is vital for health visitors. Communication skills and, in particular, listening skills are essential components that enable health visitors, or indeed others, to lead.

Offering opportunities to allow several key skills to develop is essential: for example, reflecting, making people feel valued and motivating people. This reinforces how health visitors learn to lead by application to practice and having the opportunities to try out leadership skills in practice (Curtis et al., 2011).[51,52] This would allow all health visitors to take responsibility because leadership is not title/grade-dependent but something that can be undertaken informally by all health visitors, as it has been suggested that many leadership skills/behaviours can be learnt.[44]

As highlighted at the start of this chapter, health visitors have a key role in leading on the HCP.[75] To do this, health visitors need to have the skills to do this and these skills have to incorporate extensive understanding of the Healthy Child Programme and the ability to work across professional groups and agencies.

## CONCLUSION

This chapter has explored what good leadership means for health visitors and the different leadership theories available for health visitors to use in their practice. It has suggested the use of a specifically designed leadership development model.[4] As a way of articulating and guiding leadership in clinical practice. The importance of developing a leadership as well as a professional identity has been recognised as essential if health visitors are to see themselves as leaders. Leadership development has been discussed and the importance of having opportunities to apply leadership in a safe environment with support from a mentor/manager has been highlighted.

The importance of good role models when developing leadership is essential. The specific skills relevant to health visiting leadership have been discussed and the importance of practicing these in a safe environment and for managers and others to provide leadership opportunities for health visitors to be involved in is essential if health visitors are going to reach their full potential as leaders of children's services.

## KEY LEARNING POINTS

- There are a wide range of leadership theories; however, it is important to consider how they support leadership skills in health visiting.
- Health visitors operate in complex environments; the context needs to be considered if they are to lead effectively.
- To be effective leaders, health visitors need to be outcome-focused.
- Health visitors need to be confident in their own leadership identity and have the opportunity to find their voice to support effective practice.

- Health visitors need to make a difference through leadership and be able to articulate specifically the leadership activities they have undertaken to do this.

## RESOURCES

- The Leadership Game@GameLeadership
- NHSleadershipgame.co.uk
- ihv.org.uk

## REFERENCES

1. Public Health England. (2018). Best start in life and beyond: Improving public health outcomes for children, young people and families. Guidance to support the commissioning of the Healthy Child Programme 0–19: Health visiting and school nursing services. https://assets.publishing.service.gov.uk/government/uploads/system/uploads/attachment_data/file/686928/best_start_in_life_and_beyond_commissioning_guidance_1.pdf.
2. Stansfield, K. J. (2017). Making a difference: How health visitors understand the social processes of leadership. Unpublished Thesis. Sheffield Hallam University.
3. NHS Leadership Academy. (2012). *Clinical leadership competency framework*. https://www.leadershipacademy.nhs.uk/wp-content/uploads/2012/11/NHSLeadership-Leadership-Framework-Clinical-Leadership-Competency-Framework-CLCF.pdf.
4. Stansfield, K. J. (2021). Leadership development for public health practice. In S. Cowley, & K. Whittaker (Eds.), *Community public health in policy and practice* (3rd ed.). London: Elsevier.
5. Department of Health. (2016). Delivering high quality, effective, compassionate care: developing the right people with the right skills and the right values; a mandate from the Government to Health Education England: April 2016 to March 2017. https://assets.publishing.service.gov.uk/government/uploads/system/uploads/attachment_data/file/559940/HEE_mandate_2016-17_acc.pdf.
6. Department of Health Northern Ireland. (2016). Health and wellbeing 2026: Delivering together. October 2016. https://www.healthni.gov.uk/sites/default/files/publications/health/health-and-wellbeing-2026-delivering-together.pdf.
7. NHS Scotland. (2017). Everyone matters: 2020. workforce vision. https://www.gov.scot/publications/everyone-matters-2020-workforce-vision/ https://www.workforcevision.scot.nhs.uk/wp-content/uploads/2017/12/Everyone-Matters-2020-Workforce-Vision-Implementation-Plan-2018-20.pdf.
8. Welsh Government. (2018). A Healthier Wales: Our plan for health and social care. https://gweddill.gov.wales/docs/dhss/publications/180608healthier-wales-mainen.pdf
9. Welsh Government. (2018). The parliamentary review of health and social care in Wales. A revolution from within: Transforming health and care in Wales. https://gweddill.gov.wales/docs/dhss/publications/180116reviewen.pdf.
10. Health Education England. (2015) Understanding and Maximising Leadership in pre-registration nursing. https://www.hee.nhs.uk/sites/default/files/documents/Report%20-%20Maximising%20Leadership%20in%20Pre-eg%20Curricula%20Research%202015_0.pdf.
11. Health Education England (HEE). (2018). *Maximising leadership learning in the pre-registration healthcare curricula*. Models and Guidelines for Healthcare Education Providers: 2018. Guidelines - Maximising Leadership in the Pre-reg Healthcare Curricula (2018).pdf (hee.nhs.uk).
12. Nursing and Midwifery Council (NMC). (2018). Future Nurse: Standards of proficiency for registered nurses. London: NMC. https://www.nmc.org.uk/standards/standards-for-nurses/standards-of-proficiency-forregistered-nurses/.
13. Royal College of Nursing. (2019). RCN Nurses in Leadership and Management Forum.
14. Institute of Health Visiting. (2020). *State of health visiting survey*. https://ihv.org.uk/wp-content/uploads/2020/02/State-of-Health-Visiting-survey-FINAL-VERSION-18.2.20.pdf.
15. Anandaciva, S., Ward, D., Randhawa, M., Edge, R. (2018). Leadership in today's NHS. Delivering the impossible. London: The Kings Fund. Leadership in today's NHS The King's Fund (kingsfund.org.uk).
16. Nursing and Midwifery Council (NMC). (2004). *Standards for specialist community public health nurses*. https://www.nmc.org.uk/standards/standards-for-post-registration/standards-of-proficiency-for-specialist-community-public-health-nurses/.
17. Institute of Health Visiting. (2019). *A recommended national curriculum* https://ihv.org.uk/our-work/education/recommended-national-curriculum/.
18. West, M. A., Armit, K., Loewenthal, L., Eckert, R., West, T., & Lee, A. (2015) *Leadership and leadership development in health care: The evidence base*. https://www.kingsfund.org.uk/sites/default/files/field/field_publication_summary/leadership-in-health-care-apr15.pdf.
19. NHS Leadership Academy. (2020). Developing systems leadership. https://www.leadershipeastmidlands.nhs.uk/sites/default/files/National%20Brochure%20Web%20final.pdf.
20. Scottish Government. (2017). Nursing 2030 Vision: Promoting confident, competent and collaborative nursing

for Scotland's future. https://www.gov.scot/publications/nursing-2030-vision-9781788511001/pages/0/.

21. Department of Health/Department of Children, Schools and Families. (2009). *The Healthy Child Programme: Pregnancy and the first five years of life*. London: The Stationary Office.

22. Baldwin, S. (2013). The importance of leadership development for health visitors. *Journal of Health Visiting*, *1*(1), 38–42.

23. Chartered Institute of Professional Development. (2019). *Leadership factsheet*. https://www.cipd.co.uk/knowledge/strategy/leadership/factsheet.

24. NHS. (2019). *The NHS long term plan*. https://www.longtermplan.nhs.uk/publication/nhs-long-term-plan/.

25. Bass, B. M. (1990). *Handbook of leadership: A survey of theory and research*. New York: Free Press.

26. Cummings, G., MacGregor, T., Davey, M., Lee, H., Wong, C. A., Lo, E. et al. (2010). Leadership styles and outcome patterns for the nursing workforce and work environment: A systematic review. *International Journal of Nursing Studies*, *47*, 363–385.

27. Northouse, P. G. (2018). *Leadership theory and practice* (8th ed.). London: Sage.

28. Kotter, J. P. (1996). *Leading change*. Boston: Harvard Business School Press.

29. Marquis, B. L., & Huston, C. J. (2017) *Leadership roles and management functions in nursing: Theory and application*. Lipincott, Williams and Wilkins.

30. Ahmed, Z., Nawaz, A., & Khan, I. (2016). Leadership theories and styles: A literature review. *Journal of Resources Development and Management*, 16.

31. Yukl, G. (2013). *Leadership in organisations* (8th ed.). Essex: Pearson.

32. Cottey, L., & McKimm, J. (2019). Putting service back into health care through servant leadership. *British Journal of Hospital Medicine*, *80*(4), 220–224.

33. Bass, B. M., & Avolio, B. J. (1993). Transformational leadership and organizational culture. *Public Administration Quarterly*, *17*(1), 112–121.

34. Curtis, E., & O'Connell, R. (2011). Essential leadership skills for motivating and developing staff. *Nursing Management (Harrow)*, *18*(5), 32–35. doi: 10.7748/nm2011.09.18.5.32.c8672.

35. Gilmartin, M. J., & D'Aunno, T. A. (2007). Leadership research in healthcare: A review and roadmap. *The Academy of Management Annals*, *1*(1), 387–438.

36. West, M., et al. (2014) *Developing collective leadership for healthcare*. https://www.kingsfund.org.uk/sites/default/files/field/field_publication_file/developing-collective-leadership-kingsfund-may14.pdf.

37. Mckergrow & Bailey. (2016). *Host six new roles of engagement for teams, organizations, communities and movements*. Solution Books.

38. Donetto, S., et al. (2013). Health visiting: the voice of service users. Learning from service users' experiences to inform the development of UK health visiting practice and services. https://www.kcl.ac.uk/nmpc/research/nnru/publications/reports/voice-of-service-user-report-july-2013-final.pdf.

39. Institute of Health Visiting. (2019). *Health Visiting in England: A vision for the future* https://ihv.org.uk/news-and-views/news/ihv-launches-health-visiting-in-england-a-vision-for-the-future/.

40. Cowley, S., Whittaker, K., Malone, M., et al. (2015). Why health visiting? Examining the potential public health benefits from health visiting practice within a universal service: A narrative review of the literature. *International Journal Nursing Studies*, *52*(1), 465–480.

41. Stansfield, K. J. (2018). *Final Report for the Burdett Nursing Trust – To pilot and implement a targeted leadership development model for Health Visitors/School Nurses to strengthen their collective clinical leadership skills (funded)*. Institute of Health Visiting.

42. Day, D. V., & Harrison, M. M. (2007). A multilevel, identity-based approach to leadership development. *Human Resource Management Review*, *17*, 360–373.

43. Avolio, B. J., & Gardner, W. L. (2005). Authentic leadership development: Getting to the root of positive forms of leadership. *The Leadership Quarterly*, *16*(3), 315–338.

44. Hartley, J., Martin, J., & Benington, J. (2008). *Leadership in healthcare. A review of the literature for health care professionals, managers and researchers*. Commissioned by the National Institute for Health Research (NIHR) Service Delivery and Organization (SDO) Programme.

45. Day, D. V., Gronn, P., & Salas, E. (2006). Leadership in team-based organisations: On the threshold of a new era. *The Leadership Quarterly*, *17*, 211–216.

46. Bowers, J. R., Rosch, D. M., & Collier, D. A. (2015). Examining the relationship between role models and leadership growth during the transition to adulthood. *Journal of Adolescent Research*, *31*(1), 96–118.

47. Whittaker, K., Grigulis, A., Hughes, J., Cowley, S., Morrow, E., Nicholson, C., et al. (2013). *Start and stay: The recruitment and retention of health visitors*. London: National Nursing Research Unit. https://www.kcl.ac.uk/nursing/research/nnru/publications/Reports/Start-and-Stay-report-FINAL.pdf.

48. Malone, M., Whittaker, K., Cowley, S., Ezhova, I., & Maben, J. (2016). Health visitor education for today's

Britain: Messages from a narrative review of the health visitor literature. *Nurse Education Today*, 44, 175–186.

49. Zheng, W., & Muir, D. (2015). Embracing leadership: A multi-faceted model of leader identity development. *Leadership and Organisational Development Journal*, 36(6), 630–656.

50. Lord, R. G., & Hall, R. J. (2005). Identity, deep structure and the development of leadership skill. *The Leadership Quarterly*, 16(4), 591–615.

51. Cameron, S., Harbison, J., Lambert, V., & Dickson, C. (2011). Exploring leadership in community nursing teams. *Journal of Advanced Nursing*, 68(7), 1469–1481.

52. Brigham, L., Maxwell, C., & Smith, A. (2012). Leading in practice: A case study of how health visitors share and develop good practice. *Community Practitioner*, 85(5), 24–28.

53. NHS Leadership Academy. (2013). The Healthcare Leadership Model. Leeds: NHS Leadership Academy. https://www.leadershipacademy.nhs.uk/wp-content/uploads/2014/10/NHSLeadership-LeadershipModel-colour.pdf.

54. Greening, K., & Haydock, D. (2014). Delivering a health visiting leadership programme. *Community Practitioner*, 87(3), 35–37.

55. Bandura, A. (1977). *Social learning theory*. London: Prentice Hall.

56. Gibson, D. (2004). Role models in career development: New directions for theory and research. *Journal of Vocational Behaviour*, 65, 134–156.

57. Murray, C. J., & Main, A. (2005). Role-modelling as a teaching method for student mentors. *Nursing Times*, 101(26), 30–33.

58. Brown, M. E., & Trevino, L. K. (2014). Do role models matter? An investigation of role-modelling as an antecedent of perceived ethical leadership. *Journal of Business Ethics*, 122, 587–598.

59. Ogunfowora, B. (2014). It's all a matter of consensus: Leader role modeling strength as a moderator of the links between ethical leadership and employee outcomes. *Human Relations*, 67, 1467–1490.

60. Brown, M. E., Trevino, L. K., & Harrison, D. A. (2005). Ethical leadership: A social learning perspective for construct development and testing. *Organizational Behavior and Human Decision Processes*, 97(2), 117–134.

61. Bennis, W. A. (2003). Six qualities of leadership. http://changingminds.org/disciplines/leadership/articles/bennis_qualities.htm.

62. Paterson, K., Henderson, A., & Trivella, A. (2010). Educating for leadership: A programme designed to build a responsive health care culture. *Journal of Nursing Management*, 18, 78–83.

63. Dixon-Woods, M., Baker, R., Charles, K., Dawson, J., Jerzembek, G., Martin, G., et al. (2014). Culture and behaviour in the English National Health Service: overview of lessons from a large multimethod study. *British Medical Journal*, 23, 106–115.

64. Wong, C. A., & Giallonardo, L. M. (2013). Authentic leadership and nurse-assessed adverse patient outcomes. *Journal of Nursing Management*, 21, 74–752.

65. Machin, A. I., Machin, T., & Pearson, P. (2011). Maintaining equilibrium in professional role identity: A grounded theory study of health visitors' perceptions of their changing professional practice context. *Journal of Advanced Nursing*, 1526–1537.

66. *Delivering the impossible*. London: Kings Fund. https://www.kingsfund.org.uk/sites/default/files/2018-07/Leadership_in_todays_NHS_summary.pdf.

67. Ham, C., et al. (2011). The future of leadership and management in the NHS: No more heroes https://www.kingsfund.org.uk/sites/default/files/future-of-leadership-and-management-nhs-may-2011-kings-fund.pdf.

68. Supporting paper for RCN congress fringe event 2019 – Everyone's a leader. https://www.rcn.org.uk/get-involved/forums/nurses-in-management-and-leadership-forum/our-work.

69. Poulton, B. (2009). Barriers and facilitators to the achievement of community-focused public health nursing practice: a UK perspective. *Journal of Nursing Management*, 17(1), 74–83.

70. Goleman, Daniel & Boyatzis, Richard & McKee, Annie. (2002). Primal Leadership: Realizing the Power of Emotional Intelligence.

71. Ham, C. (2014). Reforming the NHS from within. Beyond Hierarchy, Inspection and Markets. London: Kings Fund.

72. West, M., Eckert, R., Collins, B., Chowla, R. (2017) Caring to change How compassionate leadership can stimulate innovation in health care. London: The Kings Fund. Caring_to_change_Kings_Fund_May_2017.pdf (kingsfund.org.uk).

73. NHS Leadership Academy. (2017). Developing systems leadership. Interventions, Options and Opportunities. Developing-Systems-Leadership-July-2017.pdf (leadershipacademy.nhs.uk).

74. Scottish Government. (2013). Everyone matters: 2020 health workforce vision. Edinburgh: Scottish Government Accessible from: https://www.gov.scot/publications/everyone-matters-2020-workforce-vision/.

75. Department for Children Schools and Families (2009) Departmental Report. London: The Stationary Office. DCSF-Annual_Report_2009.pdf (publishing.service.gov.uk).

# 9

# TECHNOLOGY AND HEALTH VISITING PRACTICE

RITA NEWLAND

## CHAPTER CONTENTS

WHAT DOES TECHNOLOGY MEAN?

EXAMPLES OF TECHNOLOGY

THE POLICY CONTEXT FOR TECHNOLOGY AND HEALTH VISITING PRACTICE

CHARACTERISTICS OF A DIGITALLY ENHANCED HEALTH SERVICE

IMPLICATIONS FOR HEALTH VISITING PRACTICE

THE WORKFORCE STRATEGY

CORE DIGITAL ABILITY

ESSENTIAL DIGITAL SKILLS FOR HEALTH VISITORS

HEALTH VISITING PRACTICE

RECORD-KEEPING AND DOCUMENTATION

RECORD KEEPING AND THE LAW

TO CREATE A SLIC RECORD, THE HEALTH VISITOR SHOULD

IN ORDER NOT TO CREATE A SLAC RECORD, THE HEALTH VISITOR SHOULD

CONCLUSION

## LEARNING OUTCOMES

*To:*

- Discuss and describe the policy context for the use of technology in health visiting practice
- Outline and critically consider the principles of record keeping and documentation for health visiting practice in a digitally influenced era
- Appraise and critically discuss the priorities for health visitors striving to meet the challenges for health visiting practice and service provision in the Information Age

## WHAT DOES TECHNOLOGY MEAN?

Technology means different things to different people. Essentially, it refers to methods, tools and systems. We use technology to help us to do things quicker and more effectively.

Technology is dynamic and changes in response to emerging needs and demands. Operating in the Information Age of the 21st century, health visitors require technological advancements to enable them to collect, collate, apply and store information. Health visitors therefore use technology in several areas of their practice, including when they:

- communicate with others (i.e. written, verbal and audio-visual)
- facilitate the learning of others including clients, other professionals and students
- facilitate personal learning, education and professional development
- share information with others
- record and document information about client care needs, provision and outcomes

- record and document information about service delivery, provision, quality and outcomes
- securely store information.

If used well, technology will benefit health visitors' practice. However, used incorrectly or maliciously, it has the potential to harm health visitors and clients alike.

### Case study 9.1: An example of poor use of technology in health visiting practice

Claire is a health visitor employed by an NHS Community Trust. In the last 6 months the trust has implemented virtual working and Claire has been given a laptop and a mobile phone. She no longer has a desk or a work base and in the past 3 months has only seen her fellow health visitors on three occasions during sector meetings.

Claire is 'allowed' to work from home and does not need to report daily to the team leader. Claire describes herself as a 'pen and paper girl' because she did not have computers when she was at school. She types with two fingers and finds it difficult to see the small laptop screen clearly. It seems to take her such a long time to access her calendar, let alone 'write up her notes'. Since the onset of virtual working, Claire's working day has been extended by 2 hours as she tries hard to keep up with the record keeping and documentation after a full day of home visits or clinic contacts.

Claire is exhausted, and this has got worse in the past 2 weeks because three members of the six-person team have been away from work because of sickness.

Claire feels that she would have benefited from having time before the onset of virtual working to learn how to use the laptop. She also wishes that she had created time to talk and meet with her colleagues in between the monthly team meetings because she feels lonely and has no one to share her concerns with or talk to when she has had a bad day.

### Case study 9.2: An example of a good use of technology in health visiting practice

Peter has worked as a health visitor in the same trust for 6 years and started working virtually 4 years ago. He uses a laptop for each activity. He likes it because it means that he can easily access information about the clients on his caseload, deal with enquiries and keep an eye on the progress he is making towards his monthly targets using the online dashboard. Before virtual working, he often stayed late at work to complete his record keeping and documentation. This, in addition to a 90-minute commute, meant he was often not home before 7pm. Now he can plan his visits from home, complete the record keeping and documentation during each visit/client contact and finish his working day by 5 pm or 6 pm on days when he starts at 10 am.

The Trust provided IT training before virtual working went 'live', which helped Peter to develop his typing skills and knowledge of the Electronic Patient Record system. He was also able to attend training about time management and making effective use of the electronic calendar.

Peter was part of the virtual working pilot and chaired the health and well-being working group. They implemented a system of 'social spaces' before virtual working began and aligned each health visitor to a hub where they can meet with the same group of health visitors. Each group uses WhatsApp (group chat) to share concerns and workload if needed and each health visitor meets with at least one of their colleagues every day, even if this is for a short period of time.

The standard operating policy for virtual working states that each health visitor can work from home and complete record keeping and documentation at home between the hours of 8am and 6pm. The system is unavailable after 6.30pm in the evening so that the backup process can take place. This means that each health visitor cannot engage in workload activity after 6.30pm each day.

Since commencing virtual working, productivity has increased by 30% and the sickness absence rate has decreased by 10%. The monthly team meetings are well attended and there is usually a vibrant discussion.

## EXAMPLES OF TECHNOLOGY

### Information technology

This section includes the tools needed to store, transfer and process information. Health visitors use Information Technology to enable them to provide the right people with the right information at the right time.

**This involves:**

1. **transferring** information from one department in an organisation to another. This facilitates decision-making within an organization because it allows the information to be available to different people at the same time. For example, it may include information about the number of consultations a health visitor completes each day, the care programme the client/family has been allocated following consultation with the health visitor, care plans and email communication between members of the multidisciplinary team.

2. **providing a management information system**: This allows the health visitor to manage information so it is accessible and available and promotes accuracy and service efficiency. For example: a dashboard is a tool which organises and presents information about the supply, demand and delivery of the service over time. The information is presented in a way that makes it visible, easy to read, understand and explain. This means that, when using the dashboard, the health visitor will be able to see progress towards an outcome: for example, the achievement of key performance indicators (KPIs) and monthly outcome targets.

## Communications technology

Communications technology includes the design, construction and maintenance of communication systems and tools. This technology is used to transmit information from one person or place to another. It allows health visitors to convey ideas, exchange information, and express emotions, using the telephone, the computer, email and text messaging tools. All these tools facilitate the flow of information in the workplace, and help health visitors,

their managers and leaders to make decisions, address client needs and requests and promote efficient and effective service delivery. Examples include the electronic patient health record.

## THE POLICY CONTEXT FOR TECHNOLOGY AND HEALTH VISITING PRACTICE

The four UK countries have developed policy and strategy to increase the use of technology in all aspects of the health and care service provision.[1–5] For health visiting services responsibility for implementing these developments lies with Local Government (England) or local Health Boards (Scotland, Northern Ireland and Wales), in line with the national policy agenda and changes to primary legislation, which seeks to decentralise decision-making and budget responsibility across all areas of health and care provision.[1–5] Health visiting service design and provision across the UK is therefore influenced by different organisations, including:

1. National Government bodies – oversee the planning, provision and quality of the service.
2. Local Government or Health Boards – commission the health visiting service.
3. The Nursing and Midwifery Council (NMC) – as the UK health regulator, ensures the protection of public safety.

All the UK Governments have published policies which detail their commitment to creating a digitally enhanced health and care service.[1–5] This is because the use of technology is seen to be a positive move forward. The assumption is that increasing the use of technology in health and social care will make services quicker, automatic and less labour-intensive. Technology-enhanced services are also seen to be more cost-effective and efficient.

## CHARACTERISTICS OF A DIGITALLY ENHANCED HEALTH SERVICE

1. **Clients/patients have access to health information**

   UK Governments plan to use technology to provide all patients, clients and their carers with access to personalised treatments, improved access to care and a clinician who can manage their health and condition(s).[1–5] Using a range of APPS and Internet links, clients can also access information about specific health related subjects. This information will help them to develop expertise, knowledge and understanding of their health and care situation.[6] This digitally enhanced service is available whenever the client chooses to access it. It is also possible for the client to access the information as many times as they need to. It does not require them to attend a face-to-face appointment.

### THINKING SPACE

a. Using the links below consider how health visitors can use the existing Technology provisions in the NHS to positively influence their practice and service delivery.

   - **NHS Digital:** this site contains information about how the NHS is using data and technology to improve health and social care services https://digital.nhs.uk/
   - **NHS APP Library:** the APPS library houses health and well-being apps that have been assessed to be clinically safe and secure to use https://www.nhs.uk/apps-library/
   - **The Child Protection Information Sharing Project:** a system which allows practitioners in health and social care organisations to securely share information about children who are vulnerable and in need of protection. The interactive map presents details of organisations that are currently using the system https://digital.nhs.uk/services/child-protection-information-sharing-project
   - **The Digital Red Book pilot:** part of NHS England's strategy for using technology to modernise the child health information system. In time it is envisaged that each child will have access to an electronic personal child health record (the e-Red Book) https://digital.nhs.uk/services/digital-red-book-pilot-toolkit
   - **Baby Buddy:** an APP that provides information about pregnancy and the first 6 months of a child's life https://www.nhs.uk/apps-library/baby-buddy/
   - **Ready, steady, baby:** produced by NHS Inform, this is part of the Scottish Government's strategy for using technology to enhance women's knowledge and understanding of pregnancy, labour, delivery and the first 8 weeks of parenthood https://www.nhsinform.scot/ready-steady-baby
   - **Ready, steady, toddler:** this suite of information is one of three produced by NHS Inform and focuses on the health, well-being and care needs of the toddler http://www.readysteadytoddler.org.uk/
   - **Parent club:** this third package from NHS Inform provides information to parents about early years provision for children up to and including nursery and primary school https://www.parentclub.scot/
   - **Parenting – give it time:** produced by the Welsh Government, this package supports parents to parent their children by providing information about child development, behaviour management and service provision https://gov.wales/parenting-give-it-time
   - **Parenting NI:** produced by Northern Ireland Parenting, a leading registered charity in Northern Ireland, this package provides information about all aspects

of parenting and child care https://www.
parentingni.org/
b. As a health visitor/student health visitor, consider
the elements of your practice that require you
to use a pen and paper? How will you continue
to complete your health visitor practice in these
areas without using pen and paper?

2. **Health visitors have electronic access to client health and care information**

Government policy aspires to creating a situation where all clinicians, including health visitors, will have access to and be able to interact with patient records and care plans wherever they are located.[1–5] The aim is to create full digitalisation and a paper-free service within the next 5 to 10 years (2024–2030).[1–5]

This will make it possible for health visitors to access client information through the electronic health record within or outside the work base. Indeed, many organisations are creating virtual working mechanisms where health visitors work from hubs rather than a specific office and work within a 'hot desk' system.

Many organisations have chosen to adopt different electronic patient record systems. These include SystmOne, EMIS, RIO, Care Notes, Attend Anywhere, The Welsh Community Care Information System (WCCIS) and The Northern Ireland Electronic Care Record (NIECR). However, the systems share certain characteristics including:

a. the system contains a series of templates or screens which require specific information about each client, the consultation, and the plan for ongoing care/intervention

b. the system contains a separate record for the child and the parent

c. the system makes it possible to link information about parents, children and people living in the same household

d. the system contains specific read codes, which make it possible to categorise, analyse and audit information

e. the system is usually available and accessible to other health members of the multi-professional team (this is not currently the case for social care members of the multi-professional team)

f. the system allows access to people with specific authorisation and allows access to different levels of information depending on the role and responsibility of the person. Access is usually via a password or specific form of identification including smartcard which is linked to the employment tracking system (Electronic Staff Record (ESR).

3. **Health visitors have access to a technologically enhanced Child Protection and Safeguarding system**

Health visitors work with the multi-agency team to safeguard and protect children. Technology provides an important mechanism for enhancing information sharing and communication during multi-agency working. An example of this is provided by the Westminster government in England. Here the government aspires to improve the child protection system by 2022. In doing so, the aim is to create an integrated child protection system which will replace the individual systems that are currently in place. Once the organisation has the system in place, they will have real time up-to-date information.[7] The child protection information sharing project contains information about all children who have a child protection plan and are Looked After by the Local Authority. It uses the NHS SPINE, a system which links more than 23,000 health care Information Technology (IT) systems in more than 20,000 organisations, to ensure that the information is updated daily. The NHS 'Spine' is the central point which allows information to be exchanged across local and national NHS IT systems. For health visitors in England this means that they will have access to up-to-date information about children who are vulnerable or in need of protection. Health visitors will also be able to access information about the child protection plan as well as all episodes of unscheduled or hospital care in emergency or minor injuries departments. The Child Protection Information Sharing System will help health visitors to gather information by[7]:

a. alerting the health team that the child has a child protection plan in place
b. allowing the health team to access the contact details for the child's social care team
c. automatically notifying the social care team, not just the health care team
d. sharing the previous 25 visits that the child has made to unscheduled care settings in England, not just scheduled care settings. This is important because we know that children who are vulnerable and at risk of harm are taken to different care settings and may not engage with scheduled care provision. A system like this will therefore make it possible for health visitors to link information and thereby make sense of the context in which the child is living.

https://digital.nhs.uk/services/child-protection-information-sharing-project (accessed December 29, 2019).[7]

## IMPLICATIONS FOR HEALTH VISITING PRACTICE

### Technological changes for health visiting practice and service delivery

1. The use of video conferencing packages to complete face-to-face synchronous consultations with clients when the health visitor and client are not co-located
2. Electronic Patient Record which the health visitor can access from anywhere
3. Virtual working, using mobile devices that include laptops, tablets and mobile phones
4. Automated routine tasks allowing health visitors to deliver client focused specialist care
5. A paper-free service.

### Integrated digital child protection system

The health visiting profession and service delivery is largely predicated on the fact that it is a people-focused provision. Its foundations are in the ability of health visitors to build therapeutic, trusted relationships with people and engage them sufficiently to encourage them to access the service when needed. It is not a service based on illness or specific health conditions and so does not benefit from the ability to design linear referral or discharge criteria. Rather, it seeks to engage people (usually, but not exclusively, mothers) in order to gain access to their children and monitor growth, development and well-being over the 5 years from birth to school entry. This means that health visitors work with mothers, parents and children over time and at different stages of their lives. This complexity is not open to linear, algorithmic, cause-and-effect situations, which suggests that any technology-enhanced service must be able to accommodate differences and deal with subsequent complexity.[8]

The emerging health policy and strategy for creating an increasingly digitally enhanced health service means that health visitors will be working more and more with technology to deliver their service. They must therefore be capable of working with technology in different ways.

Digitally enhanced health visiting services may be characterised by:

a. A reduction in the number of co-located face-to-face consultations between health visitors and their clients

b. An increased use of APPS and Internet sources of information by health visitors to enable clients to develop their knowledge of specific health care and conditions

c. An increasing need for health visitors to be familiar with Internet sources of information and the rigour of the evidence on which the information is based

d. An increasing need for health visitors to explain the value and danger of Internet sources of information to clients in order to be assured that they are making informed decisions/choices.

Health visitors will increasingly work in a health care system where clients actively use digital sources to gather information, rather than face-to-face contact. This situation was thrust upon health visitors in the UK during the COVID-19 pandemic in 2020, which necessitated a national lockdown and social distancing measures. This meant that the health visiting service was unable to deliver traditional face-to-face or home-based consultations. Instead, the service was delivered remotely using virtual and digital methods, including video conferencing, as well as contact by phone, email or chatroom.

---

**Examples of technology to facilitate virtual consultations**

a. Microsoft Teams (MS TEAMS): https://www.microsoft.com/en-gb/microsoft-365/microsoft-teams/free

b. Attend Anywhere/ NearMe (NHS Scotland): https://www.vc.scot.nhs.uk/attendanywhere/

c. ZOOM: https://www.techradar.com/uk/news/what-is-zoom-how-does-it-work-tips-and-tricks-plus-best-alternatives

d. SKYPE: https://www.skype.com/en/

e. WHATSAPP: https://www.whatsapp.com/

f. BLUEJEANS: https://www.bluejeans.com/

---

## Consultations using digital technology

Technology-assisted consultations using video conferencing packages provide an opportunity to simultaneously see and talk to clients when the health visitor and client are not co-located. Furthermore, as illustrated during the National COVID-19 pandemic these technologies allow synchronous communication in real time.[9]

Evidence about the success or otherwise of video conferencing as a mechanism for synchronous consultations is in its infancy.[9] A review completed by the Early Intervention Foundation (EIF) suggests that the addition of specific verbal and non-verbal communication techniques makes it possible to maximise the potential of video conferencing for synchronous communication between the health visitor and the client.[9]

a. Use the technology to offer a person-to-person consultation in real time, rather than merely providing a video for the client to watch alone

b. Provide unambiguous meeting and joining instructions

c. Arrive early for the appointment and be ready to admit the client into the virtual meeting room. This will allow the client to feel you (the health visitor) are expecting them and is ready for the consultation

d. Create a structure including a start and end time, agreed content, an action plan and information about future appointments

e. Allow additional time for the consultation because it may take longer to gather information and develop a rapport with the client

f. Allow the client time to relax into the consultation at the beginning, by using general day-to-day (chit-chat) conversation, e.g. the weather, to replicate the start of a co-located real-time conversation

g. Engage in turn-taking as you would do during a co-located consultation. It is even more important to actively listen to the client, allow them time to speak and feel that they are being heard

h. Ask questions because this is a way to clarify understanding and avoid misunderstanding

i. Take care with non-verbal communication, including facial expressions, eye contact and posture. The health visitor must create an environment where the client feels that they are the only thing s/he is thinking about

j. Allow time between appointments to resolve problems with Internet connectivity.

However, not all clients will be able to use technology. In a study by Deloite[10] in 2015, 75% of the UK population used the Internet to access information. In the same study 23% of the population readily used APPS to gather information about their symptoms and medical condition.[10] This means that health visitor consultations in 2020–2021 will be very different to those in 2029. However, any future service design must also accommodate the needs of people who choose not to use technology. Deloite suggests that this may account for up to 25% of the population.[10]

The advances in technology and the increasing range of information source place the health visitor in a pivotal position to help clients understand the information, respond to questions and challenge myth in favour of research. Parents are increasingly accessing online communities and networks for help, advice and information. Many, including NETMUMS and MUMSNET, are not listed in the NHS Digital Library, and so are not 'approved' by the NHS scheme. However, they remain popular and provide a source of information in addition to health visitors and other NHS sources.

- NETMUMS: An online community for parents https://www.netmums.com/info/about-us

- MUMSNET: An online network for parents to share and receive information https://www.mumsnet.com/info/about-us

## THINKING SPACE

For every 100 clients you see as a health visitor, 25 clients will not be able to use technology to engage with the service.

Using a model of reflection, consider how health visitors can continue to provide an accessible and available health visiting service to all clients.

**Hints:**

1. What factors would make you think a client could not use technology?
2. How will you provide the health visiting service to this client?
3. What action is needed to make your strategy fit with your employer's service model?

## THE WORKFORCE STRATEGY

The strategic vision for health and social care is one which includes increasing amounts of technology and automation and less labour-intensive activity. Health visitors, as part of the NHS workforce, will need to be able to deliver this vision.[1–5] They will need to engage with an emerging culture in which digitally supported care is the norm, rather than the exception.

Health visitors therefore need the skills and knowledge to enable them to use technology effectively as an integral part of their work. The health visitor role will increasingly require them to be able to manage the data, as well as the technological and clinical elements of service delivery. This is because future service delivery will use technology to automate care provision and delivery, as well as to improve the organisation, delivery and productivity of health visiting services.[1–5,11]

In order to work in a data rich, technologically supported health and social care system, health visitors must have a core level of digital ability.

## CORE DIGITAL ABILITY

In 2018, the Department for Education in England defined the core level of digital ability that people would need for life and work in terms of five skill categories. It stated that people would need to be able to use technology to communicate, solve problems, handle information, complete transactions and to use technology in a safe and legal way.[12] This sentiment is also reflected in the strategies for Scotland, Northern Ireland and Wales.[2–4,12–14]

> ### Core Digital Ability
>
> 1. Communicating
> 2. Handling information and content
> 3. Transacting
> 4. Problem-solving
> 5. Being safe and legal online
>    (Department for Education[12])

## ESSENTIAL DIGITAL SKILLS FOR HEALTH VISITORS

In order to operate effectively and efficiently in 21st century health visiting practice, all health visitors need to call on these core skills daily.[12,13] For example,

| Activity | Skills required |
| --- | --- |
| **Communication** | |
| Share information with others | ▪ Send, respond to an email and manage an email account<br>▪ Share documents with others, via email<br>▪ Create and use PDF and WORD formats<br>▪ Develop, use and maintain the security of passwords<br>▪ Use video conferencing applications including Skype and Face Time<br>▪ Manage a professional networking account (i.e. LinkedIn) |

| Activity | Skills required |
| --- | --- |
| Lone working | Use devices for personal safety e.g. SKYGUARD (personal safety services for lone workers), WHATSAPP<br>Keep devices in working order (i.e. charged and ready for use) |
| **Handling information and content** | |
| Information governance | Understand and conform with the organisation's IT policy<br>Synchronise and share information across different devices, including laptops, tablets and mobile phones |
| Virtual working | Manage an electronic calendar, appointments, workload<br>Manage workload allocation and delegation |
| Record keeping and documentation | Maintain electronic patient health records (record the information, explain its meaning, record, problems, patterns, and priorities for action)<br>Record the care planned and delivered, and all changes in the client's condition |
| **Problem solving** | |
| Answer questions and challenge myth in favour of research | Search for information using different search engines including Explorer, Firefox and Chrome<br>Search for information using different databases (e.g. EBSCO, CINAHL, MEDLINE)<br>Search for information using research-based Internet sites (i.e. NICE, BNF) |
| **Transacting** | |
| Manage employment<br>Professional regulation | Submit requests for annual leave<br>Manage the online pay slips<br>Manage an online account with the health regulator (e.g. NMC ONLINE) |
| **Problem solving** | |
| Present information to others | Use presentation software applications (i.e. Microsoft PowerPoint) |

| Activity | Skills required |
|---|---|
| Domiciliary visiting | Use Internet route planner applications to plan home visiting activity |
| Identifying community health needs | Use Internet data sources (e.g. Public Health England, public health data: https://fingertips.phe.org.uk/) |
| *Being safe and legal online* | |
| Maintaining confidentiality and information security | Use the organisation's social media policy<br>Change Passwords<br>Keep Passwords secure |

## THINKING SPACE

Read the Department for Education[12] Essential Digital Skills framework and in a small group consider Claire's situation, presented in Case Study 9.1.

1. List the core digital skills that you think Claire may have.
2. Which two core skills should Claire prioritise to help her feel confident and competent as a health visitor in her organisation?

## HEALTH VISITING PRACTICE

Health visitors, as Specialist Community Public Health Nurses, are regulated by the Nursing and Midwifery Council (NMC). They work autonomously with children and families in the community and homebased settings. As regulated health professionals their priority is to keep the public safe and they do this in line with the requirements of the NMC Code of Professional Standards, Practice and Behaviour.[15]

Using evidence-based programmes of support, starting in pregnancy, through the early weeks of life and throughout childhood, health visitors contact all women during pregnancy and maintain contact for the first 5 years of the child's life. They are part of a universally offered service, predicated largely on client choice. Health visiting practice is explained using four process statements, which are collectively known as the Principles of Health Visiting.[16] These four statements (the search for health needs, the stimulation of awareness of health needs, the influence on policies affecting health and the facilitation of health-enhancing activities), detail the knowledge and skills required by health visitors to undertake health visiting practice.

### The principles of health visiting[16]

1. **Search for health needs**
   Health visitors are aware of the health needs of the population they are working with. They use technology to find information about client, family and community health and social needs so they can organise their activities and deliver needs-based care.

2. **The stimulation of an awareness of health needs**
   Health visitors integrate information from research- and NHS-approved APPS into their consultations with parents and children to help them learn about their health, well-being and care needs.

3. **The influence on policies affecting health**
   Health visitors access research-based databases to identify information for local policies and guidelines. This enables them to positively influence the learning, development and understanding of other members of the health visitor team. It also helps them to positively influence the health care knowledge and understanding of parents, families and children.

4. **Facilitation of health enhancing behaviours**
   Health visitors work with clients and other members of the health and social care team to facilitate activity that will benefit the child. technology to communicate with others to initiate activity on behalf of the child, parents and families.

## RECORD-KEEPING AND DOCUMENTATION

### What is a record?

A record is anything that refers to a client (i.e., in health visiting practice this may be a parent, child or a family).

### Examples of a record in health visiting practice

a. Electronic patient health record
b. Personal child health record (PCHR)
c. Care plans (action plan)
d. Emails
e. Electronic or paper diaries
f. Message books
g. A register of clinic attendees or births
h. Letters from members of the multi-professional team
i. Incident report and statements.

### Why have records?

The record acts as a tool to assist communication in several ways including to:

- communicate information about the client to other professionals involved in the delivering of care
- share information about any changes in the client's condition or the priorities for action
- demonstrate the professional practice used to deliver care
- identify any problems or changes in the client's condition or situation.

Record-keeping and documentation are an essential component of health visiting practice. The health visitor maintains records for:

a. The mother/parents
b. Each child in the family

These are two different but related records. Technology allows the health visitor to access both records simultaneously and cross reference information in real time. This helps them to see the whole picture. It also allows the health visitor to present the information so that related issues are linked together. This means that the reader will see the whole picture and is better able to understand the context, as well as any issues or concerns that the health visitor has documented.

Health visitors may be working with electronic or paper records or a combination of the two. However, the principles for practice remain the same. The information recorded in a client's record must be:

- accurate, containing information which is based on facts, not assumptions or hearsay
- presented in a logical and systematic way so it is easy to understand
- clearly written and not contain jargon or abbreviations
- concise so that the important points are visible and easy to see
- complete with no information missing.

A legally sound record has three important characteristics. It must have information about the care planned, the care delivered and any changes in the client's condition. This is important because care planned is frequently descriptive information. By contrast, care delivery is analytical and requires the author to explain what the information means to the child, in the context in which the child is living. Sidebotham et al (2016) describe this in terms of what it feels like for the child and suggest that this level of analysis requires the author (i.e., the health visitor) to consider the information in depth rather than on a superficial basis.[17] The health visitor must organise and reorganise the information. This takes time, is hard to complete and requires knowledge and understanding. It is, however, essential to produce a legally sound record. This is important to remember because, in the eyes of the law, an action/activity that is not recorded has not taken place.

### Components of a legally sound record

The record must contain information about:

- the assessment
- the care plan (care that is planned and has been provided)
- the client's condition (changes as well as no change)
- all contacts (even when there is no change in the condition or situation, when there is no access, or the client has not attended an appointment).

Health visitors must work with the prescribed format of the electronic patient record to ensure that all required information is included. They must also think carefully about the free text entries so that the information recorded builds a cohesive picture. It is important to avoid duplication, as well as missing out information from the record.

Technology allows the health visitor to record and organise information in a timely way (i.e., input the information into the electronic record during the consultation with the client and effectively use the cut and paste facility). It also provides the health visitor with opportunities to review the content of the record before it is authorised through the validation process.

### Essential content of health visitor records

- Frequency of intervention
- Actions taken when a problem is identified
- Date and time of care delivery
- Analysis of all information collected
- Date and version of policies and guidelines used to justify actions.
- All assessments and care plans
- All care plan revisions considering new information
- All care provided
- All referrals made
- All referrals accepted
- All communication between professionals
- All care given and the outcome
- All contacts made, even when no access is achieved, or the client did not attend the appointment

The technology of the electronic patient record provides the health visitor with a further opportunity to demonstrate that the information is legally sound. This is because it automatically records the date of the entry. It is important to demonstrate that the information within the record has been collated contemporaneously, or as near to the event at possible. Technology allows the time of the entry to be recorded but requires a free text entry denoting the date and time of the consultation or event. Any time lag between the event and record must be accompanied by information which describes the approach the health visitor has taken to provide an accurate account of events. The legal standing of the information recorded will be possible only if the health visitor can demonstrate that the information they have recorded is not reliant on their memory.

### Case study 9.3: An example of poor use of technology in health visiting practice

Claire works part-time. Her working days are Tuesday, Wednesday and Friday. On Fridays she must leave at 5pm to collect her son from school.

Claire is not good at typing and doesn't like the computer because she says it prevents her from maintaining eye contact with her clients. She therefore makes notes during each consultation and types them up after the clinic.

She is responsible for leading the child health clinic on a Friday afternoon from 2 to 4 pm. Claire is often the only health visitor and may see up to 20 clients. Most people come during the last 90 minutes, which means the clinic does not finish until 5 pm. If it finishes on time, she has 45 minutes to type up her records; but when it finishes at 5 pm, she cannot complete the records before she leaves.

Claire plans to complete the records the following Tuesday (4 days later) when she is next on duty.

**Issue one: Claire is not complying with the legal or regulatory requirements for a client record. She is not:**

- producing contemporaneous records
- assuring the reader that the information recorded is not based on her memory

8.3 keep colleagues informed when you are sharing the care of individuals with other health and care professionals and staff (*practice effectively*)[15]

8.6 share information to identify and reduce risk (*practice effectively*)[15]

10.1 complete records at the time or as soon as possible after an event, recording if the notes are written sometime after the event (*practice effectively*)[15]

### Possible solution

- Claire should demonstrate that she is not relying on her memory to complete the records. She could do this by scanning the hand-written notes, made during the consultations, into the electronic patient health record. The scanned notes should be labelled with the patient's name, NHS number, the date and time of consultation and Claire's signature.

**Issue two: Claire is not meeting the requirements for NMC registration.[15] She is failing to:**

- keep the public safe because she will not share client information with other members of the team for 4 days
- tell her manager that she is unable to fulfil her responsibilities in a way that will keep the public safe
- develop her skills and knowledge to help her provide safe and effective care.

16.3 tell someone in authority at the first reasonable opportunity if you experience problems that may prevent you working within the Code or other national standards, taking prompt action to tackle the causes of concern if you can (*Preserve safety*)[15]

22.3 keep your knowledge and skills up to date, taking part in appropriate and regular learning and professional development activities that aim to maintain and develop your competence and improve your performance (*Promote professionalism and trust*)[15]

### Possible solutions

- Claire should access training to learn how to use the computer during her consultations with clients
- Claire should consider amending the position of the computer so that she can type and look at the client at the same time

### Case study 9.4: An example of good use of technology in health visiting practice

**Issue One: Peter is complying with the legal requirements for a client record because he is:**

- producing contemporaneous records (he is recording the information as near to the consultation/event as possible)
- assuring the reader that the information recorded is not based on his memory (the date and time that the information is recorded is the same as the date and time of the entry into the computer system)

10.1 Complete records at the time or as soon as possible after an event, recording if the notes are written some time after the event (reference 15)

**Issue Two: Peter is meeting the requirements for NMC registration.[15] His actions help him to:**

- keep the public safe because he is sharing client information with other members of the team as it becomes available
- create a system for keeping in touch with others, including his manager, so that changes can be made to his workload when he is busy
- he has also access training to help him manage his time and use the computer effectively. This means that he can fulfil his responsibilities in a way that will keep the public safe, even when he is busy.

## RECORD KEEPING AND THE LAW

Record keeping and documentation is governed by specific legislation. This legislation protects the access, security and content of the record.

### 2018: General Data Protection Regulation (GDPR)

- The Act regulates personal data
- The Act requires the individual to 'opt' into data sharing arrangements rather than 'opt out'
- The Act has been in place since May 2018 and represents the first major change in data protection regulation for 20 years.

### 2018: Data Protection Act

- The purpose of the Act is to maintain confidentiality in the digital age
- The Act applies the requirements of the GDPR
- The Act allows practitioners to share a child's personal information without consent in order to keep the child safe
- The Act states that a 13-year-old child no longer needs their parent's consent to process data online.

### 2000: The Freedom of Information Act

- The Act deals with all information in the public arena
- The Act aims to prevent secrecy
- People can apply to see information (via a Freedom of Information Request)
- The Act means that Information may be scrutinised some time after it was first recorded.

### 2016: Records Management: NHS Code of Practice

- Electronic and paper records
- Records must be retained for up to 26 years.

Health visitors' records contain information about more than one aspect of a child's health and well-being. It is therefore essential that all information collected is collated in a way that the reader will understand. The reader must understand not only what is happening to the child but also the significance of what is not happening. Sometimes the important information in a health visitor's record is that which tells the reader what is not happening and the impact it has or will have on the child. Collating this information is complex because it may come from several sources and address different periods of time. Furthermore, at the time of recording the health visitor may not have all the information because it may not be available. This means that health visitors must revisit the content of the record once more information comes to light. Importantly, health visitors may also need to revisit the decisions and judgements made considering new information and record the impact that this has had on the care/action plan.[18]

By using a consistent approach to recording information, the health visitor will provide a complete account of events. In the past 20 years the health visiting profession has adopted the Department of Health,[19] Framework for the Assessment of Children in Need and their Families, commonly known as the 'assessment triangle' (or in Scotland 'My World Triangle). This framework provides a logical and systematic approach which helps the health visitor collate the information. Its content is based on the ecological model of child development outlined in the work of Bronfenbrenner,[20] which identified the influence that the environment and societal factors have on a child's development, health and well-being. The framework for assessment requires the health visitor to collect and collate information about:

- The child's growth and development
- The environment in which the child is living
- The capacity of the child's parents to keep them safe.

Technology allows this framework to be reproduced and used by health visitors wherever they are located. By being available when needed, the health visitor can use the framework accurately and consistently to record the information. It therefore helps the health visitor to:

a. present information succinctly and concisely by making the point, supporting it with evidence from their assessment and stating the impact on the child and the implication

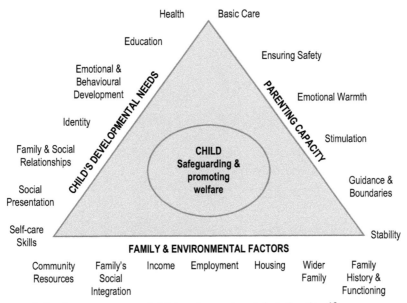

Figure 9.1 ■ Framework for the assessment of children in need and their families.[19]

for the child's ongoing health, growth, development and well-being

b. avoid including information not considered as part of the assessment framework and thereby not relevant to the child

c. avoid using 'standard phrases' that don't relate to the child.

### Characteristics of succinct information

- contains pertinent points
- contains the facts (i.e., what is seen, not seen and evidence of the impact on the child)
- may be presented as bullet points in a list
- relates directly to the issue being presented in the record.

### Summarising information

Summarising information in a record requires the author to choose to include only information that will help others to understand the message being shared. The message will be easier to understand if the information:

- is separated into chunks
- presents the most important points first
- uses clear language not jargon
- includes all judgements (this could be happening because…)
- includes all decisions (an explanation for the chosen actions).

All records must contain **SLIC** entries and health visitors must take care to avoid producing **SLAC** records.[21]

| SLAC RECORDS | SLIC RECORDS |
|---|---|
| ■ S…. Selective entries | S…. Succinct |
| ■ L…. Lengthy | L…. Legally sound |
| ■ A…. Any time | I…. Informative |
| ■ C…. Careless | C…. Contemporaneous |

## TO CREATE A SLIC RECORD, THE HEALTH VISITOR SHOULD

### Succint information

- Position the most important information at the beginning
- Ensure the content is jargon free and does not contain any abbreviations
- Make the sentences short and focus the content directly on the issue under discussion.

### Legally sound information

- Outline the care planned
- Outline the care delivered
- Outline any changes in the client condition or situation.

### Informative information

- Only include facts
- Include information that will help the reader learn more about the client or the situation.

### Contemporaneous information

- Record the information as near to the event as possible
- Include additional information that illustrates the content is not produced from memory.

## IN ORDER NOT TO CREATE A SLAC RECORD, THE HEALTH VISITOR SHOULD

### Selective entries

- Avoid including information that does not increase the readers, knowledge and understanding about the client or situation
- Avoid including information that does not directly relate to the client or situation.

### Lengthy entries

- Ensure the record does not contain irrelevant information
- Ensure the record does not contain jargon
- Ensure the record does not contain abbreviations
- Ensure the record does not contain confusing information that does not make sense.

### Written at any time

- Avoid delaying the recording of the information
- Avoid recording information from memory.

### Careless

- Avoid recording information in a random way that does not have a beginning, middle or an end
- Avoid missing out information
- Avoid repeating information.

## CONCLUSION

Technology is omnipresent in health visiting practice. This chapter has presented the national policy and strategy for technology advancement and the ways in which this is integrated into health visiting practice.

Technology helps health visitors to work in different ways depending on the context and the client group. In many cases, technology allows the health visitor to work more effectively and efficiently. However, this is not always the case and requires careful planning and investment.

The health visitor's record keeping and documentation activity continues to be heavily influenced by the introduction of the electronic patient health record and the development of digital mobile devices. These all have the power to change the design of health visiting service delivery and enable the health visitor to embrace the opportunities that arise from the Information Age.

### KEY LEARNING POINTS

- Increased understanding of the policy context for using technology in health visiting practice.

- Increased understanding of how to use technology and meet the legal and regulatory requirements for safe and effective health visiting practice.
- Increased understanding of the strategies/actions needed to prepare for health visiting practice in the Information Age.

## REFERENCES

1. Health and Social Care Act. (2012). London. TSO.
2. Health and Social Care Board (2015). *e-Health and care strategy for Northern Ireland*. Belfast: Health and Social Care Board.
3. Welsh Assembly Government (2010). *Delivering a digital Wales*. Cardiff: Welsh Assembly Government.
4. Scottish Government (2017). *A Digital strategy for Scotland*. Edinburgh: The Scottish Government.
5. NHS England (2019). *The NHS long term plan*. London: NHSE.
6. Castle-Clarke, S. (2018). *What will new technology mean for the NHS and its patients?* London: The Kings Fund.
7. NHS Digital (2019). Child *protection – information sharing project*. London: NHS Digital. https://digital.nhs.uk/services/child-protection-information-sharing-project. Accessed December 29, 2019.
8. Greenhalgh, T., Wherton, J., Papoutsi, C., Lynch, J., Hughes, G., A'Court, C., et al. (2018). Analysing the role of complexity in explaining the fortunes of technology programmes: empirical application of the NASSS framework. *BMC Medicine, 16*(66), 1–15. https://doi.org/10.1186/s12916-018-1050-6. Accessed August 18, 2020.
9. Martin, J., McBride, T., Masterman, T., Pote, I., Mokhtar, N., Oprea, E., & Sorgenfrei, M. (2020). *Covid-19 and Early intervention evidence: Challenges and risks relating to virtual and digital delivery*. London: Early Intervention Foundation.
10. Deloitte (2015). *Connected health: How digital technology is transforming health and social care*. London: Deloitte.
11. NHS (2019). *The interim people plan*. London: NHS.
12. Department for Education. (2018). *Essential digital skills framework*. London: Department for Education.
13. Department for Education (2019). *National standards for essential digital skills*. London: Department for Education.
14. NHS England.(2019). *A Health and care digital capabilities framework*. London: NHS England.
15. Nursing and Midwifery Council (2018). *The code*. London: NMC.
16. Council for the Education and Training of Health Visitors (1977). *An investigation into the principles of Health Visiting*. London: CETHV.
17. Sidebotham, P., Brandon, M., Bailey, S., Belderson, P., Dodsworth, J., Garstang, J., et al. (2016). *Pathways to harm, pathways to protection. A triennial analysis of serious case reviews 2011-2014*. London: Department for Education.
18. Munro, E. (2011). *The Munro review of child protection: Final report, a child-centred system*. London: Department for Education.
19. Department of Health (2000). *Framework for the assessment of children in need and their families*. London: DH.
20. Bronfenbrenner, U. (1979). *The ecology of human development: Experiments by nature and design*. USA: Harvard College.
21. Newland, R. (2007). *Record keeping and documentation. principles into practice*. London: CPHVA.

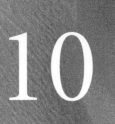

# 10

# FACILITATING HEALTHY BEHAVIOUR – AN EMPOWERMENT APPROACH

KAREN ADAMS ■ MICHELLE CLARK

## CHAPTER CONTENTS

INTRODUCTION

THE HISTORY OF BEHAVIOUR CHANGE

REDUCING THE INTENTION-BEHAVIOUR GAP–TAKING ACTION AND MAINTAINING IT

FACILITATING HEALTHY BEHAVIOUR: EMPOWERING INDIVIDUALS AND THEIR FAMILIES, GROUPS AND COMMUNITIES

EVALUATING THE IMPACT OF HEALTH VISITOR INTERVENTIONS

CONCLUSION

## LEARNING OUTCOMES

*To*:

■ summarise the historical and more contemporary approaches to promoting health and facilitating healthy behaviour

■ discuss different mechanisms of behaviour change

■ critically consider how health visitors can work with individuals and their families, groups and communities to promote health and facilitate healthy behaviour

■ Evaluate the outcomes of health visitor interventions that aim to promote health

## INTRODUCTION

This chapter provides an overview of the science and the art of facilitating health-promoting behaviour, why it is important and what this looks like in health visiting practice. We begin by reflecting on the history of behaviour change in health and care services and how this has changed over the years. We then look at what these changes and a growing evidence base mean for the way health visitors work with individuals, families and communities. Finally, we consider how health visitors can evaluate the interventions they design and deliver to improve outcomes for the communities they support.

## THE HISTORY OF BEHAVIOUR CHANGE

### What is behaviour?

Firstly, this may seem like an unusual question, but it is useful to define at the outset what we mean by behaviour when supporting people to change it. According to the American Psychological Association, behaviour is,

*An organism's activities in response to external or internal stimuli, including objectively observable activities, introspectively observable activities, and nonconscious processes.*[1]

We generally accept behaviour to be responses which are observable; i.e. actions and speech. This means that *everything* we *do* is a behaviour, and from a health point of view, certain behaviours can be judged positively, neutrally or negatively, based on our knowledge of the risks to health and well-being. The behaviours that are most often thought about when talking about health are smoking, drinking too much alcohol, diet and physical activity. However, it is unhelpful to think about health behaviour in these narrow terms, as each one can be broken down into lots of other behaviours that lead to the 'unhealthy' behaviour. For example, changing from eating an unhealthy to a healthy diet involves changing what you buy at the shop, possibly changing how you cook or prepare food and eating the 'healthier' food. All these behaviours are influenced by different factors (determinants). There are also behaviours which may not be directly related to the target behaviour, but when changed, can result in the desired change being achieved. For example, a family receiving support to find a different energy provider which saves them money each month, then allows them to afford to purchase more fresh food in their weekly shop. It may help to keep this in mind as you go through this chapter, as the behaviours which may seem obvious targets for change, may not be the most helpful or appropriate.

## Pre- and post-1950s

From a public health perspective, it is now generally accepted there are behaviours or activities which, when carried out by enough people and become the 'norm', can have a large negative influence on the health of the population: smoking, drinking too much alcohol, poor diet, lack of physical activity have been identified as the most harmful.[2] However, it has not always been this way. The focus on 'non-communicable diseases' – conditions such as coronary-artery disease, cancer and diabetes – which are in part caused by lifestyle factors, and therefore can be reduced by adopting healthy lifestyle behaviours, only occurred after the 1950s. Prior to this, health policy focused on infectious diseases such as tuberculosis, as the leading cause of death and reduced life expectancy. The introduction of childhood immunisation in the 20th century all but eradicated infectious diseases such as poliomyelitis, diphtheria and measles. Advances in sanitation, provision of clean water and nutrition, led to dramatic increases in life expectancy, leaving non-communicable diseases to become the main cause of mortality. From the 1960s onwards, health-related behaviour was viewed as a risk factor for diseases, such as coronary artery disease and cancers resulting in early mortality.[3] Consequently, policymakers have sought to improve the populations' health by advocating support for people and communities to change their health-related behaviour.

However, supporting people to change their behaviour has always been a challenge. Assumptions about health, disease and illness, and how individuals make decisions about their health, have over the years shaped the way we have supported people to change. Three related developments of note relate to:

(i) The move away from the biomedical model – prior to 1960, the dominant model in medicine was the biomedical model, which took a purely physiological view of disease.[4] With the introduction of the biopsychosocial model,[5] and more recently, with the move towards socio-ecological models[6] and person-centred care,[7] this view changed to take into account the impact of psychological and social factors on how health, disease and illness are defined, understood and experienced.

(ii) The patient-practitioner relationship and the model of health-related decision-making – the paternalistic model was also dominant during the 'reign' of the biomedical model. Health care practitioners assumed the role of the expert and made decisions on the patient's behalf and in the patient's best interest based on their expertise.[8,9] Although paternalism was always rooted in doing what was best for the patient, the hierarchy involved creates a power imbalance and leaves patients as passive recipients of the expert's knowledge and care. In the UK, there has been a transition towards practitioners and patients sharing the decision-making process, with the understanding that the patient is the expert in their own life, and that health and well-being outcomes are improved when the relationship takes the form of a partnership with information and decision-making being shared between practitioner and patient.[9] This change in relationship also acknowledges that the often-well-meaning advice given by practitioners undermines that partnership, and instead of telling people what to do, patients can be supported to find their own ways to address health concerns, which make sense in the context of their lives.

(iii) The effectiveness of providing information to change behaviour – many individual and population-based behaviour change interventions in the past were based on an assumption rooted in the field of traditional economics: that people make decisions based on a rational evaluation of the costs and benefits of an action in order to achieve the best outcomes.[10,11]

This assumption may explain the practice of telling people which behaviour is unhealthy (e.g. smoking), the health consequences of their behaviour (e.g. cancer, coronary heart disease, gum disease) and telling them how to change (e.g. set a quit date, wear nicotine patches). Once people know what the risks are and the consequences, it is assumed they will change their behaviour to avoid those consequences. As this chapter will go on to discuss, we now know there is more involved than simply telling people what to do.

## Instrumental theories and the 'intention-behaviour gap'

The book *ABC of Behaviour Change Theory*[12,13] lists 83 individual theories which relate to explaining and influencing behaviour, and can be used in the design of behaviour change interventions. Theories and models are useful to understand why the people we support act in the way they do. When we understand what may lie behind someone's behaviour, it can help us to be more compassionate and empathetic towards them, which in turn helps them to feel listened to and validated. Many of the most commonly researched theories and models used to design interventions to support behaviour change (see Fig. 10.1 for examples of these prominent behaviour change theories) were based on the assumptions of 'utility maximisation' and, as a result, aimed to change behaviour by influencing beliefs and attitudes about risk and consequences, leading to direct behaviour change. To date, these theories have mainly demonstrated that changing peoples' beliefs and attitudes will support a person's intentions to change a behaviour, but will not necessarily lead to direct changes in behaviour, which has become known as the 'intention-behaviour gap'.[14]

This is important, as behaviour change, whether at an individual or community level, involves a process of initiating change but then

**Theory of Planned Behaviour** [23] – This model, based on the earlier Theory of Reasoned Action[24] **keep comma after 'Action' is based on the premise that behaviours are directly influenced by the person's intentions to carry out the behaviour. The intentions are in turn influenced by attitudes, social norms and the person's perceived behavioural control, for example, what they think about the behaviour, what other important people think about the behaviour and the person's belief that they are able to carry out the behaviour. However, many studies[25] have found that intentions do not guarantee that the behaviour will occur – as we know, just intending to stop smoking doesn't mean that the person will be successful.

**Stages of change (Transtheoretical Model (TTM))**[26] – The stages of change part of this model has been used extensively across health and social care services, beginning with smoking cessation services. There are six proposed stages that people go through in relation to change, from precontemplation, contemplation, preparation, action, maintenance and termination. A review of the effectiveness of the TTM in supporting health behaviour change found a lack of evidence for its use, despite the model making conceptual sense to people.[27]

**Health Belief Model**[28] – Developed in the 1950s, this model proposes that there are six predictors of behaviour; beliefs about perceived susceptibility, perceived seriousness of condition or risk, perceived benefits of behaviour, perceived barriers, however, in a review analysing the effectiveness of the model to predict behaviour, there were mixed results.[29]

**Protection Motivation Theory**[30] – This model has been used to develop and assess persuasive communication, mainly focusing on fear or threat messages, which are assumed will motivate the individual to act to reduce the fear caused by the message. On receiving the message, the individual appraises it on two levels: in relation to threat (based on how severe the threat is, and how vulnerable the person judges themselves to be to the threat) and in relation to coping (belief that taking action will remove the threat, and that they have a high level of self-efficacy). The result of these appraisals is either adaptive (successful at removing the threat) or maladaptive (does not directly alter the threat) responses.[31]

Figure 10.1 ■ Influential behaviour change theories.[23-31]

also maintaining it. The common occurrence of the 'intention-behaviour gap' suggests that being motivated and intending to change is an important requirement but not enough; something else is getting in the way of changing the behaviour. Some reasons for this include:

- Intentions are not always stable – a person may have an intention to change at one point, but this changes
- Barriers in the environment to carrying out and maintaining the behaviour – these can be barriers from the physical, social or emotional environment

A scoping review by Davis et al[15] highlighted that other models of behaviour change – for example, those based on control theory (Powers 1973/2005)[16] – had more evidence for their effectiveness. This theory, and others, such as Bandura's[74] Social Learning Theory or Deci[75] and Ryan's Self determination Theory, focuses on how we regulate our behaviour (volitional or regulatory process) when we carry out a behaviour.[17]

## REDUCING THE INTENTION-BEHAVIOUR GAP–TAKING ACTION AND MAINTAINING IT

As the Davis et al review[15] and Dombrowski et al (2012) meta-analysis suggest, theories or models which incorporate both a 'motivational phase' (increasing intentions/motivation) as well as a 'volitional' phase (the doing part) of the change process have more evidence of their efficacy in supporting behaviour change in research trials.

Understanding why and how we regulate our behaviour is important. We need to control our behaviour in order to successfully live and navigate our way through society. This wouldn't work if everyone responded instinctively and emotionally to every internal or external impulse or cue in the same way animals do.

## Current thinking on supporting healthy behaviour at an individual and community level

In conjunction with an understanding that influencing knowledge, beliefs and attitudes helps people to increase their motivation or intention to change, current thinking also recognises the importance of helping people to self-regulate their behaviour.

Self-regulation is the process of actively controlling behaviour by resisting and overriding dominant and automatic behaviours, urges, emotions or desires, and replacing them with behaviours which are consistent with achieving a goal. Self-regulation of our behaviour requires three things: the goal or desired end result, monitoring and operating.[18] A feedback loop is created whereby we establish a goal and monitor where we are in relation to that goal. If there is a discrepancy between where we are and where we want to be, we respond (or operate) in a way that closes the gap. The outcome of these responses is further monitored to gauge whether or not we've achieved the goal. If not, we make more changes – and so on until we have achieved our goal. Once there is no discrepancy between where we are and where we want to be, we 'exit' the feedback loop. The things that we do in order to respond to the discrepancies are called 'self-control' and the overall process is called self-regulation.

Linked to this process is the current prominent view of the internal systems that control our behaviour, which are described as 'dual processing' models.[76] The brain is constantly presented with information which it processes and responds to in the form of actions, thoughts and feelings. When information is repeatedly presented, the brain saves effort and resources by automating its responses: whenever the same information is presented, it acts as a cue for the same response to occur. The information and the behaviour become paired (e.g. finishing a meal acts as a cue to crave and reach for a cigarette). This is how habits are formed, governed by the fast, automatic and unconscious thinking system. The other process is characterised by slow, deliberate, conscious thinking, which requires more effort and resources. It occurs, for example, when we are learning a new skill, or performing an action in an unfamiliar environment. In this case, we need to deliberately concentrate on what we are doing, which takes time and effort. However, if done repeatedly in the same circumstances, this new behaviour will become automatic, fall under the control of the fast thinking system and be carried out without much effort.

Up until now, these theories and models have tended to focus on individual behaviour change. However, it is crucial to appreciate that our behaviour does not occur in isolation; it is influenced by, and influences, others' behaviour. In order to promote lasting change to the health and well-being of the population, it is essential that communities are supported to identify their own needs and to develop their own strategies to address those needs. On the face of it, it may seem that an individualistic behaviour change approach and an empowerment approach are at odds with each other. Indeed, some have argued that a health promotion goal, which aims at behaviour change, could be perceived as ethically problematic for health visitors in that it lends itself to paternalism, stigmatising and victim-blaming, and disregards the individual's or the community's perceptions of their priority health needs.[19] In addition, the individual approach can often ignore the wider social determinants that influence health behaviours, such as education, housing and access to health care etc. An empowerment approach sits more comfortably where the aim is for individuals and communities to have a measure of control over the determinants of their quality of life.[19] Strategies to increase autonomy have the potential to reduce inequality and lead to better health outcomes since individuals and communities are more likely to achieve their goals if they have determined their own priorities.[19]

Laverack and Pratley (2019) describe an empowerment model of society and health.[20] It is a model which can bring both approaches together by suggesting that community empowerment begins with the individual making a change in order to achieve a goal that they value, and through the process of empowerment, can support further change within families and communities.

So, what does this look like in practice? The next section of the chapter looks at the approaches that health visitors can, and already do, embrace in order to increase both community and individual capacity through empowerment.

## FACILITATING HEALTHY BEHAVIOUR: EMPOWERING INDIVIDUALS AND THEIR FAMILIES, GROUPS AND COMMUNITIES

Recently, there have been calls from England's chief medical officer for a '5th Wave' in public health[21,22] that will support embedding health and well-being at a cultural level. The main focus of this 5th wave is to *promote the active participation of the population as a whole, and to renew focus on working towards health as a common good*,[22:1889] so that valuing health and taking responsibility for your health become the 'norm' (see Chapter 1 for more detailed information on this '5th Wave in Public Health').

Accordingly, the four nations of the United Kingdom and Northern Ireland have highlighted the need to take a 'whole systems' approach. An example of this is the policy document published by Public Health England, in conjunction with other representatives and organisations from the behavioural and social sciences, to support the implementation of evidence from these fields into public health practice.[32] This document acknowledges that a purely individual approach to behaviour change is insufficient to address the main issues affecting the health of the population. In order to achieve a 5th wave in public health, the 'whole systems' approach involves incorporating the contributions of both social and behavioural science, and an amalgamation of 'bottom up' (empowerment-based) and 'top down' (individual responsibility-based) health promotion planning approaches to address the social, cultural, political and economic determinants of health.[20,33] Given that relationships with individuals and families are developed during repeated home visits, regular groups and community events, health visitors are well placed in the community to deliver interventions which are informed by this evidence.

### Community level/empowerment approaches

The next part of the chapter explores the influence of community on the way people act and the strategies health visitors can draw upon to successfully promote health and empower communities. If we can understand the capabilities (or assets) that exist within communities at an individual, community and organisational level,[34] then we are better placed to support the development of community leadership, which in turn promotes empowerment, which can support behaviour change (if that is identified as a priority by the individual or community).

### Building community capacity

Building Community Capacity, as a term, really came to prominence for health visitors during the Health Visitor Implementation Plan[35] and signalled a renewed commitment to community participation, development and empowerment. Contemporary health visiting practice involves a responsibility to identify and lead in the development of resources (capital) within a defined community to meet the needs of children and families.[35:9] Health visitors have a key role in identifying assets and supporting the development of networks within the communities that they work with and sign posting parents to early years services and parenting groups. They are ideally positioned to do this, as they are able to draw on existing partnership with other key stakeholders, including local government, early years services, children's centres, education settings, school nurses and voluntary organisations (PHE, 2016).

## Why should health visitors build capacity?

There is good evidence to indicate that a lack of social support and social networks can adversely affect health.[36] Social isolation is a common experience for new parents and is known to be a contributory factor in the aetiology of depression with subsequent consequences for attachment and parenting capacity, which can extend across generations.[37] The networks created through capacity building can thus have a positive influence on mental health and parenting capacity.

Capacity refers to the capabilities that exist within communities to identify their own health priorities and take action to address them. For capacity building to be meaningful to a community, the process of defining their own needs is important. Capacity building is a significant element in terms of effective health promotion practice. '*It improves both the ability of individuals to take action, and the capacity of groups, organisations or communities to influence the determinants of health*'.[38:5] Building community capacity refers to the development of knowledge, skills, commitment, structures, systems and leadership

to provide a foundation for effective and sustainable health promotion practice. It relates to the strengths that individuals or groups of individuals collectively contribute to improving health in their own communities. These communities might be defined geographically or may share a common affinity, such as a religious or ethnic group, being a new parent or a breastfeeding mother.

### THINKING SPACE

What challenges are associated with involving communities and determining priorities?

### The challenges

Government policy shapes services and determines priorities in a 'top down' manner,[39] and this compromises opportunities for communities to determine and act on their own identified priorities in their own way and at their own pace. Health visitor workloads are challenging, and the need to deliver what has been commissioned inevitably forces health visitors to prioritise interventions more amenable to shorter term measurement such as delivering the Healthy Child Programme.[40] Building community capacity takes time, and outcomes are less straightforward to quantify. To progress 'bottom up' projects, it can be tempting for health visitors to take the lead, however, this defeats the object of capacity building and has consequences for sustainability. To be successful, health visitors must take a step back and support the emergence of leaders from the community itself. The community must be substantially involved in determining their own priorities, and this takes time. The health visitor's role necessarily needs to be facilitative, and relationships of trust need to be created over time before any other work can take place.

### Individual approaches

Even when we are empowering people to make changes to their own lives, or to become leaders in their community, this ultimately results in individuals developing new skills, knowledge and attitudes. As a result, the way health visitors 'are' with the people they support and the techniques they use are important to ensure relationships, which are conducive to empowerment, are created, and that learning is successful. This next section will look at communication skills and behaviour change techniques and frameworks that bring both community and individual approaches together.

## Being facilitative and develop trusting, empowering relationships

Although health visiting comes from a place of advocacy and enablement, behaviour change can sometimes spark 'the righting reflex' in us, and it becomes easy to fall into the trap of believing that we know what is best and how the person can achieve the changes we want them to make – which we do! But we also know that change will be easier and more likely to be maintained when the person is supported to understand their behaviour and to change in a way that is relevant to their life and to their needs and values. When we find ourselves making suggestions about things a person can do to change (when they haven't asked for suggestions), we put ourselves in the position of the expert and can damage the relationship we have with them. Understanding the person and the context in which their behaviour is occurring is crucial when navigating challenging conversations; without this knowledge, we will never know what specific 'barriers to change' they face, or, indeed, what matters to them the most.

One approach which supports practitioners to develop advanced communication skills and demonstrate person-centred care in practice is Motivational Interviewing (MI).[41] This counselling approach was not initially borne from theory, instead, from the observation of therapist style and clinical approach in the alcohol addiction field. The approach describes an empathic and person-centred style when responding to client speech, focusing on the client's verbalisations of motivation to change (change talk) and giving empathetic responses to 'sustain talk'; i.e., verbalisations against change and encouraging the client to express their own reasons for change as opposed to the therapist recommending change and how to achieve it.[42] Various techniques, such as active listening, OARS (open questions, affirmations, reflections, summaries), avoiding the 'righting reflex', asking permission before giving information and the 'elicit-provide-elicit' technique all convey the underlying ethos of MI, which is person-centred, respectful, compassionate and non-judgemental. Described as a 'way of being' with a person, demonstrating these values using these techniques helps build trust and rapport, which is the foundation of any supportive relationship. By 'stepping back' and avoiding the 'righting reflex', health visitors can build those trusting relationships in which the people they support are able to grow in confidence and self-efficacy.

Another area of recent development has been the creation of the Behaviour Change Technique Taxonomy.[43] This list of 93 specific evidence-based behaviour-change techniques (BCTs), which have been identified from interventions from the behaviour change literature, describes how the technique should be used in order to be counted as evidence-based. Some techniques are used by the practitioner only when supporting others, for example, modelling a 'skill' such as how to give medicine to a baby, or providing information on the health consequences of a behaviour. Other techniques are more effective when the practitioner supports the person, family or community to learn the technique for themselves to carry out without the practitioner's support. For example, setting goals, action-planning, problem-solving, self-monitoring and reviewing goals are all behaviour change techniques that practitioners can support the person to learn and do themselves and which have been shown to make change more likely and to support maintenance of the behaviour.[44] The behaviour-change techniques work in different ways to result in changes in behaviour. This is referred to as the 'mechanism of action'.[45] For example, when demonstrating how to give medicine to a baby (which is the BCT: Instruction on how to perform a behaviour) helps to change behaviour by increasing the parent/carer's confidence in their capabilities as well as increasing their knowledge.[46,47] However, what is also known is that there are many other variables which may help or hinder the technique from being fully effective in changing behaviour.[48] One of these variables is the approach and 'interpersonal style' of the practitioner.[49] A behaviour change technique such as 'action planning' or 'problem-solving', used by a practitioner whose style is supportive of the individual's autonomy and choice, has a better chance of being effective than when by a practitioner whose style is authoritative and grounded in 'the righting reflex'. Therefore, it is important to reflect on both the approach or style we take when supporting a person, family or community, as well as the behaviour change techniques we use to provide that support.

## Frameworks to guide intervention design

How can the 'bottom up' and 'top down' approaches be combined when planning a health promotion intervention. The past 10 years has seen the development of intervention design frameworks which do just that. For example, 'Intervention Mapping',[50] 6 Steps for Quality Intervention Development (6SQuID)[51] and 'The Behaviour Change Wheel',[13] which is referenced in the PHE document,[52] are examples of frameworks which guide practitioners, service providers and policy-makers through the process of combining both approaches with the aim of improving health by empowering people and communities to change their behaviour.

The frameworks advocate many of the methods used by health visitors, such as community consultations and focus groups, in helping individuals, communities and other relevant stakeholders to identify their own needs, as well as needs which have been identified through epidemiological studies. Once the needs of the relevant groups are identified, these frameworks help identify what needs to change (the mechanism(s) of action) to achieve the desired outcomes, which techniques or approaches can be used to empower each stakeholder group to make changes and in which format the change intervention will be delivered. For example, a study by Fassier et al[53] used this framework to plan an intervention to support women with breast cancer return to work.

### Case study 10.1: Parents group in West Yorkshire – BCC success story (Adams, 2001 Unpublished)

The health visiting team was approached by a small group of parents of 1-year-olds seeking a group that they could access following the completion of a new parents' programme that had been initiated and run by the health visiting team. The parents were concerned regarding the potential loss of valuable social networking opportunities that supported their mental well-being. The health visitors worked with the parents to clarify their needs, and then subsequently supported them to create this new group themselves. Whilst the parents initially lacked the confidence and skills to take on this responsibility, the health visitors successfully facilitated the development of the parents, enabling them to take the lead in establishing the group. Through their well-established networks, the health visitors were able to put the parents in touch with services that could support them with accessing funding, insurance, premises and equipment. They were subsequently available to offer ongoing guidance and support when required. Evaluation of the group in the short, medium and longer term indicated that it was still active and well attended more than 2 years later. Additional outcome data indicated a growth in confidence, knowledge and skills of the participants themselves that had benefits that extended beyond group facilitation and leadership.

### Case study 10.2: Wisbech Knit and Natter – BCC success story[54]

Migrant mothers are at a high risk of social isolation,[55,56] and this has potential consequences for the development of depression and associated attachment disorders between mothers and their infants (Murray, 1992).[57] Isolation and loneliness are also key issues impacting on the health and well-being of older people.[58,59] A group of mainly migrant mothers in the community highlighted their feelings of social isolation, and local health visitors recognised a significant number of isolated elderly people living in the same geographical area. The two groups had not previously interacted with one another possibly as a consequence of cultural and generational differences.

A Knit and Natter group was proposed in order to respond to the expressed needs of community members. Younger women wanted to learn new skills, whilst older women wanted to teach them. Having something practical to do at the group provided a common purpose, which helped overcome language barriers and reduce social isolation. Health visitors identified a young migrant mother willing to run the group and liaised with local agencies to identify a venue and act as a collection point for donations of wool and needles. They also helped publicise the new group locally. Although health visitors supported the development of the group and assisted group members in developing new social networks, it is now successfully run by members of the community.

Evaluation data indicated that the group had addressed needs expressed by community members to improve personal and social support networks and reduce social isolation. In the longer term, this has the potential to improve mental health outcomes and break down generational and cultural barriers, and thus build community capacity.

As well as adopting person-centred communication skills, health visitors need knowledge and skills in building community capacity, developing

social capital, building social networks and understanding communities.[35] But what does this all mean? As lead public health practitioners, an understanding of how to affect change in human, social, political and cultural capital is essential and is often included in intervention design frameworks.

### Cultural capital

Cultural capital was defined by Bourdieu in the 1970s and refers to the social assets that bond a community together. It may include heritage, language, mannerisms, preferences, qualifications and who we feel comfortable with, as well as economic wealth and social class.[60] Cultural capital influences the ways in which individuals and groups define and access other forms of capital and helps individuals to network with others who have similar knowledge and experience. Health visitors can contribute to the development of cultural capital by first of all seeking an understanding of the community's assets and challenges and the community's collective efficacy. Health visitors routinely undertake community profiling and needs assessment and thus have privileged access to rich data. Case study 10.2 is a good example of how health visitors bridged generational and cultural differences and built cultural capital.

### Political capital

Political capital is important for driving forward community projects. It's about an individual or a community having a voice and the ability to influence the allocation of resources.[61] In Case study 10.1, for example, when faced with losing a parenting group that they valued, a group of parents used political capital to form an alliance and lobbied health visitors to develop something new to address their needs.

### Human capital

Health visitors are skilled in the 'facilitation of health-enhancing activities'[62] and are thus ideally placed to identify opportunities to work in partnership with others to build human capital. Human capital refers to the knowledge, skills and attributes of individuals or communities that influence their productive capacity.[63] Health visitors can support growth in human capital by drawing on their networks to support individuals and community groups to access learning opportunities that reflect their own priority needs. This may be raising awareness and supporting access to education, such as a cooking class or leadership training, or may be about supporting access to networking opportunities where individuals or groups can learn how to draw on resources and services that may be required to, for example, set up a new group or service themselves.

## Social capital

Social capital is about the value of social networks, social norms and reciprocity to individuals and society.[64] It is a key component of building and maintaining democracy and creating a sense of social cohesion, personal investment and mutual trust in the community. Where a good level of social capital exists, it can facilitate individual or collective action to change behaviour and improve health. In Case study 10.1, for example, social capital supported collective action in the development of a parents' group. Health visitors helped increase social capital by identifying a group member who they could support to develop their leadership skills and manage the project. This enabled the group to develop new bonds among themselves and new bridges among the community groups with whom they interacted.

Whilst good levels of social capital can have a positive influence on health outcomes (and behaviour change), these same networks can cause harm.[65] The social norm of smoking or getting drunk, for example, can restrict individual freedom or place excessive demands on certain group members, thus impinging upon their capacity to change. At a community level, high levels of social capital may not be health-promoting for all members. Villalonga-Olives and Kawachi[65] found that where individual members lacked trust or where individuals were of a different disposition, then this could actually be harmful to health.

## Community leadership

Identifying leaders with the potential to best represent the community and support the development of their skill set will be essential. This will mean health visitors looking beyond those who 'shout the loudest', to those who may more effectively represent and reflect the views of the wider community. Leadership is key to strong communities, and health visitors can support the development of the leaders that emerge. Health visitors need to understand the skill set that is needed in terms of building leadership in communities and make efforts to create a shared meaning of who can practice leadership in the community. Communities must recognise and develop the capacity that exists among them and nurture and support those who choose to step forward. Health visitors can contribute by helping to identify and acknowledging the skills that people have, and matching them with the tasks that need to be achieved. Community leadership seeks to widen the set of informed decision makers to be more inclusive and participatory. Community leadership education will therefore need to focus on building networks as well as skills[66,67] to facilitate distributed leadership where role-taking gives individuals the authority to exercise voice.

## THINKING SPACE

Reflect on your learning from this chapter. Select a community project or group that you have had some involvement with in practice. In what ways have the health visitors supported cultural, political, human and social capacity building?

Organisational skills – developing appropriate management strucures
Planning skills – to recruit and prepare people to become leaders
Communication skills – to establish and negotiate a role, build trust & communicate a vision
Consultation skills – to consult with community groups
Evaluation skills – process & outcome evaluation

Figure 10.2 ■ Core skills to support community leadership.

## EVALUATING THE IMPACT OF HEALTH VISITOR INTERVENTIONS

Evaluation will help you reflect and improve upon your health promotion practice, enabling you to design better health promotion programmes and develop the evidence base for health promotion. It is also valuable for capturing data on unexpected outcomes. Evaluation involves making a judgement about what has been achieved, considering critically it's worth or merit and whether it achieved the stated aims.[68] Evaluation is critical in today's efficiency-driven health care system, where evidence is required by commissioners to justify expenditure and continued funding. You will need to determine, for example, the strengths and weaknesses of the intervention, whether the intervention was efficient in terms of the resources used to achieve the stated objectives and how it could be improved.[68]

Evaluating a health promotion intervention is not without its challenges. How do we measure, for example, whether the smoking cessation advice that we offer in our 'brief interventions' with parents reduces the number of childhood asthma–related hospital admissions? To what extent can we attribute a reduction in the number of obese pre-school children in our local community to the parents cooking class that we ran? How can we evaluate the extent to which our parenting group supports capacity building? Health promotion occurs in settings where a whole range of variables may be impacting upon the health behaviour of the population. We cannot control the setting or the multitude of factors that may

be influencing health behaviour, and this creates challenges in terms of demonstrating the success or otherwise of our health promotion practice. This should not dissuade us from conducting an evaluation and learning what we can, however, we must recognise its limitations.

### Types of evaluation

It is important to be clear about what you are evaluating, why you are evaluating it and for whom, as this will determine the approach that you take. Evaluating both the process and the outcome are important.

### Outcome evaluation

Outcome evaluation describes what happens subsequent to delivery of the programme and assesses whether the programme can be said to have caused the outcome. It seeks to determine the immediate impact of the intervention (e.g. a change in knowledge or attitude), as well as the longer-term outcomes (such as a lifestyle change) and estimates the costs associated with it.[69]

The most obvious reason to evaluate an intervention is to establish whether it has achieved its stated aims, such as a change in knowledge, skills or behaviour.[68] A behaviour change, however, may not be immediately evident; for example, a decision to quit smoking may have been influenced by the smoking cessation advice that you offered, but the behaviour change may not occur until well after you have completed and evaluated your intervention. If the only valued outcome was behaviour change, we might assume that our intervention was not successful or worthwhile.

We therefore need to consider carefully what other information our evaluation needs to capture to help determine the worth of the intervention. The impact of an intervention, such as a change in knowledge around the dangers of passive smoking, may also be a valued outcome: it has the potential to shift attitudes towards passive smoking and may influence a behaviour change at some point in the future.

Health promotion interventions can also have unexpected or unintended outcomes, and it is important that evaluation strategies capture this too.[70] For many new parents, for example, the benefits of participation and partnership in terms of developing new friendship networks (think back to your reading on capacity building) through attending a parenting group may far outweigh the facilitators, aim which might have been to develop parenting capacity.

Health visitors have a key role in reducing health inequalities[35] and may thus wish to determine the extent to which a health promotion intervention achieved this. Higgerson et al[71] for example, evaluated the impact of providing free leisure facilities on inequalities in physical activity and found that it could increase population levels of physical activity while also reducing inequalities. This is important since some interventions, whilst seeking to improve the health of the most disadvantaged, might inadvertently increase inequality if those attending are not those that the organisers sought to target.[72]

## Process evaluation

In addition to outcome data, we need to look at what went on during the implementation of the programme. We can then use the data to strengthen or improve the programme. This is known as process evaluation and may ask questions such as whether it is was done as cost-effectively and quickly as possible, whether the quality was as good as intended, whether the appropriate methods and materials were used.

Organisations need to weigh up whether expenditure can be justified and therefore input data need to be captured. If the cost in terms of health visitor hours to facilitate the baby café are high, and perhaps attendance figures are low, it may be judged more cost effective to consider alternative approaches to supporting these mothers.

## Strategies/techniques to evaluate health promotion interventions

Evaluation needs to be planned from the outset of the health promotion intervention. This will enable you to collect the relevant information to inform your evaluation as the programme progresses.

### Evaluating the process

*Measuring the input*

You will need to measure and record everything that went into your health promotion initiative, for example, time, money and materials. You can then make a judgement about whether the outcome was worth the cost.

*Be reflective*

Think critically and constructively about what you did well and what you would like to change. How could you improve it next time?

*Feedback*

Capture feedback from others, including peers and parents. Try using suggestion boxes and asking directly for feedback. Observe what is happening – do participants look interested, bored or anxious?

### Evaluating the outcomes

Outcomes might include changes in health status, health awareness, knowledge, attitude and behaviour.[68] They might also include changes to local or national policy, or changes to the physical environment. At our cooking skills class, we will therefore want to gather information on the characteristics of those attending, how many attended and how often. We will also want to understand what sort of skills and knowledge the parents wanted to develop and whether the group was successful in developing this. We will also want to capture unanticipated outcomes, for example, the development of new networks and friendships.

Changes in health awareness might be demonstrated through changing levels of interest shown by consumers or changes in demand for health-related services. Analysis of media coverage, use of questionnaires, interviews, discussion and observations of individuals and groups are useful in capturing data on changing levels of health awareness. Changes in knowledge and attitude might be detected through discussion and observation of how a client applies knowledge in real-life situations, observing how clients demonstrate their knowledge and newly acquired skills, written tests or questionnaires. Are there changes in what clients say and do, for example, choosing a healthy option on a menu or in the supermarket? Through an interview or discussion, you might capture data regarding newly acquired knowledge and changing attitudes towards, for example, exposing children to passive smoking. Behaviour changes can be evaluated by observing what clients do and recording behaviour; for example, an immunisation campaign might be evaluated in part by measuring the uptake of immunisations both before and after the campaign. Changes in health status could be captured through, for example, blood pressure monitoring, cholesterol levels monitoring or weight monitoring.

At a community level, change might be identified through policy statements and plans, for example, making healthy eating choices available in schools, legislative changes such as restrictions on tobacco advertising and changes in availability of health promotion products and facilities.

## THINKING POINT

Your objective is to evaluate the impact of a cooking class aimed at parents of pre-school children living on a local social housing estate. The aim of the project is to develop parents, cooking skills to enable them to prepare simple, nutritious and economical family meals. The facilitator used practical demonstrations and other learning strategies to deliver cooking skills education over an 8-week period. The NHS Eatwell Guide (PHE, 2016) was used to support the teaching. This tool simply indicates, in the format of a plate, how much of what we eat overall should come from each food group to achieve a healthy, balanced diet.

**What strategies could you use to** evaluate **changes in knowledge, skills and attitudes towards healthy eating? How could you evaluate whether any behaviour changes had occurred (participants actually cooking simple nutritious economical meals on a regular basis for their families)? How could you determine the extent to which your intervention had reduced health inequalities?**

## Evaluating community capacity building

Evaluation of capacity-building activities is particularly challenging. How can health visitors measure an increase in social capital? To what extent can we attribute increased cultural capital, for example, to the capacity-building activity that health visitors were engaged in? Evaluation of health promotion activities have tended to focus on outputs such as numbers of people that attended rather than the wider impact of the project. Alternative approaches are required if health visitors are to evidence the value of capacity building activities to service commissioners.

Capacity-building activities seek to be sustainable once external resources have been withdrawn. Evaluation will thus need to capture the extent to which capacity has developed. The World Health Organisation (1998) proposed that health promotion should be empowering, participatory, holistic, intersectoral, equitable, sustainable, multi-strategy, and this has the potential to inform the development of a tool for evaluating the extent to which community projects might have built community capacity. We discussed earlier how building human, social, political and cultural capital were essential to sustainable health promotion practice. Designing an evaluation tool based on these principles has the potential to capture meaningful data,[73] for example, devised a survey instrument which consisted of five domains. It evaluated participation, local leadership, available resources, networking and local cooperation. Look back at the earlier section on capacity building, and you will notice how well these relate to its key principles. Importantly, Nickel et al[73] describe how evaluation data were gathered over a 10-year period, from 2001 until 2011, in order to identify trends. Evaluation of such projects must inevitably be conducted over an extended period since capacity building takes a considerable amount of time. A lengthy evaluation period, however, does pose additional problems in relation to demonstrating whether the changes identified in the evaluation are attributable to the intervention. The environment cannot be controlled in either the short or longer term, and so it is always possible that other projects or interventions might be occurring simultaneously and influencing outcomes. Evaluation strategies should seek to capture broader data about the changing characteristics of the environment to inform data interpretation as the project progresses.

Arnstein's ladder of participation (Arnstein,[77] 1969) is a hierarchical typology denoting degrees of community participation, from non-participation through to citizen control. It can be used to help you reflect on the extent to which the community participated in each aspect of the project (including its evaluation) to help you determine

to what extent the project was successful in building capacity.

8 Citizen control
7 Delegation
6 Partnership
5 Placation
4 Consultation
3 Informing
2 Therapy
1 Manipulation

## THINKING POINT

Reflect on your learning from this chapter. Select a community project or group that you have had some involvement with in practice. How could you evaluate the extent to which health visitors supported cultural, political, human and social capacity building in this project? Review Arnstein's typology (1969) and determine the degree of community involvement.

## CONCLUSION

This chapter has provided an overview of the art and science of behaviour change in relation to health visiting practice and what this means for the way in which health visitors work with individuals, families and communities. We have critiqued the assumptions made and the behaviour change approaches used in the past, and we have proposed an empowerment approach that more appropriately reflects the way that health visitors work with families and communities. Strategies are presented that health visitors can draw upon to identify community leaders who can support sustained activity that can promote health, build capacity and support behaviour change at an individual and community level. Finally, in today's efficiency driven health care system, we acknowledge the importance of evaluating our interventions and propose some key ideas to inform an approach to evaluation.

## KEY LEARNING POINTS

■ You should now have a good understanding of historical and more contemporary approaches to facilitating healthy behaviour and empowering individuals and their families.

■ You should be able to discuss different mechanisms of behaviour change and describe how health visitors can work with individuals and their families, groups and communities to promote health and facilitate healthy behaviour.

■ You should now be able to apply the key concepts of process and outcome evaluation to your health promotion practice as a health visitor.

## REFERENCES

1. American Psychological Association. (2020). *APA Dictionary of psychology – Behavior*. Retrieved October 24th, 2020, from https://dictionary.apa.org/behavior.

2. Marmot, M., Allen, J., Goldblatt, P., Boyce, T., McNeish, D., Grady, M., & Geddes, I. (2010). *Fair society healthy lives (The Marmot Review)*. London: The Marmot Review.

3. Office for National Statistics. (2017). *Causes of death over 100 years*. Retrieved October 23rd, 2020, from https://www.ons.gov.uk/peoplepopulationandcommunity/birthsdeathsandmarriages/deaths/articles/causesofdeathover100years/2017-09-18.

4. Farre, A., & Rapley, T. (2017). The new old (and old new) medical model: four decades navigating the biomedical and psychosocial understandings of health and illness. *Healthcare, 5*(4), 88.

5. Engel, G. (1977). The need for a new medical model: A challenge for biomedicine. *Science, 196*, 129–136.

6. Dahlgren, G. & Whitehead, M. (1991). *Policies and strategies to promote social equity in health*. Stockholm, Sweden: Institute for Futures Studies.

7. Stewart, M. (2001). Towards a global definition of patient centred care. *BMJ, 322*, 444–445.

8. Komrad, M. (1983). A defence of medical paternalism: Maximising patients' autonomy. *Journal of Medical Ethics, 9*, 38–44.

9. Sandman, L. M. & Munthe, C. (2010). Shared decision-making, paternalism and patient choice. *Health Care Analysis, 18*, 60–84.

10. Crossman, A. (2020). 'Rational Choice Theory'. ThoughtCo. Retrieved September 12th, 2020, from https://www.thoughtco.com/rational-choice-theory-3026628.

11. Friedman, M., & Savage, L. J. (1948). The utility analysis of choices involving risk. *Journal of Political Economy, 56*(4), 279–304.

12. Michie, S, West, R., Campbell, R., Brown, J., & Gainforth, H. (2014). *ABC of behaviour change theories: An essential resource for researchers, policy makers and practitioners*. Bream: Silverback Publishing.

13. Michie, S., Atkins, L., & West, R. (2014). *The behaviour change wheel: A guide to designing interventions*. London: Silverback Publishing.

14. Sheeran, P. W., & Webb, T. L. (2016). The intention-behaviour gap. *Social and Personality Psychology Compass, 10*(9), 503–518.

15. Davis, R.C., Campbell, R., Hildon, Z., Hobbs, L., & Michie, S. (2015). Theories of behaviour and behaviour change across the social and behavioural sciences: A scoping review. *Health Psychology Review, 9*(3), 323–344.

16. Powers, W. T. (1973/2005). Behavior: The Control of Perception. New York: Hawthorne.

17. Dombrowski, S.U., Sniehotta, F.F., Avenell, A., Johnston, M., MacLennan, G., & Araújo-Soares, V. (2012). Identifying active ingredients in complex behavioural interventions for obese adults with obesity-related co-morbidities or additional risk factors for co-morbidities: A systematic review. *Health Psychology Review, 6*(1), 7–32.

18. Carver, C., & Scheier, M. (1982). Control Theory: A useful conceptual framework for personality—social, clinical, and health psychology. *Psychological Bulletin, 92*(1), 111–135.

19. Tengland, P. A. (2016). Behavior change or empowerment: On the ethics of health-promotion goals. *Healthcare Analytics, 24*, 24–46.

20. Laverack, G., & Pratley, P. (2019). *The empowerment model of society and health 166*. From https://www.researchgate.net/publication/334001145_The_empowerment_model_of_society_and_health.

21. Hanlon, P., Carlisle, S., Hannah, M., & Lyon, A. (2011). Making the case for a 'fifth wave' in public health. *Public Health, 125*, 30–36.

22. Davies, S. C., Winpenny, E., Ball, S., Fowler, T., Rubin, J., & Nolte, E. (2014). For debate: A new wave in public health improvement. *Lancet, 384*, 1889–1895.

23. Ajzen, I. (1985). From intentions to actions: A theory of planned behavior. In J. Kuhl, & J. Beckman (Eds.), *Action-control: From cognition to behavior* (pp. 11–39). Heidelberg: Springer.

24. Fishbein, M., & Ajzen, I. (1975). *Belief, attitude, intention and behaviour: An introduction to theory and research*. Reading, MA: Addison-Wesley.

25. Sniehotta, F., Presseau, J., & Araujo-Soares, V. (2014). Time to retire the theory of planned behaviour. *Health Psychology Review, 8*(1), 1–7.

26. Prochaska, J., & DiClemente, C. (1983). Stages and processes of self-change of smoking: Towards an integrative model of change. *Journal of Consulting and Clinical Psychology, 51*(3), 390–395.

27. Littell, J., & Girvan, H. (2002). Stages of change: A critique. *Behavior Modification, 26*(2), 223–273.

28. Rosenstock, I. M. (1966). Why people use health services. *Millbank Memorial Fund Quarterly, 44*, 94–124.

29. Jones, C., Smith, H., & Llewellyn, C. (2014). Evaluating the effectiveness of health belief model interventions in improving adherence: A systematic review. *Health Psychology Review, 8*(3), 253–269.

30. Rogers, R. (1983). Cognitive and physiological processes in fear appeals and attitude change: A revised theory of protection motivation. In J. Caccioppo, & R. Petty (Eds.), *Social psychophysiology: A sourcebook* (pp. 153–176). New York: Guilford.

31. Floyd, D., Prentice-Dunn, S., & Rogers, R. (2000). A meta-analysis of research on protection motivation theory. *Journal of Applied Social Psychology, 30*(2), 407–429.

32. Public Health England. (2018). *Improving people's health: Applying behavioural and social sciences to improve population health and well-being in England.* London: Public Health England.

33. Laverack, G., & Labonte, R. (2000). A planning framework for community empowerment goals within health promotion. *Health Policy and Planning, 15*(3), 255–262.

34. Foot, J., & Hopkins, T. (2010). *A glass half full: How an asset approach can improve community health and well-being.* London: Improvement and Development Agency.

35. Department of Health and Social Care (DHSC). (2011). *Health visitor implementation plan: A call to action.* London: The Stationery Office.

36. Leigh-Hunt, N., Bagguley, D., Bash, K., Turner, V., Turnbull, S., Valtorta, N., & Caan, W. (2017). An overview of systematic reviews on the public health consequences of social isolation and loneliness. *Public Health, 152*, 157–171.

37. Kritsotakis, G. E., Vassilaki, M., Melaki, M., Georgiou, V., Philalithis, A. E., Bitsios, P., et al. (2013). Social capital in pregnancy and postpartum depressive symptoms: A prospective mother-child cohort study (the Rhea study). *International Journal of Nursing Studies, 50*(1), 63–72.

38. World Health Organisation. (1997). Jakarta declaration on leading health promotion in 21st century. WHO Seyfzadeh et al 2019, Holwerda et al 2014.

39. Craig, G. (2007). Community capacity-building: Something old, something new …? *Critical Social Policy, 27*(3), 335–359.

40. Shribman, S., & Billingham, K. (2009). *Healthy child programme: pregnancy and the first five years of life.* Department of Health.

41. Miller, W., Rollnick, S., & Butler, C. (2008). *Motivational interviewing in health care: Helping patients change behavior.* New York: Guilford Press.

42. Miller, W., & Rose, G. (2009). Toward a theory of motivational interviewing. *American Psychologist, 64*(6), 527–537.

43. Michie, S., Richardson, M., Johnston, M., Abraham, C., Francis, J., Hardeman, W., Eccles, M.P., Cane, J., & Wood, C.E. (2013). The behavior change technique taxonomy (v1) of 93 hierarchically clustered techniques: building an international consensus for the reporting of behavior change interventions. *Annals of Behavioral Medicine, 46*(1), 81–95.

44. Kwasnicka, D., Dombrowski, S., White, M., & Sniehotta, F. (2016). Theoretical explanations for maintenance of behaviour change: A systematic review of behaviour theories. *Health Psychology Review, 10*(3), 277–296.

45. Carey, R., Connell, L., Johnston, M., Rothman, A., de Bruin, M., Kelly, M., et al. (2019). Behavior change techniques and their mechanisms of action: A synthesis of links described in published intervention literature. *Annals of Behavioral Medicine, 53*(8), 693–707.

46. Centre for Behaviour Change. (2020). *The theory and techniques tool.* Retrieved November 13, 2020, from https://theoryandtechniquetool.humanbehaviourchange.org/.

47. Johnston, M., Carey, R., Connell Bohlen, L., Johnston, D., Rothman, A., de Bruin, M., Kelly, M. P., Groarke, H., & Michie, S. (2020). Development of an online tool for linking behavior change techniques and mechanisms of action based on triangulation of findings from literature synthesis and expert consensus. *Translational Behavioral Medicine, 11*(5), 1049–1065.

48. Hagger, M., Moyers, S., McAnally, K., & McKinley, L. (2020). Known knowns and known unknowns on behavior change interventions and mechanisms of action. *Health Psychology Review, 14*(1), 199–212.

49. Hagger, M., & Hardcastle, S. (2014). Interpersonal style should be included in taxonomies of behavior change techniques. *Frontiers in Psychology, 5*, 254.

50. Eldredge, L., Markham, C., Ruiter, R., Fernandez, M., Kok, G., & Parcel, G. (2016). In *Planning health promotion programs: An intervention mapping approach* (4th ed.). San Francisco: Jossey-Bass.

51. Wight, D., Wimbush, E., Jepson, R., & Doi, L. (2016). Six steps in quality intervention development (6SQuID). *Journal of Epidemiology and Community Health, 70*(5), 520–525.

52. Public Health England. (2019). *Achieving behaviour change: A guide for local government and partners.* London: Public Health England.

53. Fassier, J., Lamort-Bouché, M., Broc, G., Guittard, L., Peron, J., Rouat, S., Carretier, J., Fervers, B., Letrilliart, L., & Sarin, P. (2018). Developing a Return to Work Intervention for Breast Cancer Survivors with the Intervention Mapping Protocol: Challenges and Opportunities of the Needs Assessment. *Frontiers in Public Health, 6*(35). doi: 10.3389/fpubh.2018.00035.

54. Gilmour, J., Lakes, S., Whiting, J., Harvey, R., Mills, S., & Wallace, H. (2014). *Building community capacity: Health visiting case studies.* Health Education East of England.

55. Fellmeth, G., Fazel, M., & Plugge, E. (2016). Migration and perinatal mental health in women from low- and middle-income countries: A systematic review and meta-analysis. *International Journal of Obstetrics and Gynaecology.*

56. Gonidakis, F. (2012). Postpartum Depression and Maternity Blues in Immigrants. In M. G. R. Castillo (Ed.), *Perinatal Depression* (pp. 117–138). Rijeka, Croatia: InTech.

57. Eastwood, J., Jalaludin, B., Kemp, L., Phung, H., Barnett, B., & Tobin, J. (2012). Social exclusion, infant behaviour, social isolation, and maternal expectations independently predict maternal depressive symptoms. In *Brain and Behavior.* Wiley Periodicals, Inc.

58. Seyfzadeh, A., Haghighatian, M., & Mohajerani, A. (2019). Social isolation in the elderly: The neglected issue. *Iran J Public Health, 48*(2), 365–366.

59. Holwerda, T. J., Deeg, D. J., Beekman, A. T., van Tilburg, T. G., Stek, M. L., Jonker, C., & Schoevers, R. A. (2014). Feelings of loneliness, but not social isolation, predict dementia onset: results from the Amsterdam Study of the Elderly (AMSTEL). *J NeurolNeurosurg Psychiatry, 85*(2), 135–142.

60. Kamphuis, C. B. M., Jansen, T., Mackenbach, J. P., & Van Lenthe, F. J. (2015). Bourdieu's cultural capital in relation to food choices: A systematic review of cultural capital indicators and an empirical proof of concept. *PLoS One, 10*(8), e0130695. doi:10.1371/journal.pone.0130695.

61. Jacobs, C. (2011). Community capitals: Political capital. Extensions Extra. Paper 522. South Dakota State University Open PRAIRIE: Open Public Research Access Institutional Repository and Information Exchange. http://openprairie.sdstate.edu/extension_extra/522.

62. Nursing Midwifery Council. (2004). *Standards of proficiency for specialist community public health nurses.* London: NMC.

63. Keeley, B. (2007). *Human capital: How what you know shapes your life.* OECD Publishing.

64. Elgar, F. J., Davis, C. G., Wohl, M. J., Trites, S. J., Zelenski, J. M., & Martin, M. S. (2011). Social capital, health and life satisfaction in 50 countries. *Health and Place, 17,* 1044–1053.

65. Villalonga-Olives, E., & Kawachi, I. (2017). The dark side of social capital: A systematic review of the negative health effects of social capital. *Social Science & Medicine, 194,* 105–127.

66. Emery, M., Fernandez, E., Gutierrez-Montez, I., & Butler Flora, C. (2009). Leadership as community capacity building: A study on the impact of leadership development training on community. *Community Development, 38*(4), 60–70.

67. Kirk, P., & Shutte, A. M. (2004). Community leadership development. *Community Development Journal, 39*(3).

68. Scriven, A. (2017). *Promoting health: A practical guide.* (7th ed.). Elsevier.

69. Naidoo, J., & Wills, J. (2009). *Foundations for health promotion.* Bailliere Tindall.

70. Benning, T. M., Alayli-Goebbels, A. F. G., Aarts, M. J., Stolk, E., De Wit, G. A., Prenger, R., et al. (2015). Exploring outcomes to consider in economic evaluations of health promotion programs: What broader non-health outcomes matter most? *BMC Health Services Research, 15,* 266.

71. Higgerson, J., Halliday, E., Ortiz-Nunez, A., Brown, R., & Barr, B. (2018). Impact of free access to leisure facilities and community outreach on inequalities in physical activity: A quasi-experimental study. *Journal of Epidemiology and Community Health, 72*(3).

72. Hart, J. T. (1971). The inverse care law. *Lancet, 1,* 405–412. doi:10.1016/S0140-6736(71)92410-X pmid:4100731.

73. Nickel, S., Sub, W., Lorentz, C., & Trojan, A. (2018). Long-term evaluation of community health promotion: Using capacity building as an intermediate outcome measure. *Public Health, 162,* 9–15.

74. Bandura, A. (2004). Health promotion by social cognitive means. *Health education & behavior, 31*(2), 143-164.

75. Deci, E. L., & Ryan, R. M. (2012). Self-determination theory in health care and its relations to motivational interviewing: a few comments. International Journal of Behavioral Nutrition and Physical Activity, 9(1), 1–6.

76. Strack, F., & Deutsch, R. (2004). Reflective and impulsive determinants of social behavior. Personality and social psychology review, 8(3), 220–247.

77. Arnstein, S. R. (2019). A ladder of citizen participation. Journal of the American Planning Association, 85(1), 24–34.

# PART 3

# Health Visitor Practice-Focused Interventions

PART OUTLINE

11  CHILDHOOD ADVERSITY AND TRAUMA

12  BUILDING EFFECTIVE SAFEGUARDING SKILLS: A SHIFT FROM THE 'WHAT' TO THE 'HOW' IN PRACTICE

13  PERINATAL MENTAL HEALTH

14  EMOTIONAL AND MENTAL HEALTH WELL-BEING AND DEVELOPMENT OF INFANTS AND CHILDREN

15  COMMUNICATION AND LANGUAGE DEVELOPMENT

16  MANAGEMENT OF COMMON CHILDHOOD AILMENTS AND ACCIDENT PREVENTION

17  TRANSITION TO SCHOOL

# 11

# CHILDHOOD ADVERSITY AND TRAUMA

BERNADETTE BRADLEY ■ JAMES MCTAGGART

## CHAPTER CONTENTS

INTRODUCTION

OUTLINE CONCEPTS AND DEFINITIONS

TRAUMA, ADVERSITY, HEALTH AND WELL-BEING

PHYSICAL ENVIRONMENT

RESOURCES

ATTACHMENT

MODERATE AND RESOLVED STRESS

STIMULATION

ASSESSMENT, ANALYSIS AND INTERVENTION

REFLECTIVE PRACTICE

CONCLUSION

## LEARNING OUTCOMES

*To:*

- examine the different kinds of trauma and adversity and how they impact on children's outcomes both short and long term

- examine how trauma and adversity might present in health visiting practice, including disguised ways

- explore frameworks for assessing and analysing the impacts of adversity and trauma to support holistic intervention

- analyse the effects of working with trauma and adversity on the health visitor and how to prevent and address these

## INTRODUCTION

Trauma and adversity are common experiences in childhood[1] and the effects can last into adulthood. This has three important implications for health visiting. Firstly, there is much that we can do to prevent trauma and adversity, to help children have better outcomes even if they do have such experiences, and to build resilience for children and families against future adversities. There is consensus in the research literature that the first 1001 days of life are of particular importance for brain development.[2] While there is also evidence that intervention can be effective later in childhood, health visitors are therefore engaged with children and families at a period of maximum potential for long lasting change. Secondly, health visitors are highly likely to be working with parents and other family members who will have experienced significant trauma and adversity. To support health visitors in practice there are also some basic principles for trauma-informed practice that can enhance the benefits of a health visiting service for all families. Thirdly, working with families experiencing adversity can be challenging for anyone, and health visitors need to be aware of when they may be experiencing secondary traumatisation and the steps they can take to address it.[3]

Health visitors have the core and additional skills and knowledge required in their role to address adversity and trauma. These are discussed in other chapters, including establishing therapeutic relationships, providing leadership and assessment and prioritising early intervention, as well as partnership working and promoting clear, family friendly, communication. As will be discussed below, the holistic approach that health visitors bring to early brain development is a key strength in both addressing and preventing trauma and adversity. They can also contribute an understanding of development in context, where aspects of the environment, rather than skills or willingness, may impact on the ability of parents to provide what their children need to build resilience.

Adversity and trauma are real and affect many families. Different forms of adversity and trauma can be found in any walk of life or locality. Deprivation and poverty increase the risks of encountering trauma and adversity,[4] as will be explained below, but health visitors need to avoid assumptions about particular families or populations.

This chapter will begin with clarification about definitions and a brief survey of evidence about the prevalence of trauma and adversity. It will then set this in the context of childhood development and how health visitors may become aware of the signs of adversity and trauma and respond to those signs, as well as discuss concerns and ways forward with parents and families. Lastly, since working with traumatised and stressed families can be itself traumatising for workers, the chapter briefly covers essential self-care.

## OUTLINE CONCEPTS AND DEFINITIONS

This is a field with a wide range of terminology, often used imprecisely or interchangeably. It is important that health visitors are clear about what they are seeing and assessing, so as to be able to speak sensitively and effectively with families about ways forward. This section therefore offers some clarification of main terms, at least as they are used in this chapter. In particular, adversity is a broader concept than psychological trauma, and each can be encountered without the other. The concept of adverse childhood experiences (ACEs) is in some ways helpful, but also confusingly understood in many different ways, with considerable controversy around the different meanings. This chapter suggests a pragmatic approach that can take into account the breadth of experiences and needs of children and families.

### Psychological trauma and triggers

A traumatic event is something that threatens, or seems to threaten, the life of an individual or that is so emotionally painful that it overwhelms their ability to cope.[5] Many people recover fully after traumatic events, especially with support from close friends or family, while some develop persistent and intrusive memories of the event that do not fade over time. They may experience flashbacks, or strong feelings when reminded of the traumatic event and may have strong urges to fight, flight, or freeze responses. Traumatic memories seem to be stored not just verbally, but as intermixed strong feelings, body states and actions. For adults, traumatic memories often have cognitive elements that may relate to cultural background, such as doubt in the self or the future, or that one is to blame or lacking, or even being punished.[6]

Traumatic memories can be triggered by events or experiences that are in some way like the original event. For example, someone who was in a road accident may feel high levels of fear at junctions, or when encountering certain colours or sounds. One author (JM) for years felt highly anxious in supermarket checkouts – the trigger here was the 'beeps' of the checkout machine that brought back an early memory of visiting his father in hospital surrounded by beeping machines. A triggered memory feels very real, as though it is actually happening. Talking about it sometimes does not help, and should never be forced.

When a traumatic memory is triggered, a person may vividly experience aspects of the original trauma – strong feelings, a desire to escape or hide, negative thoughts or body sensations. Children will most likely show this via their behaviour as described below.

### Simple trauma

Simple trauma refers to single events which were soon over, or which were not repeated often.[7] An example for a young child might be having a big scare when lost in a park, or being in a car accident. After such events, children can become emotional when they encounter traumatic triggers, or may be more generally clingy or have disrupted sleep or eating. They may develop avoidances, such as a reluctance to go to the shop or get in the car.

It is important to realise that adults may not always be aware that children have experienced trauma or that they have found an event traumatic. One of us (JM) has worked with children who were terrified by a sudden sound of a vacuum cleaner and developed avoidances as a result, and others who were distressed by fire safety commercials on television – both unknown to their parents. Where children display behaviour that seems well explained by strong feelings of terror, anger or numbness, or where their behaviour patterns suddenly change, simple trauma is worth considering. Health visitors can help parents understand the possible feelings underlying repetitive play or questions, avoidances or developmental regressions such as sleep issues or becoming clingy.

Even very young babies and children can develop traumatic memories.[8] It does not matter if they are 'old enough to understand' or not. This is because much of a traumatic memory is stored as feelings, body states and uncompleted actions rather than as words or narrative. Health visitors should also be aware that traumatic memories do not necessarily fade over time – just because something was a long time ago does not mean it is not still impactful for child or parent.

After a simple trauma, most children recover with extra love and care, and gentle encouragement to try things again. Some will develop more lasting reactions, and if concerns remain after a few weeks, then specialist advice should be sought. Many children's and mental health charities produce useful resources to help support children who have experienced trauma, and health visitors should be aware of the resources recommended by mental health specialists in their localities.

### Complex or developmental trauma

Complex or developmental trauma refers to overwhelming and frightening experiences that are repeated or on-going, such that they have a deeper impact on the way the child's brain develops.[9] If children are exposed to repeated high levels of stress during their early years, then they will develop long-term brain and physical adaptations designed to maximise their chances of survival. This includes strong stress reactions so as to react effectively to danger, and higher levels of inflammatory response so as to be ready for action and for repairing wounds. Conversely, development may not be so strong in other areas that appear to be less needed for immediate survival, such as cognition and language.

Because the first few years from conception onwards are times of significant changes in the brain as different functions develop and start to coordinate, developmental trauma can have life-long effects on basic physiology as well as emotional functioning.

### Adverse childhood experiences

In the last few years, this has become a widely known concept for trying to understand the long-term impact of developmental trauma. The term derives from a family of epidemiological studies originating in the United States. The ACE research design is fairly simple, which is its main strength and source of weakness. The studies find associations between high levels of traumatic experiences in childhood and increased risks of poorer health and other outcomes in adulthood.[10] There is also emerging evidence that this risk can be significantly reduced if children also experience high levels of supportive care from adults.[11] The associations are now well established, along with the buffering effects of adult care, but it is less clear what they mean, both theoretically and in practice.

A main concern for health visitors is to avoid misapplication of the ACE ideas, and to use their professional standing to influence good practice (a spirited discussion of the issues is provided by White et al. 2019).[12] Firstly, the ACE studies use as a measure a common list of experiences that include neglect, sexual abuse, having an incarcerated relative, divorced parents. The list (sometimes called 'the ten ACEs') is a research measure, not an assessment tool. It is obvious that not all potentially adverse experiences are included, and also that, for a given family the experiences listed may not be traumatic. For example, many parental separations are amicable, or handled in such a way as to minimise impact for children. There is a lack of persuasive evidence to support the ACE research measure as a screening tool, or that screening for ACEs is advisable or effective in the current UK context.[13]

Secondly, the studies show a 'dose-related' effect, whereby the more adverse experiences the greater the risk of poorer outcomes. This is a population-level finding, and it does not mean that an individual's so-called ACE score has any such meaning. While it can be very helpful for individuals to become aware that their present difficulties may well be due to significant amounts of childhood adversity, counting and scoring is less helpful, and should never be used as a criterion for intervention or access to services. The aim, instead, is to understand families' individual situations and how they can be helped. Not all families are alike, and nor are all trauma and adversities the same. Just as we cannot simply 'add up' the amount of trauma as though all experiences have the same impact, nor can we say that a given event has the same impact for every family, or for every child within that family. There is even balancing evidence that the key variable is not the amount of adversity, but the amount of nurturing support available to a child.[14]

Finally, the ACE studies sit within a much wider and well-developed research literature on adversity. Each kind of ACE has its own body of knowledge and different pathways of impact on children and families. In particular, ACEs occur within social and economic contexts – poverty and deprivation are also key factors that impact on child development and adult outcomes in similar ways to the ACEs in the studies. The next subsection sketches out the wider concept of adversity as a foundation for discussing how health visitors can assess and analyse its impact and work with families to ameliorate and prevent it.

### Adversity

A richer and more actionable analysis can be gained from seeing adversity in terms of two dimensions.[15] The first is how *stressful* it is, as this can affect the developing stress system and metabolism. The second is how *depriving* it is, how far the experience reduces the availability of needed resources and stimulation for the developing child. For example, a child growing up in a home where there is a lot of violence is exposed to high levels of continuing or repeated stress. But it is also possible that, for example, a parent experiencing violence may themselves be too stressed to talk much to their baby, or feel confident enough to take their toddler to the park to play. If we only think about the stress then our assessment and analysis will fail to be sufficiently holistic – but also, we will miss opportunities for intervention for the child and parent.

Additionally, there are factors that can be called adversity that are not necessarily traumatic in themselves. Living in a neighbourhood with poor transport links, or a lack of accessible public services, both can impact directly on a child's development and indirectly on a parent's ability to provide what they need.[16,17] Lack of money might, for example, mean fewer toys, less opportunity for developmental experiences, and also indirectly, pressures of time and attention on parents.

Clear and nuanced assessment of child development and its context will lead to more effective and acceptable intervention. The broad goal of this is to increase the child and family's resilience, and this important concept will be described first before the next main section gives more detail on how adversity and trauma, in their many forms and interactions, can be identified.

### Resilience

This final concept is another that can have a wide range of meanings, with different ones being used interchangeably. In day-to-day speech, resilience often refers to qualities such as toughness or grit. We talk of towns being resilient to floods, or people being resilient to infections. In human development, the concept is different in important ways. It refers to an outcome, whereby people survive, maintain well-being or even flourish, in conditions of adversity. Some of this will be due to their own abilities – for example, a parent who is skilled at seeking help, and has the confidence and language to do so. However, much is due to the environment and the stance of others – for example, that same parent will be less resilient if help is not available, is hard to access or is stigmatising or inflexible. Resilience is therefore an ecological concept[18] where individual capacities interact, and are affected by, available relationships and sources of

coping, environmental facilities and neighbourhood characteristics,[19] including the quality of relationship, understanding and strengths-based assessment provided by health visitors.

### THINKING SPACE

By yourself, or in a small group, think about some of the small challenges of life you have coped with. This might be learning to drive, going to live in a new place, starting a new job. What helped you to manage this? Make as long a list as you can, and put all your lists together. Now, can you divide those things into three groups – things about you, things that others did to help, and things about the environment or resources you had?

Now think about some of the families you have worked with. What resilience factors do they have or not have in each of the three groups? How can services help them find what they need?

## TRAUMA, ADVERSITY, HEALTH AND WELL-BEING

### Child development as adaptation

Unlike other mammals, humans are born early in the process of brain development.[20] Compared to other animals we are born with very few abilities to regulate ourselves or survive independently. Health visitors are privileged to witness many journeys of maturation with families, and this experience underlines how long it takes human children to develop the capacities and skills to manage independently.

Babies are born with almost the number of brain cells (neurons) that they will have for the rest of their lives. We do not in general develop by growing new neurons. Instead, what happens is that the connections (synapses) between the neurons gradually become more efficient. We are born with many connections, but as we experience more and more of the world, these are gradually 'pruned' so that we end up with just the brain circuits and networks that we need. One interesting example of this in action is speech sounds. Babies are born able to recognise the speech sounds of any human language, but by about one year old they have lost this ability and retain only the sounds of the language(s) they have heard.[21]

There are two reasons why human beings are born so far before development is complete. The first is anatomical, in that walking upright places constraints on hip size and other aspects of anatomy. This means that there is a limit on how large a baby's head can be to be safely born. The second is about adaptation. Being born with incomplete brain development allows the baby and child to adapt to the world around them.[22] For example, in a world where there is considerable danger and food resources are scarce, the child can develop high vigilance and quick reactions for detected and responding to danger, and a metabolism that can cope with low or occasional nutrition. By contrast, a child born into a resource rich and relatively safe and reliable environment will develop so as to do well in that context.

Development involves choices, however, since the brain is expensive to build and costly to run, absorbing a large proportion of the body's energy. Prioritising one aspect of development, such as a vigilant stress system, has a cost in terms of reduced priorities for other developmental areas that are less vital for survival in the particular context of danger, such as focussed attention or language. There are also longer-term costs, as the ACE studies show, for health and well-being – the mechanisms for these, and how health visitors can help disrupt them, are described below.

### How adversity impacts on development

Routine health visiting assessments may well highlight concerns about a child's development, or issues in a parent's life that may have an impact on the family's well-being. Practitioners also need to have a preventive stance that can be aware of risk factors for future problems. Timely intervention before a problem develops, or before impacts are seen in delayed or atypical development, will be both more effective and more acceptable to families since any suggestion of blame can be more easily avoided.

An essential step is to reflect carefully on possible underlying processes that lead to the assessed need, or that might give rise to a need in the future. Sometimes this is simple – we know, for example, that children's rate of language development is partly related to how often they are talked with and exposed to new experiences (see Chapter 15). Alternatively, poor housing conditions might clearly be unsafe for child and family, and a likely source of stress for both. Often, however, more in-depth analysis may be needed to ensure that the most effective and respectful approaches are suggested to caregivers.

Adversity has its effects through at least five different aspects of the developmental environment. In practice, this can be quite complex with direct and indirect impacts, and each aspect can interact with the others. The five are as follows and can be remembered using the mnemonic PRAMS:

**P**hysical environment
**R**esources
**A**ttachment
**M**oderate and resolved stress
**S**timulation

Each of these is now considered in turn, with an emphasis on how they might be observable and assessed.

## PHYSICAL ENVIRONMENT

All humans need a minimum of physical care in order to survive. For adults, much of this is through self-care, though greatly enhanced if in a social context. We can decide for ourselves when and what to eat, how warm we want the house to be, when it is time to sleep or – harder – get out of bed. For young children physical needs are met almost entirely through caregivers, usually a parent.

Physical needs can impact on child development, and on later adult well-being, in two ways. Firstly, a minimum of nutrition, sleep, warmth and so on are necessary for healthy growth and biological functioning. Secondly, the regularity with which physical needs are met gives messages to the developing brain as to what kind of world it is growing up into, and the brain and body will adapt accordingly.[23] For example, if feeding is insufficient or inconsistent, the implication is that survival will need more self-reliance and getting what you can when you can – so developing impulse control and trust in others becomes less important.

It is important to recognise that the early physical environment has a key role in shaping brain development as the young human adapts to the world as they find it. The impact is not simply psychological but is found in the development of basic brain systems that underpin behaviour and well-being.

## RESOURCES

Resources are vital to meeting the physical needs of children. For example, young humans (and older ones) need to be able to move about, explore and take risks. If children are growing up in a neighbourhood that has few safe play spaces, this is more difficult for caregivers to provide. Or if a family depends on unreliable public transport, it may be more difficult to find time to play and talk together or to keep necessary medical appointments. They may have to depend on smaller, local, shops with higher prices and fewer healthy choices available.

Poverty has a key role in adversity.[16] It impacts directly on children's development, and also indirectly through reducing what caregivers can provide and increasing the stresses on the whole family. Other aspects of the physical environment are also linked to poverty and can have an impact on healthy development, including housing quality and security, noise and air pollution and access to services. There is also potential for a vicious circle, where a resource-poor environment leads to high stress, leading to higher risk of trauma – which then impacts on ability to manage or gain resources, thus leading to further poverty.

## ATTACHMENT

The concept of attachment is covered in Chapter 14, but its relation to adversity and trauma is both important and sometimes misunderstood, meriting a short recapitulation here.[24,25] Early work on the construct included using an experimental procedure called the Strange Situation to classify child-parent pairs according to the degree of security observed in the relationship. The procedure tapped into the balance of autonomy and help-seeking that children need and how parents provide this through a balance of giving space and providing support. Like two halves of a see-saw, these cannot be seen separately. Attachment is sometimes over-interpreted as an intrinsic feature or trait of the child – for example, focussing solely on whether they are 'securely attached' or 'have' disorganised attachment. In fact, children can show different attachment patterns with different people and in different situations, and a life-course perspective suggests that these patterns can change over time with intervention.

What matters in attachment are three aspects of care-giving. The first is *reflective functioning* by the parent. This is sometimes called mind-mindedness or mentalising, and comes down to thinking of the child, and his or her behaviour, as having to do with thoughts and feelings. It is called reflective functioning because it involves taking space to think about why a child might be doing what they are doing, and to respond to this, rather than simply reacting. For example, a baby may be crying because of hunger, heat, cold, tiredness, boredom or simply through overflow of feelings. Each of these needs a different response – simply picking up and feeding may be the right response, but might not.

Reflective functioning is important because it helps with *attunement*, the second key element. This is the way that caregivers can align their feelings and behaviours to their children. When this happens, the child feels understood and contained, but also can use the caregiver's response to grow their own understanding of self. Attunement is also a key part of co-regulation which will be described more in the subsection on moderate and resolved stress.

The third key part of attachment is *sensitive care*, a timely response to the needs of the child as understood by the caregiver. Attachment is a practical business, not just a feeling. The sense of being loved, included and wanted is conveyed to an infant through responsive care. For example, many infants dislike being changed. From a mind-minded perspective, we can understand this as we would not ourselves like to be suddenly turned upside down and undressed. If a caregiver understands this for their child, and attunes to these emotions, then they will be able to provide sensitive care through soothing sounds and actions.

The importance for brain development are the messages that the developing brain receives about whether this is a world where social relationships are important for survival, and where others can be relied upon for understanding and help – or whether one needs to develop not just independence but self-reliance and a distrust of other's reliability and intentions.

Some forms of developmental trauma and adversity can be seen as the shadow side, or negative, of attachment. This is where children do not experience sensitive care with their needs being met promptly enough. The regular rhythms of sensitive care and attunement, done in a mind-minded way, help develop brain areas that support self-regulation.

A final aspect of attachment to consider is how well supported the family is within their community. If a parent feels unincluded or marginalised – or even victimised – within their local environment, then they will experience high stress that might impact on their care for their children. Similarly, if children do not feel welcome or safe going out to play, or the family is shunned for whatever reason, this will impact on development.[18] Some researchers suggest this extends even to higher level social stigma – for example, certain groups or lifestyles that are seen as inferior, such as being a single parent or, still in many places, in a same sex relationship. Health visitors will need to be aware of the impact of marginalisation on families as this can reduce social support, access to community and public amenities as well as attitudes to services. If the family feels unsafe in its home or community, the burden of stress on the child is likely to be higher or more difficult to mitigate.

Health visitors can be very influential in helping the significant adults around the child to provide secure attachment through promoting reflective functioning, attunement and sensitive care. The section below on working with parents suggests some ideas and signposts some resources to help. Programmes to help parents and carers develop positive relationships with their children are described in depth in Chapter 14. Health visitors also have a role in seeing attachment in context and considering whether a programme is what a particular family needs. Parents may well have the desire and the skills to provide positive relationships for their children, but are trying to do so in adverse circumstances. Understanding attachment in the context of the other factors in this section is paramount, and some suggestions for how to do this are in the section on reflective practice below.

## MODERATE AND RESOLVED STRESS

As a society we place high importance on protecting children from too much stress. We grade movies and games by ages so young children are not unduly frightened or challenged, and provide soft and gentle contexts for learning. Many adults can recall a favourite stuffed animal that was a companion and friend, but also importantly a comfort and protection.

Too much stress, or stress that goes on too long, or without sufficient support to manage it can have a lifelong impact as the developing brain adapts to what seems to be a world full of danger and difficulty. What we need are fast stress reactions, with fight and flight responses ready – to act first and think later. We need to be vigilant, scanning the space around us for danger, and investment in the future can wait as the priority is to be safe now. Thus, children exposed to too much stress for too long in their early lives can present as inattentive, impulsive, aggressive, fearful, slow to learn, poor in language – because their development has prioritised other abilities.[22]

There are also physical consequences.[26] The body responds to danger through a complex cascade of processes largely controlled by the hormone cortisol. This is well known as a stress hormone, but also has a role in the immune system and in wound repair. Essentially, the body responds by getting into a state ready for rapid action, but also for defence against damage and infection. Most of the time, this is a temporary response and self-limiting. With on-going or repeated high stress, the response can become chronic. This is thought to be one of the links from early adversity to poor health in adulthood, through a state of chronic inflammation.

It is also probably the main reason for the findings that supportive care from adults can reduce the links between early adversity and poor outcomes later in life. Children who experience high levels of background stress or repeated stress will have high stress reactions. But if an adult is able to provide soothing and protection, they will act as an external regulator for the child's stress system. So instead of having to depend on their own ability to manage stress, a young child can reply on a caregiver to help them get safe and feel safe. Over time, this will help the young stress system develop its own soothing and coping mechanisms. Within the brain, what is happening is that basic survival systems found in the limbic system start to work together with higher level processes in the cortex. Long term, this means that feeling and thinking become more connected, supporting the development of planned actions, self-soothing and control of attention.[27]

The beneficial effects of manageable and resolved stress have been observed in nonhuman primates and is sometimes called 'stress inoculation'. It is a specific example of a general rule, that we need stress in order to develop.[28] Many experiences of small stressors that we can manage, or that we can manage with mind-minded and sensitive help, grow our ability to manage stress. One implication is that children who are 'over' cared for or who do not have the space to explore and experience stress and setbacks are likely to be more vulnerable to the inevitable ups and downs of life.

It is key that stress is not only manageable but that it is also resolved. This builds the pattern of stress-soothing-coping-resolution that underlies individual resilience. One example is the 'rupture and repair' cycle of daily communication. With the best will in the world, caregivers will not always be perfectly attuned to their children or may not always be prompt in meeting their needs, or even may express annoyance or impatience. If this is resolved reasonably quickly through sensitivity and soothing, then the experience is helpful for development. Even small instances are important, such as the mounting anticipation of peek-a-boo relieved by the sight of the beloved parent's face; or the encouragement to try again after our first faltering steps resulted in a fall. Exploring parental thoughts about responding to the needs of the infant can be very helpful. Some may feel that they always need to be available to the infant, engaging and entertaining them at all waking moments, with the other extreme being limited engagement with a child experienced as over-demanding. Both approaches will reduce the opportunities for rupture and repair, as well as becoming self-confirming as the child adapts to the care available.

More significantly, all children will be exposed to stress at some point in their formative years, this could be anything from reduced availability of the principal care giver or a traumatic event or the expected setbacks of growing up in a complex society amid multiple expectations. So long as these are self-limiting and managed appropriately then the long-term adverse impact can be contained and minimised – and the emerging stress system may become more resilient as a result.

## STIMULATION

At any age we human beings need interesting things to do that challenge us, and that we can share with others. The form differs by age and preference. Some adults love to ride motorbikes, while others will sit for hours fishing. Young children are born ready to explore the world and discover it all anew for themselves, and to join their culture and society and learn its ways. For this, they need stimulation as they rely on caregivers to bring the world and their culture to them. Developmentally appropriate stimulation is not just about knowledge development – it also grows confidence, creativity and the core skills of managing information and impulses. For infants and toddlers, the main source of stimulation is playing, and responsive conversations, with caregivers.

Adversity can disrupt these processes in a number of ways. Parents who are themselves stressed may find it harder to tune in to their children and to find calm and quiet times for play and talk. Households in which there are high levels of chaos or violence are not the best settings for learning language or the play sequences that underpin problem solving. Poverty, and the local environment, can limit the possibilities for stimulation, whether through toys and books or access to outdoor opportunities such as parks, libraries and museums.

Lack of developmentally appropriate stimulation can have long-term consequences that are covered in Chapters 13, 14 and 15. It can also impact on the development of stress regulation since children may lack the language skills to express needs or access help; as well as having less effective self-soothing strategies such as self-talk. Alternatively, a lack of cultural knowledge about sources of help, or how to access them, can prolong a situation of toxic stress that could otherwise have been resolved. For example, the understanding that adults will help, and you can ask for it, develops in part through shared play experiences as simple as child and caregiver working together to find the right-sized building block.

### Case Study 11.1

*You undertake an assessment in the clinic of a two-and-a-half-year-old girl and it is evident that her speech language and communication is not age and stage appropriate. Her mother also complains that she has become very difficult to manage over the last year, with frequent tantrums, and sometimes hiding in her room when it is time to go out.*

*What might be the reasons for what you are seeing and hearing in terms of each of:*

*Physical environment*
*Resources*
*Attachment*
*Moderate and resolved stress*
*Stimulation*

*How might you work with the family to address any of those issues?*

*Who would you refer to and why?*

*Community nursery nurse*

*Nursery*

*Speech language and communication – at which point?*

## ASSESSMENT, ANALYSIS AND INTERVENTION

### Presenting issues and touchpoints

There are many situations that health workers encounter where the presenting issues match the underlying need in a clear way, and where action is not needed unless an issue arises. We cannot treat a chest infection until it occurs, and the signs and symptoms are easily linked with the problem and its management.

Adversity and trauma differ in two ways from these kinds of issues. Firstly, we need to work to build resilience even before a child and family has experienced any trauma or adversity. Difficult things can happen in any life, circumstances can change, and if health visitors work with families to help them with the PRAMS factors above, then they are in a sense providing 'inoculation' against future adversity and potential health and wider consequences.

Secondly, families may sometimes present health visitors with information about adversity and trauma. They may complain about their housing situation, the safety of their neighbourhood, or disclose traumatic experiences such as house fires or domestic violence. Sometimes, however, what is presented instead are some of the consequences or correlates of adversity and trauma, and sensitive conversations are needed to help families assess what is happening.

Some of the most common presenting issues include difficulties with a child's behaviour, beyond the usual and developmentally expected occasional sleep issues, toddler dysregulation, or sharing problems in preschool. Health visitors can be vigilant for when a child's behaviour might be a manifestation (or communication) of strong underlying feelings, such as fear or rage. Similarly, when, for example, a developmental assessment indicates delayed development of concern in any area, this may be an intrinsic biological issue, or it may be related to the family's circumstances or how they are, or are not, providing stimulation and reflective care.

The different nations of the UK have different frameworks with respect to routine enquiry about some potential sources of adversity and trauma, such as domestic violence and alcohol use. In terms of more specific routine enquiry about adversity and trauma, there is at present a lack of evidence as to its effectiveness, and health visitors should not do this without appropriate training. Actual screening for adversity and trauma is more controversial and there is not at present evidence to recommend it.[13]

Exploring touchpoints might be helpful here.[29] A touchpoint is a moment in the development of a child when parents and carers are most reflective about what is happening and most likely to be willing to engage in conversations about issues. There are obvious change moments where this is so – such as antenatal appointments, or soon after birth, or as children become toddlers, or prepare to go to school. Also, every family will differ in providing other touchpoints where a health visitor can develop conversations about adversity and trauma. These may be as simple as anxiety over the expense of a new buggy, struggling to attend appointments, or a child who won't stay in bed. Contact with parents or carers at these moments is ideal for introducing the key ideas about brain development, and the environment that supports it, and how adults can have an optimal role in this. Reframing parental anxiety, helplessness or frustration as an expression of care can turn a difficult moment into a touchpoint.

It is important that health visitors engage with families on these issues since in their role, they have unique influence and knowledge of each family. The health visitor is ideally placed, not only for supporting the parents or carers to support their child, but also to give some consideration to the level of resilience that the parents or carers have. Engaging in discussion around resilience, adversity and trauma provides the health visitor with an understanding of the parents' own experiences of being parented. All of this enables the health visitor, alongside the parents or carers, to identify any additional support they may need to promote resilience in their child and establishing the level to which the child is supported, promoted and safeguarded. Facilitating this level of enquiry and interaction requires the health visitor to utilise an array of skills, and in particular communication: verbal and nonverbal.

Communication is considered to be essential to all nursing practice, and continues to be key in health visiting. While this may seem obvious and fundamental, communication is consistently identified in significant case reviews as compromised or ineffective, both with families and interagency. This reinforces that learning and development of communication skills is not only ongoing professional development, but essential to support health visitors to build professional confidence to engage in meaningful and quality communication. An example of this is probing and open-ended questioning, which some practitioners may avoid out of concern that they may not be equipped to manage the information that is disclosed and shared (BB, anecdotal from students & peers).

## THINKING SPACE

By yourself, or in a small group, imagine (or remember a time when) you've made a mistake at work – just a small one, not life threatening! Your supervisor needs to talk to you about it. How would you want them to do this – what could they say, how could they ask questions? How you would want it done – what kind of setting, what kind of timing? And how would you want them to talk about it to others, if that was needed?

Now think about when you are talking to parents about potential or actual trauma or adversity. Just as above, how do you think you should do this so it is an effective but also comfortable conversation for them and for you?

Through building relationships and active and respectful listening, health visitors can be effective in eliciting the lived experience of parents even where there is a high level of trauma and abuse.[30] For this to happen the health visitor needs to be confident and competent in their role and be familiar of the resources that are available, both to families and themselves, following disclosure. This is reflected within six Cs of nursing; compassion, care, competence, communication, commitment and courage, all of which are significant; however, courage can be emphasised in relation to probing and opening questioning.[31] Furthermore, contemporary practice and evidence advocates that the voice of the child is also heard and acknowledged. One can helpfully think of a triad of communication, when the child, the parent(s) and the professional interact to establish a care plan for the child.[32] How this evolves will be dependent on capacity and capability of the child, however, provision still needs to be made to support the child's voice through age and stage appropriate engagement. This again requires practitioner confidence and courage and also reflects the requirement that nurses need to consider individual abilities and capabilities.[33]

### Ecological and holistic approaches

Many forms of adversity and developmental trauma are to do with reduced adult sensitivity and care, or even active causing of harm – such as physical or emotional neglect, sexual abuse, or the high levels of stress consequent on high levels of violence or disorder in the home. Health visitors must have child protection or safeguarding considerations at the front of their minds always and act quickly according to local guidelines to address these issues. Chapter 12 provides more detail on safeguarding and the health visitor role.

However, many parents and carers are trying to do their best to raise their children in circumstances that make this difficult to do – whether this be personal circumstances such as drug dependence, mental or physical health issues; or factors outside the family such as poverty or neighbourhood facilities. The section above emphasises the importance of taking a holistic view of adversity and offers a PRAMS mnemonic to assist. Table 11.1 below gives some examples of how the different factors may be seen in assessment to support analysis. Some issues can be resolved through health visitor support, and the following section will give more detail on how health visitors can work with parents. Others lie beyond a health visitors direct power to bring change, but health visitors can be very effective in working with others to advocate for, and support the delivery of, improvements in the environment in which children and families are living and growing. For example, health visitors might have an important input when local services, such as health or play facilities, are being planned, to ensure that planning takes account of the needs of young children and their families.

### Case study 11.2

*Afiya Magunda aged 32 arrived in the UK six weeks ago from Uganda seeking asylum. She has three children: Amina, her 12-year-old daughter, and her two sons Akiki, aged four, and Sanyu, aged 27 months. Afiya is also four months pregnant. She is fleeing violence and had to watch as her husband was brutally murdered in front of her and the children. She was then repeatedly raped, as was her daughter Amina.*

| TABLE 11.1 | |
|---|---|
| **Adversity factors** | **Sources of assessment information** |
| Physical | Parents or carers may raise issues about housing, transport, accessibility of needed services, play spaces, shops, etc |
| | Health visitors can build up local knowledge of area |
| | Child development assessments may show delays or gaps |
| Resource | Demographic information about family, eligibility for benefits, etc |
| | Parents may raise money or other resource issues, such as fuel poverty |
| | Tactful enquiries based on visual assessment of home environment |
| | Local knowledge of prices and costs – e.g., only a corner shop, no bus routes |
| Attachment | Assessments of social and emotional development |
| | Observations of interactions |
| | Parents raising issues of behaviour, or of their own concerns about bonding |
| | Discussions with parents about their own sources of support in family and community |
| | Knowledge of whether family is likely to be experiencing stigma or marginalisation – social, race, sexual orientation, gender, poverty, immigration, etc |
| Moderate & resolved stress | Assessments of social and emotional development |
| | Observations of interactions |
| | Parents raising issues of behaviour, or of their own concerns about bonding |
| | Sensitive conversations with parents (or disclosures) about their burden of stress and available supports |
| Stimulation | Developmental assessments showing gaps or delays |
| | Parents may voice concerns |
| | Assessment of home environment, and also of neighbourhood facilities |

*Afiya is struggling with her mental health and manifests this through signs of anxiety and depression, all exacerbated by the trauma. She is also self-harming and has already attempted suicide.*

*Amina is struggling to settle in school and comes home crying every day and Afiya has also caught Amina self-harming.*

*Akiki, aged four, has a nursery place but Afiya does not want him to go to nursery as she does not want to go out. All of Akiki's teeth are rotten, he does not speak, is still in nappies, can't hold a pen, throws and destroys his toys and won't engage with his mum reading to him. He constantly hits Afiya and Sanyu.*

*Sanyu is 27 months old and only takes formula milk, refuses food. He is also very underweight and does not seek out interaction.*

*The family live in a two-bedroom multistorey block on the 12th floor, which is provided through UK border agency and located in an area of deprivation. She feels well supported by her local community. However, female genital mutilation (FGM) is customary in the community and Afiya has disclosed that the elders are insisting on her compliance with this.*

*Overall, the family have little English language.*

*Can you use the material in this chapter to map out the issues for the family and prioritise the help they could be offered? How do you, as a practitioner, avoid being overwhelmed?*

The following table provides some broad ideas for assessment and analysis based on different pathways through which adversity can impact on child development. Bear in mind that more than one of these will be the case at any one time, and that they overlap and interact with each other.

## Working with parents and carers

There is an emerging research consensus that the early years of life are of particular importance in shaping outcomes over a lifetime, since this is a period when most brain development occurs. There are other periods of significant brain development, such as early adolescence, where intervention can be particularly effective, and the brain remains plastic throughout life. However, the early years, sometimes called 'the first 1001 days', but extending beyond that, is of critical importance.

Health visitors are therefore a key profession to deliver primary and secondary prevention through helping families build their resilience and that of their children and to reduce the impacts of adversity and deprivation. There is abundant evidence that this kind of intervention can be effective. For example, children whose mothers experience very high levels of stress while they are still in the womb tend to have poorer outcomes for cognition and emotional regulation – unless those children experience high levels of nurturing care in their first few months after birth, in which case outcomes are not poorer.[34] Other studies have shown how effective health visitors can be in reducing the physical abuse of babies through supporting parents with attachment and stimulation.[35]

These opportunities are reflected nationally, and while the different countries of the UK work to different policies, standards and legislation, all prioritise early intervention and child-centred approaches.[36–39] In the entire UK, there is recognition of the importance of promoting healthy brain development and the impact this can have on lifelong development and well-being, and has been further enhanced by the introduction of an antenatal health visiting contact in all of the countries in the UK.[40]

This antenatal contact is ideal for supporting parents to understand their role in promoting baby brain development for their child. Through accessing reliable and evidence-based resources, such as those provided by the Harvard Center on the Developing Child,[41] the health visitor can support parents to understand the fundamentals of brain development, and in particular support them to understand the response of the brain to sustained stress. With the increased opportunities for contact through the four national approaches, there are increased opportunities for assessment and early intervention. The four national approaches also enhance the anticipatory role of the health visitor, where primary intervention is just as, if not more important as secondary intervention.

Amidst all this opportunity, health visitors need to be aware of the amount of information that parents of babies and young children are given and sensitive to how much they can take on board and put into action. Throughout, a strengths-based and respectful approach is needed in order to empower caregivers and to maximise the likelihood of interventions being both acceptable and effective. Being a parent is complex, and doing so in adverse circumstances can be overwhelming. Fortunately, the research on trauma and adversity converges on findings that although all aspects of adversity are important, if adults can provide positive relationships and sensitive care for their children then this is often effective in offsetting many of the impacts.

Even in the face of overwhelming complexity, or adversity that is engrained in large scale social or economic processes, it is important that health visitors do not feel helpless. Encouraging, modelling, supporting and reinforcing parents to provide what they can of sensitive care, attuned interactions, and to reduce or resolve the stresses on the child – all of which can have a positive impact on the health and wellbeing of the child and family that may last a lifetime.

## REFLECTIVE PRACTICE

### Secondary stress and self-care

Secondary trauma (sometimes called vicarious trauma) develops when workers are exposed to actual or described trauma experienced by others.[3,42] It is somewhat misnamed as 'secondary' trauma is just as real, and can be as impactful, as primary trauma. Typical examples include a health visitor or social worker who witnesses abuse of a child, or hears it described by the child or another. But typing up notes or letters, or providing support through supervision, can give rise to traumatic responses to the material. What can also happen is that staff who cope well with individual events can become gradually traumatised by experiencing many such events.

This is not a case of anyone being weak or things going wrong – it is an expected aspect of working with children and families who experience trauma and adversity. Workers can easily feel helpless and find they are taking the stress home and struggling to disconnect. The better news is that there are effective ways to prevent or reduce secondary traumatisation in the workplace and that recognising the signs of overload and taking steps to care for oneself or each other are often enough to help.

Some of the common signs that a worker is getting overwhelmed by secondary stress include:

- Being highly emotional out of context – or numbing reactions
- Trouble sleeping or relaxing
- Feeling discouraged, unusually pessimistic or hopeless
- Avoidance of tasks and issues, or clients
- Concentration and memory difficulties
- Usual recreations appeal less, or becoming less sociable
- Turning to self-medication through food intake, alcohol or other forms of comfort seeking more than usual

Evidence suggests that organisational factors can have strong effects in helping staff cope both with day-to-day stressors and with peak events. These are not just a matter for managers, even if they hold the main responsibility – everyone has a part to play in creating and maintaining a nurturing and supportive team. These factors include:

- A culture that acknowledges the impact of work on the staff
- Warm and supportive ethos among all staff
- Supervision models that prioritise reflective supervision as well as case discussion
- Managers addressing self-care issues in team meetings, and modelling responses
- Careful distributions of workload

- Personalised and 'human' workspaces
- Attention to self-care needs of staff – kitchen/staff areas, breaks together, etc
- Information for all staff about secondary trauma and self-care
- Strong, shared, sense of identity and purpose and individual effectiveness within this
- Time for social interaction and shared celebrations
- Informal and formal peer support structures
- Active development of staff competencies and skills

Self-care comes down to simple and common-sense ways of reconnecting with loved ones and enjoyable and refreshing activities. This might include:

- Maintaining positive connections with family and friends
- Allowing and encouraging enough relaxation and rest
- Maintaining physical health through good nutrition, exercise and sleep
- Putting effort into recuperative pastimes and hobbies, especially creative ones, or those with a social element
- Keeping up connections with colleagues
- Understanding that these reactions are normal and healthy and that they may persist for a while, or come and go for a bit

If teams experience a critical incident, such as the death of a child in violent circumstances, or other disasters, then a more focussed approach may be needed. Each health board or trust will have procedures in place for this that health visitors should be aware of.

### The image of the child and family

Over the last few decades, the traditional image of the family as Mum, Dad and children, has evolved to take into consideration global and socio-cultural developments. Definitions of a family have changed from being considered as a unit within the same household,[43] to acknowledging that members of a family can be in different locations and countries and still be considered a unit.[44,45] However, consideration of this growing diversity of what constitutes a family unit is rarely reflected in the assessment tools and documentation used nationally. That said Bronfenbrenner's ecological model[46] places the child at the centre of microsystem, exosystem and macrosystem. This ecological approach to family assessment is also supported by the increased use of ecomaps and genomaps. However, irrespective of the definition of the term family, it is paramount that all assessments remain child focused.

Health visitors need also to reflect frequently on how they are thinking about children and families. The daily stresses of working with families in difficult circumstances can gradually promote mindsets about parents as helpless or hopeless, or about children as very vulnerable or else beyond help. These mindsets can then affect practice in a vicious circle. The research and practice on adversity described in this chapter should fundamentally be a source of hope in that we see that although there is much trauma and adversity for children to cope with, there is also increased understanding of how to promote resilience through small changes and fostering positive relationships. The health visitor needs to practice in a reciprocal way – just as children need positive relationships and sensitive care from their families, so do those families need the same from the professionals who seek to help them provide it.

## CONCLUSION

This chapter has provided information on psychological trauma and childhood adversity, including a framework to assist health visitors with assessment and analysis. There has also been consideration of the impact of working with trauma and adversity on the practitioner and how this can be mitigated.

## KEY LEARNING POINTS

- Trauma and adversity are common and affect the lives of many children and families. Health visitors encounter families during a key period of development and can be very influential in ensuring resilient outcomes for children, families and communities.
- Trauma and adversity are complex phenomena which require both nuanced understanding of the evidence base and careful, respectful assessment and analysis with families.
- Health visitors need to see children and families as a whole and within the communities and socio-economic circumstances in which they live.
- Much childhood trauma is preventable, especially through good safeguarding processes, but much is not preventable. Health visitors can work with parents and carers to support the provision of the physical environment, resources, attachment relationships, experiences of moderate and resolved stress and developmentally appropriate stimulation that children need.
- In order to do this well, health visitors need to attend to their own well-being, both as individuals and as teams, with an awareness that secondary stress is not a sign of weakness and can be addressed through workplace and lifestyle adjustments.

## REFERENCES

1. Ferrara, P., Corsello, G., Basile, M. C., et al. (2015). The economic burden of child maltreatment in high income countries. *The Journal of Pediatrics*, 1457–1459.
2. Leach, P. (2017). *Transforming infant well-being: Research, policy and practice for the first 1001 critical days*. Routledge.
3. Dmytryshyn, A. L., Jack, S. M., Ballantyne, M., et al. (2015). Long-term home visiting with vulnerable young mothers: An interpretive description of the impact on public health nurses. *BMC Nursing*.
4. Marryat, L., & Frank, J. (2019). Factors associated with adverse childhood experiences in Scottish children: A prospective cohort study. *BMJ Paediatrics Open*, 3(1).
5. Perrotta, G. (2019). Psychological trauma: Definition, clinical contexts, neural correlations and therapeutic approaches. Recent discoveries. *Current Research Psychiatry Brain Disorder*. CRPBD-100006 Routledge.
6. van der Kolk, B. A., Burbridge, J. A., & Suzuki, J. (1997). The psychobiology of traumatic memory. Clinical implications of neuroimaging studies. In R. Yehuda, & A. C. McFarlane (Eds.), *Annals of the New York Academy of Sciences. Vol. 821. Psychobiology of Posttraumatic Stress Disorder* (pp. 99–113). New York Academy of Sciences.
7. Taylor, S., Asmundson, G. J., & Carleton, R. N. (2006). Simple versus complex PTSD: A cluster analytic investigation. *Journal of Anxiety Disorders*, 20(4), 459–472.
8. Spiel, S., Lombardi, K., & DeRubeis-Byrne, L. (2019). Treating traumatized children: Somatic memories and play therapy. *Journal of Infant, Child, and Adolescent Psychotherapy*, 18(1), 1–12.
9. D'Andrea, W., Ford, J., Stolbach, B., et al. (2012). Understanding interpersonal trauma in children: Why we need a developmentally appropriate trauma diagnosis. *American Journal of Orthopsychiatry*, 82, 187–200.
10. Hughes, K., Bellis, M. A., Hardcastle, K. A., et al. (2017). The effect of multiple adverse childhood experiences on health: A systematic review and meta-analysis. *The Lancet Public Health*, 2(8), e356–e366.
11. Bellis, M. A., Hughes, K., Ford, K., et al. (2018). Adverse childhood experiences and sources of childhood resilience: A retrospective study of their combined relationships with child health and educational attendance. *BMC Public Health*, 18, 792.
12. White, S. Edwards, R., Gillies, V., et al. (2019) All the ACEs: A chaotic concept for family policy and decision-making? *Social Policy and Society*, 18(3), 457–466.
13. Finkelhor, D. (2018). Screening for adverse childhood experiences (ACEs): Cautions and suggestions. *Child Abuse & Neglect*, 85, 174–179.
14. Hambrick, E. P., Brawner, T. W., Perry, B. D., et al. (2019). Beyond the ACE score: Examining relationships between timing of developmental adversity, relational health and developmental outcomes in children. *Archives of Psychiatric Nursing*, 33(3), 238–247.
15. McLaughlin, K. A., & Sheridan, M. A. (2016). Beyond cumulative risk: A dimensional approach to childhood

adversity. *Current Directions in Psychological Science,* 25(4), 239–245.

16. La Placa, V., & Corlyon, J. (2016). Unpacking the relationship between parenting and poverty: Theory, evidence and policy. *Social Policy and Society,* 15(1), 11–28.

17. Blair, A., Marryat, L., & Frank, J. (2019). How community resources mitigate the association between household poverty and the incidence of adverse childhood experiences. *Int J Public Health,* 64, 1059–1068.

18. Ungar, M. (2015). Practitioner review: Diagnosing childhood resilience – A systemic approach to the diagnosis of adaptation in adverse social and physical ecologies. *Journal of Child Psychology and Psychiatry,* 56(1), 4–17.

19. Masten, A. S. (2015). *Ordinary magic: Resilience in development.* Guilford Publications.

20. Johnson, M. H. (2001). Functional brain development in humans. *Nature Reviews Neuroscience,* 2(7), 475–483.

21. Best, C. T. (1993). Emergence of language-specific constraints in perception of non-native speech: A window on early phonological development. In *Developmental neurocognition: Speech and face processing in the first year of life* (pp. 289–304). Springer: Dordrecht.

22. Ellis, B. J., & Del Giudice, M. (2019). Developmental adaptation to stress: An evolutionary perspective. *Annual Review of Psychology,* 70, 111–139.

23. Pears, K. C., Kim, H. K., & Fisher, P. A. (2008). Psychosocial and cognitive functioning of children with specific profiles of maltreatment. *Child Abuse & Neglect,* 32(10), 958–971.

24. Sroufe, A. (2005). Attachment and development: A prospective, longitudinal study from birth to adulthood. *Attachment & Human Development,* 7(4), 349–367.

25. Meins, E., Fernyhough, C., de Rosnay, M., et al. (2012). Mind-mindedness as a multidimensional construct: Appropriate and non-attuned mind-related comments independently predict infant–mother attachment in a socially diverse sample. *Infancy,* 17(4), 393–415.

26. Berens, A. E., Jensen, S. K., & Nelson, C. A. (2017). Biological embedding of childhood adversity: From physiological mechanisms to clinical implications. *BMC Medicine,* 15(1), 135.

27. Hughes, D. A., & Baylin, J. (2012). *Brain-based parenting: The neuroscience of caregiving for healthy attachment (Norton Series on Interpersonal Neurobiology).* WW Norton & Company.

28. Lyons, D. M., Parker, K. J., Katz, M., et al. (2009). Developmental cascades linking stress inoculation, arousal regulation, and resilience. *Frontiers in Behavioral Neuroscience,* 3, 32.

29. Brazelton, T. B. (1992). *Touchpoints: Your child's emotional and behavioral development.* Reading, MA: Addison-Wesley Publishing Company, One Jacob Way.

30. McFeely, C. W. (2016). The health visitor response to domestic abuse (Doctoral dissertation, University of Glasgow). http://theses.gla.ac.uk/8063/.

31. NHS England. (2012). *Introducing the 6Cs.* https://www.england.nhs.uk/6cs/wp-content/uploads/sites/25/2015/03/introducing-the-6cs.pdf.

32. Shapcott, J., & Gault, I. (2017). Essential communication skills: Building blocks for good communication. In I. Gault, J. Shapcott, A. Luthi, & G. Reid (Eds.), *Communication in nursing and healthcare: A guide for compassionate practice* (pp. 15–26). London: Sage.

33. Nursing and Midwifery Council (NMC). (2018). The code: Professional standards of practice and behaviour for nurses, midwives and nursing associates. https://www.nmc.org.uk/globalassets/sitedocuments/nmc-publications/nmc-code.pdf. Accessed 30 January 2020.

34. Bergman, K., Sarkar, P., Glover, V., et al. (2008). Quality of child–parent attachment moderates the impact of antenatal stress on child fearfulness. *Journal of Child Psychology and Psychiatry,* 49(10), 1089–1098.

35. Bugental, D. B., Ellerson, P. C., Lin, E. K., et al. (2002). A cognitive approach to child abuse prevention. *Journal of Family Psychology,* 16(3), 243.

36. Scottish Government. (2015). *University health visiting pathway in Scotland: Pre-birth to pre-school. [online].* https://www.gov.scot/publications/universal-health-visiting-pathway-scotland-pre-birth-pre-school/. Accessed 11 February 2020.

37. Welsh Government. (2016). *Healthy Child Wales Programme. [online].* https://gov.wales/sites/default/files/publications/2019-05/an-overview-of-the-healthy-child-wales-programme.pdf. Accessed 7 February 2020.

38. Northern Ireland Government. (2010). *Healthy child healthy future. [online].* https://www.health-ni.gov.uk/publications/healthy-child-healthy-future. Accessed 7 February 2020.

39. Government UK. (2009). *Healthy Children Programme: Pregnancy and the first five years of life. [online].* https://www.gov.uk/government/publications/healthy-child-programme-pregnancy-and-the-first-5-years-of-life. Accessed 10 February 2020.

40. Cross Party Manifesto. (2014). *The 1001 critical days: The importance of conception to aged two period.*

41. Harvard Child Development Centre. (2020). *The brain architecture. [online].* https://developingchild.harvard.edu/science/key-concepts/brain-architecture/. Accessed 11 February 2020.

42. Newell, J. M., & MacNeil, G. A. (2010). Professional burnout, vicarious trauma, secondary traumatic stress, and compassion fatigue. *Best Practices in Mental Health, 6*(2), 57–68.

43. Sonawat, R. (2001). Understanding families in India: A reflection of societal changes. *Psicologia: eoria e Pesquisa, 17*(2), 177–186. http://www.scielo.br/pdf/ptp/v17n2/7878.pdf.

44. Sharma, R. (2013). The *Family and Family Structure Classification Redefined for the Current Times. Journal of Family Medicine and Primary Care*, 306–310. https://www.ncbi.nlm.nih.gov/pmc/articles/PMC4649868/.

45. Gennarini, S. (2016). *UN report: 'There is no definition of the family'.* https://c-fam.org/friday_fax/un-report-no-definition-family/. Accessed 11 February 2020.

46. Bryans, A., Cornish, F., & McIntosh, J. (2009). The potential of ecological theory for building an integrated framework to develop the public health contribution of health visiting. *Health & Social Care in the Community, 17*(6), 564–572.

# 12

# BUILDING EFFECTIVE SAFEGUARDING SKILLS: A SHIFT FROM THE 'WHAT' TO THE 'HOW' IN PRACTICE

JANE HATT ■ ALISON J. HACKETT

## CHAPTER CONTENTS

INTRODUCTION

THE PATH TO ACHIEVING 'UNCONSCIOUS COMPETENCE' IN PRACTICE

CONCLUSION

## LEARNING OUTCOMES

*To:*

- recognise the need to be better prepared with the skills to 'read' complex situations and dynamics and build strong relationships with children and their families

- appreciate the importance of inter-cultural competency in communicating with parents and carers about their perceived identity, personal and family history, their experience of being parented and their approaches to parenting

- acknowledge professionals' need to challenge their own beliefs and attitudes to improve working with non-engaging/non-compliant families and increase their professional confidence to challenge disguised compliance

- understand the importance of safeguarding supervision in supporting competent, accountable, contained practice

## INTRODUCTION

In the UK, health visitors visit children and families in their homes; consequently, they are afforded unusual access to the home environment and have a key role in supporting the more vulnerable families on their caseloads, where issues such as domestic abuse, substance misuse and mental ill-health can lead carers to, intentionally or unintentionally, harm or neglect their children. Such families are often complex in nature. The aim is for early intervention and anticipatory care with all families,[1] though research suggests that health visitors need to be better prepared with skills to interpret and respond to potentially harmful situations to children.[2,3]

Chapter 11 described adverse childhood experiences that can significantly impact parenting capacity. It provides an important background

231

context to safeguarding children and should be read in conjunction with this chapter. The current chapter will argue the importance of health visitors' ability to 'read' complex situations and dynamics with and within families. Alongside building and sustaining relationships with families, health visitors should have the professional confidence to engage in difficult conversations with parents and carers' about issues such as alcohol use, mental health or domestic abuse. According to Astbury et al,[4] positive relationships and shared decision-making with parents can improve outcomes for children and families. At the time of writing this chapter, measures introduced by the UK government and the devolved administrations to curb the spread of the Covid-19 virus have had a significant financial and social impact on many families; vulnerable and high risk families in particular. The implications and challenges of virtual working with families of concern will be reflected upon.

This chapter will focus on the learning processes leading to achieving the level of perception and professional judgment necessary for proficient child safeguarding practice. The role of 'unconscious competence' in expert professional judgments will be also be considered, drawing on the pedagogical themes of narrative and drama dynamics. Professional judgments can be vulnerable to predictable types of error, consequently the significance of safeguarding supervision in providing the critical challenge necessary to maintain safe practice will be explored. The chapter includes a number of individual learning activities, which can also be tailored to group activities, to augment learning.

## Safeguarding skills: a shift from the 'what' to the 'how'

To protect children and young people from harm and help improve their well-being, all healthcare staff must have the competencies to recognise child maltreatment, identify opportunities to improve childhood well-being and take effective action as appropriate to their role. The 'Safeguarding children and young people: roles and competencies for healthcare staff' framework details the mandatory child protection training requirements for all healthcare staff in the NHS, ranging from non-clinical staff to experts.[5] This is the guidance used in England and in Wales. However, within Scotland, the 'National Framework for Child Protection Education and Development in Scotland 2012'[6] is used. This framework describes the competencies, knowledge and skills required by *all* workers who have direct or indirect contact with children, young people and their families, not just healthcare workers. Moreover, Health Trusts (England), Health Boards (Wales and Scotland) and Health and Social Care Trusts (Northern Ireland) have a duty to ensure staff are provided with training opportunities to gain the knowledge and skills to fulfill their child protection role. Health visitors are required to have completed and regularly updated mandatory child protection training in accordance with the[5] document and if working in Scotland, the national framework.[6] Mandatory safeguarding/child protection training is essential and should provide health visitors with knowledge:

- To know how to work effectively on an interprofessional and interagency basis when there are safeguarding concerns about children, young people and their families.
- To know how to advise other agencies about the health management of individual children in child protection cases.
- To know how to work with children, young people and families where there are child protection concerns as part of the multidisciplinary team and with other disciplines, such as adult mental health, when assessing a child or young person.
- To know how to effectively manage diagnostic uncertainty and risk.[5,6]

There is a real distinction between the knowledge provided by 'training' and the deeper learning that arises from narrative or discovery-based teaching. Training usually has a more specific focus, helping someone master a specific skill or skill set whilst narrative learning seeks to instil a deeper and more sustainable knowledge over a longer period.[7] Whilst the course content in mandatory child protection training concentrates on the 'what' of safeguarding, developing the core skills needed to work with complex families requires focus on the 'how' in practice. Role-play, small group work and simulation-based learning aims to develop the relationship and communication skills necessary for the health visitor role, built around themes such as *asking sensitive questions* and *working with resistant families*. In learning the 'how' of practice, the focus of learning shifts from content to process and relationship.[8]

## The importance of understanding the dynamics between child, family and worker

The need for professionals to be well prepared with the skills to respond to complex situations and dynamics and build strong relationships with children and their families is well supported by research.[3,9,10] Trevithick[11:402] suggests nonverbal, unspoken or hidden aspects are almost always present in a particular situation or personal encounter. This can be particularly pertinent to the encounter between the practitioner and service user during the initial home visit, as both bring to the relationship a personal history likely to shape the encounter.[12] When an experienced health visitor meets a family, he or she can intuitively pick up an awareness of the state of the dynamics in the family. Intuition takes advantage of the evolved capacities of the brain and is based on rules of thumb that enable us to act fast and with astounding accuracy; shown, for example, in our ability to recognise faces.[13]

Polany[14:4] described the term *tacit knowledge*, suggesting *we know more than we can tell*. In practicing intuitively, the health visitor focuses less on the detail of the situation, more on the whole effect of the situation, thereby considering the meaning of the situation, rather than the detail. To facilitate this reasoning process, experienced practitioners are known to use multiple *heuristics* which have been defined as informal reasoning strategies, rules of thumb, or methods of processing large amounts of data to reduce cognitive strain.[15-17] Health visitors develop heuristics as part of a raft of intuitive skills to interpret the state of the dynamics within families they encounter – the warmth of the relationship between family members, or the level of fear felt by a child.

Intuition is sometimes presented as a mysterious or mystical process, but the features of the process are well understood. Munro[18] called for those working in child protection to be given more scope to exercise professional judgment in deciding how best to help children and their families. She emphasises the centrality of relationship skills, drawing attention to the roles of intuitive understanding and emotional responses,

> *an unconscious process that occurs automatically in response to perceptions, integrating a wide range of data to produce a judgment in a relatively effortless way.*[18:89]

Serious Case Reviews and Significant Case Reviews (SCRs) following the death or serious injury to a child have, time and time again, highlighted poor understanding on the part of professionals of the dynamics within the family as a contributory factor.[2,3,19] Brandon et al[2] conducted a biennial retrospective analysis of the SCRs in England and Wales and cited the work of Sroufe (2007), who suggests a major predictor of poor parenting is a lack of understanding of the psychological complexity of children, especially babies, by their carers. Brandon et al[2] also refer to a lack of understanding on the part of the professionals of the dynamics of interactions between children, carers and agencies as a contributory factor to child fatalities.

An improved understanding of family dynamics may emerge from adopting an ecological transactional approach (ETA) to assessment, which can provide a dynamic, rather than static understanding of children and their families.[20] ETA focuses on carers' experiences of being parented themselves and the history of their own relationships with family, peers, partners and professionals which influences their sense of themselves and others. These emotional histories, cognitive models and current life stressors will affect carers' states of mind and the way they understand and interpret the needs and behaviour of their children. A dynamic ecological explanatory view of parent-child interaction could assist practitioners to spot and act upon warning signs at an earlier stage. The Framework for the Assessment of Children in Need and their Families[21] is used across agencies in England and Wales. Whilst in Northern Ireland 'Understanding the Needs of Children in Northern Ireland (UNOCINI) (Department of Health Northern Ireland, 2011) is utilised and Scotland uses the GIRFEC National Practice Model.[22] Each of these models are underpinned by ecological systems theory and emphasise the importance of recognising the presence of multiple risk and protective factors and their possible interactions. The Framework for the Assessment of Children in Need and their Families[21] and the GIRFEC National Practice Model[22] neatly capture this in the form of a triangle with sides representing a child's developmental needs, parenting capacity, and family and environmental factors.

Cicchetti and Valentino[20] risk analysis framework encourages professionals to consider the dynamic interaction between children, carers and agencies, rather than having a static or fixed view of the family. The effective practitioner is one with the ability to question, with confidence, families and professional colleagues both within one's own agency and in other sectors. Inherent within this should be a degree of 'respectful uncertainty'[23:205] towards families, which is supported by the *sustained and dogged professional challenge*[9:102] inherent in effective safeguarding supervision.

## The challenge of achieving a 'dynamic' assessment of children and their families during Covid-19 pandemic

In January 2020, the Covid-19 respiratory virus was taking hold in many nations across the world, including the UK. Initially, containment measures adopted by the UK and devolved governments appeared to be working; all individuals who had tested positive were being isolated and there were widely publicised messages on the importance of handwashing to prevent infection transmission. However, the WHO declared Covid-19 a pandemic on 11 March 2020[24] and it became clear that further public health measures were necessary to control the progression of the virus. Social distancing of no less than 2 m was directed, and the government took the unprecedented step of closing schools for all children except those of key workers. During March 2020 the UK was placed in 'lock-down'; families being restricted to leaving the home only for essential shopping and limited periods of exercise.[25] Those able to work from home were directed to do so. The 'lock-down' measures introduced across the UK led to an increase in family stress for households facing additional financial and social pressures. Many families experienced financial hardship arising from the economic fallout of the pandemic through being furloughed or losing their jobs, low-income families appearing to be more adversely affected by the financial squeeze.[26,27]

The national charity Refuge released a statement warning that the Covid-19 crisis had the potential to aggravate pre-existing abusive behaviours by perpetrators and that self-isolation and lockdown meant that women and children were spending concentrated time with perpetrators, potentially escalating cases of domestic abuse and further restricting freedoms.[28] Despite the increased stress in families and reduced resources and support for families, the numbers of referrals to police and children's social care, as well as referrals for Child Protection medical assessments appeared to be reduced.[87] However, in Scotland, a report by the Scottish Government[29] has highlighted that in the four weeks after Easter, domestic abuse was identified as a concern in more child protection plans when compared to the same time period in 2019. Indeed, the evidence indicates that there was a 16% increase in the number of cases where a child protection investigation was initiated by Police Scotland, Health and Social Work[29] when compared to 2019. Thus, adding to concerns regarding the safety and well-being of children and young people during the lockdown and the need for health visiting support.

In response to the Covid-19 pandemic, the NHS recommended that health visitors should cease additional mandated contacts, except for new birth contacts. Support for vulnerable and high-risk families was to continue, although this was recommended to be largely virtual in nature, using phone and text advice.[30] Significant changes were made to the way in which health visiting services operated, varying from health Trust to health Trust, including the re-deployment of staff to acute services, the implementation of virtual working and conducting face to face contact in personal protective equipment (PPE).

Children and young people in Local Authority care and on Child Protection/Child in Need Plans are already recognised as vulnerable to abuse and/or neglect and are identified as being vulnerable by virtue of their complex social and/or health needs. This group are at much higher risk of harm during the pandemic because of the increased level of stress in families, their reduced access to normal support services and the significantly reduced amount of professional and community oversight.[31]

Moreover, a particularly concerning group are those children and young people who are vulnerable to abuse and/or neglect but had not yet been recognised or referred. As a group they have proved extremely difficult to reach, and the lockdown has increased their vulnerability as they are more hidden from services. Unfortunately, the scale of the issue is difficult to estimate and indeed it may take years for the impact of lockdown to become apparent.[31]

Prior to the pandemic, Hammersley et al (2019) concluded that video conferencing may be suitable for simple problems that did not require a physical examination, although it was not as information rich as face-to-face contacts. Although telephone and video calls to parents and young people are helpful, they cannot replace home visiting. The RCPCH advise that decisions about home visiting must be informed by risk assessment for both vulnerability and illness. It is deemed essential that professionals have adequate access to appropriate PPE and are trained how to use it, in order to reassure families and children about the safety of such a visit and to protect professional staff.[31]

The literature exploring the impact of virtual working with families during Covid-19 is, at this point, limited. However, Cook and Zschomler[32] interviewed 31 child and family social workers in England from the period March to June 2020 to gain an understanding of the benefits and challenges of virtual working with at risk families. This study has relevance to the health visiting service and how it responds to the challenges of working with complex and non-engaging families.

The workers described a combination of video calls and text/instant messaging being used to keep in touch with parents and carers. Some benefits were identified by those interviewed. Virtual communication was greatly preferred by some service users, particularly by young people/adolescents who felt more comfortable with messaging and video calls than face-to-face contact. Indirect forms of communication without video (such as text/instant messaging) could be a non-threatening way into topics that were difficult to talk about in person, which led to families sharing their views more openly. This was surprising to many workers, who initially regarded text messages as a less appropriate form of contact with families.

There were, however, perceived risks of virtual engagement with families. Digital exclusion was a significant barrier to work with children and families as not all families had the Internet at home or could afford the data costs associated with video calls.

Significantly, virtual engagement was felt to be far less effective where the workers did not have a prior relationship with the child, parent or carer. The workers interviewed indicated that virtual home visits had significant limitations for initial assessments and high-risk cases where there were child welfare concerns, making it more difficult to assess the home environment and to pick up on important cues and sensory information. Virtual home visiting can work well in some circumstances but cannot adequately replace face-to-face home visits. The study concludes that there is an urgent need for research into children and families' perspectives on virtual social work and their perspectives on how this can work more effectively.[32] It is this group of children and families that challenge health visitors' use of intuitive skills to interpret the state of the dynamics within families they encounter. An additional risk is that of whether it is safe to talk, remaining mindful of the risks to the child/parent of being overheard.

## The influence of value base and culture on competency

Child protection is an emotive area; one which can and will raise difficult issues for professionals' working in this area. For example, domestic abuse can affect women and men of every age, socio-economic group, race, religion and sexuality; and Musimbe-Rix[33] contends it is 'a societal problem'. Consequently, there will be health visitors for whom domestic abuse issues will have personal resonance as a victim, but also as a perpetrator.

Total objectivity in making professional judgments is unattainable because of the emotiveness of the subject and the fact that professionals are shaped by their own experiences.[34] As individuals, professionals bring their own experiences of having been parented to how they view any family situation. These experiences may well influence how situations encountered as professionals are 'ranked', and the subsequent action taken – be that a highly anxious or a 'numbed' response.[34]

Families on health visitor caseloads reflect the diverse cultural backgrounds in terms of race, ethnicity and sexual orientation of the communities within which they practice. Health visitors should demonstrate inter-cultural competency (IC) in their work with families. IC is 'the ability to communicate effectively and appropriately in inter-cultural situations based on one's own inter-cultural knowledge, skills and attitudes'.[35:8] This includes being comfortable communicating with individuals about their personal and family history, their perceived identity, their experience of being parented and their approaches to parenting (Department of Education, Department of Health and Home Office, 2000).[21]

IC is not achieved by mere contact; workers need to reflect on the relationship of their own and other's identities and responses.[37] For inter-cultural learning to take place there should be *'learning/change in the individual: cognitive, attitudinal, behavioural change; change in self-perception; change in relationships with others, i.e., people of a different social group'*.[38:241–266]

Deardorff[38:241–266] emphasises the importance of key attitudes in IC – *respect, openness, curiosity and discovery*. Respect gives value to other cultures, openness and curiosity allows learning through withholding judgment and viewing situations from a different perspective. These creative approaches can turn differences into opportunities, allowing the possibility of seeing more than one perspective.[39]

Whilst being aware of different approaches to child-rearing within cultures, professionals should prioritise the best interests of children at all times.[40,41] Certain 'signposts' (from legislation, policy, guidance and research) about children, parenting and abuse should act as a guide and inform decision-making. For example, although individual workers might have been raised in a community that promotes and practices female genital mutilation (FGM), they operate within a legislative framework where FGM has been illegal in the UK since 1985.[41,42]

## Dangerous dynamics – the drama triangle

Policies and procedures do not always recognise the human and emotional aspects of interpretation, judgment and decision-making (Rawlings et al 2014). Karpman's[43] seminal essay on the *drama triangle* invites us to consider our own position or role in relation to that of the families with which we work. Karpman theorised that only three roles were necessary to depict the emotional reversals in any drama (or life) script, these three roles being the *rescuer, victim* and *perpetrator*. Karpman[43]

describes a *rescuer* as someone who often does not own their own vulnerability and seeks instead to 'rescue' those whom they see as vulnerable. A *victim* is someone who usually feels overwhelmed by their own sense of vulnerability or powerlessness and does not take responsibility for themselves or their own power, and therefore looks for a *rescuer* to take care of them. The position of *persecutor* uses their power in a negative way, which is frequently destructive.

Significantly, Karpman[43] does not view these roles as necessarily fixed positions, but suggests that drama will only take place when there is a switch in the roles. For example, the *rescuer* will always end up feeling the *victim*, but sometimes may be perceived by others, who are on the outside looking in, as being the *persecutor*.

### THINKING SPACE

Think of a situation with a family or with colleagues where you know you have been a Rescuer, Victim, or Persecutor…. You might have been all three at some time in the same scenario. Using that situation, ask yourself the following questions:

- Who had the power? How did I know?
- Who was taking responsibility for whom?
- Who was I taking responsibility for?
- Did I allow the other person to take responsibility for their actions?
- Did I agree to more than I wanted to?
- What did I feel about this situation?
- What did I want to feel?
- What boundaries did I need to set up?
- What was I not doing?
- What did I need to do?
- Did I use my power to take care of myself properly?
- What action did I need to take to make sure that I dealt with this so that there was best possible outcome?

## Intuitive skills within the context of narrative learning

A growing body of scholarship over the last two decades is recognising the importance of narrative or story-telling as a means of constructing reality and shaping our perception of it. Bruner[44] argued that narrative or stories are as indispensable to human experience as logic and science. According to Bruner,[44] intuitive thinking characterises human thought. By intuitive thinking he means that a person goes beyond the information they are given to find meaning and solve problems. Similar shifts in thinking are seen in the field of nursing. Whilst conscious logical thinking has quite rightly been highly valued in decision-making, since the 1980s there has been recognition of the importance of intuition in making clinical judgements in nursing. Benner et al[76] built on earlier work to provide an intriguing definition of intuition as 'understanding without rationale'. Goding[45] describes intuitive practice as an ability to see the whole problem rather than concentrating on the parts, with an emphasis on meaning rather than detail. Moreover, an ethnographic study of health visitors in one health authority in England revealed that intuition enabled health visitors to interpret and 'make sense' of complex and difficult situations, and was important in helping them to identify and prevent child abuse.[46:578]

For Bruner, a story or narrative is distinguished from a routine sequence of events by *peripetia* – a sudden reversal in circumstances. He argues that we come to expect that sudden breach in the ordinary state of affairs that accompanies any story. Narrative is how we make sense of interactions with others, and it is our natural way of identifying and talking about expectations. In a completed story, this breach in expectations is recognised and resolved. Bruner's notion of storytelling sits well with Karpman's drama triangle; through both, story or narrative can be interpreted or re-interpreted, dialogue (spoken and unspoken) being the medium through which learning and growth can occur. Like scientific discoveries, stories show us ways to cope with error and surprise in our daily lives.

## Working with families where there are dangerous dynamics at play

Both Karpman[43] and Bruner[44] assert that the balance of power is not fixed between the worker and family and has been shown to fluctuate in response to changing circumstances. Working Together to Safeguard Children statutory guidance[40] acknowledges the significance of 'power' held by the statutory safeguarding partners: the local authority, police and health. The statutory guidance proceeds on the premise that all, or most of, the power resides with the worker rather than the family.[40] However, a dilemma continues to exist between supporting the families and protecting the children. Workers are required to recognise and challenge possible abuse, whilst simultaneously having a supportive role and working in partnership with parents.[47] This requires highly competent levels of intuitive and communication skills on the part of the professional.

Working with Troubled Families guidance (2012) explores the approaches used by professionals working with families where there may be obstacles and resistance. It describes the importance of an honest, supportive approach with families which is also assertive and persistent in nature.[48] Practitioner guidance in England and Scotland advises professionals to be alert to families whose compliance is apparent rather than genuine, or who are more obviously reluctant, resistant or sometimes angry or hostile to their approaches. The child's welfare should always be paramount and where professionals are too scared to confront the family, they must consider what life is like for a child in the family[84] (WoS 2016).

Health visitors, like all workers in the field of child protection, are required to make difficult decisions with imperfect, limited and fragmented information. There are no perfect predictive tools with which to make decisions, and in some cases children will not receive the protection they need. Throughout the UK, various assessment approaches are available to assist health visitors in assessing the level of risk to children and young people. The Strengthening Families (HMG 2019)[93] approach was developed out of the model of practice originally developed by Turnell and Edwards' 'Signs of Safety'[49] and is integrated across statutory agencies across England and Wales. This model supports assessment of risk using a strength and resilience model to engage children, young people and families. Practitioners are required to undertake sound and well-structured discussions with families and other professionals and consider risk from the outset of casework, at all levels. At its simplest, Strengthening Families contains three domains and a scoring by family and practitioners that can be applied at all stages of intervention.

(i) What are we worried about? (Past harm, future risks and complicating factors)
(ii) What's working well? (Existing strengths and safety)
(iii) What needs to happen? (Future safety)
(iv) How worried are we? (On a scale of 1–10)

In Scotland, the Resilience Matrix is a component of the National Practice Model and uses the National Risk Assessment Framework comprising a three-stage approach of collection and collation of information, risk analysis and risk management (SG 2012). The National Practice Model views risk as a,

*dynamic concept that can be multidimensional, it is fluid and critically shaped and characterised by a range of events and movement in the context and setting where it occurs. (SG, 2012: 1)[6]*

Whichever assessment model is used workers should be alert to the following key messages when assessing and engaging with families on their caseload.

- 'Toxic risk combinations' – the increased risk posed by a combination of parenting factors within the household was described as early as 1986. Workers need to be mindful of the impact of factors of individual carer(s) which may not separately score highly on 'risk assessment' but which, in combination within a relationship, may lead to a real increase in potential risk.[50] The presence of issues such as mental ill health and/or substance misuse can be particularly 'toxic' if seen by both primary and secondary carers (Cleaver et al 2011).
- 'Disguised compliance' – the term used to describe when a parent or carer gives the appearance of co-operating with child welfare agencies to avoid raising concerns, to allay professional concerns and ultimately to diffuse professional intervention.[51]
- 'The rule of optimism' – describes a distorted view of the family by the worker which may occur when the worker finds the most positive explanation for occurrences within the family.[80,94] The revisiting of the 'rule of optimism' by two reviews of SCRs in England and Scotland has reinforced the view that a tendency towards over-optimistic

interpretation by professionals – in particular social workers – remains a recurring theme.[52,53] Insufficient professional curiosity combined with an overly optimistic view of parental behaviour can lead to interventions which are insufficiently authoritative and can leave children at risk of children being unprotected.[54]

■ 'Cultural Relativism' – workers subscribing to 'cultural relativism' believe every culture must be viewed in its own right as equal to all others, and it's culturally sanctioned behaviours cannot be judged by the standards of another culture.[55,92] This could result in hesitation on the part of the professional to intervene in cases that are a criminal offence in the UK, for example FGM.

■ 'Ethnocentrism' – workers subscribing to ethnocentrism believe that one's own cultural beliefs and practices are not only preferable but also superior to others'. This can lead to the pathologising of others' cultures.[55]

Shemmings et al[56] suggest that resistant or reluctant family members are likely to find considerable difficultly *mentalising* – a concept similar to empathy, derived from contemporary applications of attachment-based research. Low *mentalisation* results in family members having significant problems in understanding that other people (including their own children) have different thoughts and feelings from their own. A key implication of the findings from their research is that professionals need to work even harder to demonstrate empathy with reluctant and resistant families and aim to introduce interventions which increase the parents' *mentalising* capacities.[56]

A study by Rawlings et al[57] to investigate the barriers to learning from Serious Case Reviews, identified one key barrier as that of the workers' lack of challenge. Workers should challenge their own beliefs and attitudes and learn to *think the unthinkable*; challenge themselves to improve their working with non-compliant parents/carers, including the confidence to challenge apparent compliance.[57]

## THINKING SPACE

Exploring the significance of dangerous dynamics within child protection practice.

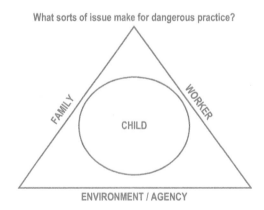

What sorts of issue make for dangerous practice?

FAMILY    WORKER    CHILD    ENVIRONMENT / AGENCY

Consider each of the Worker, Family or Environment/Agency headings separately. Ask yourself what sorts of issue may influence the dynamics within and between the family, the worker and environment/agency.

Your responses may include the following:

**The worker**

- Emotionally overwhelmed
- Overwhelmed by caseload
- Lack of self-reflection about personal beliefs, cultural views or values
- Over-identifying – objectivity becomes difficult
- Distancing from the family, a lack of empathy
- Not taking account of previous history
- Fear, paralysis, drift, stress – leading to avoidance of family (child)
- Poor professional boundaries – lack of understanding of roles
- Fearful of being accused of racism
- Poor/lack of record keeping
- Poor work/life balance
- Adult rather than child-centred focus
- 'Collusion' with family and colleagues – 'it would damage my relationship'
- Acting without an evidence base, systematic or structured approach to intervention
- Operates alone or unsupported – 'flying solo'
- The protective 'myth' of disability
- Disability or Significant harm? Sometimes difficult to distinguish
- Lack of or poor-quality supervision
- Lack of competency or training

**The family**

- Intimidating adults – threats, complaints, racist or sexual comments, overt attacks
- Lack of engagement/ contact
- Avoidant or poor engagers
- Resistant
- Chaotic
- Previous experiences with agencies/ professionals – good and bad
- Grooming of children, partners and professionals

**The environment**

- Poor quality or lack of supervision
- Poor communication/ information sharing – inter and intra agency
- Different agency thresholds
- Lack of organisational standards
- Poor provision or lack of training
- Inadequate governance arrangements – escalation/accountability
- Adult rather than child focused service (worker)
- Poorly defined boundaries of roles and responsibilities
- Absence of clear written procedures to guide intervention
- Avoidance of overt disagreement about management of cases

## THE PATH TO ACHIEVING 'UNCONSCIOUS COMPETENCE' IN PRACTICE

Several learning theories have been helpful in providing a framework on which to build the complex series of activities and processes in gaining expertise. These include Sprague and Stuart's[58] model of the four stages of development of mastery, which charts the progress to the fluid integration of clinical and intuitive competencies comprising expert professional judgment.

The fourth or final stage in their model is that of *unconscious competence*; a state in which professionals exercise the skills and knowledge in their domain so automatically and instinctively that they are no longer consciously aware of what they know or do.

Ambrose et al[59] interpret Sprague and Stuart's model to explain the process by which novices develop mastery. Novices are said to be in a state of *unconscious incompetence*, in that they have not yet developed skill in a particular domain, nor do they have sufficient skill to recognise what they need to learn. As they gain knowledge and experience, they advance to a state of *conscious incompetence*, where they are increasingly aware of what they do not know, and consequently of what they need to learn. As their mastery develops, students advance to a state of *conscious competence* wherein they have considerable experience in their domain yet must think and act deliberately and consciously. Finally, as practitioners reach the highest level of mastery, they move to a state of *unconscious competence* in which they exercise skills and knowledge in their domain so automatically and instinctively that they are no longer consciously aware of what they know or do. Westcott[60] asserted that an expert practitioner becomes able, as a result of experience, to make correct, global, professional evaluations by resorting to a great many cues of which she is, in fact, unaware.

This process, of course, may not run entirely smoothly through the stages from novice to expert. Ambrose et al[59] suggests that competence develops in a linear way, whilst consciousness may wax and wane. There is also recognition in the literature of the significance of the acquisition of key component skills on which to build expert knowledge.[61] For example, the ability to analyse a family situation where a child is at risk of harm requires component skills such as the capacity to identify the central question or dilemma of the case and recommend and justify a solution. If the practitioner lacks the critical component skills, or if their command of these skills is weak, their performance in the overall task may be weak. Introducing health visitors to the dynamics described in Karpman's *drama triangle* and, critically, the role they might adopt or be placed in, might be one of the component or foundation skills needed before embarking on more complex situations in the field. Health visitors would need to reflect on each of the drama triangle dimensions and how they might recognise and remedy a destructive dynamic within or with the family. Offering novice health visitors opportunities to apply skills

or knowledge in diverse situations could help prepare them better to transfer that skill to novel or evolving contexts.[59,61,62]

## Valuing preparation, reflection and self-awareness for difficult conversations

As no two encounters are alike there is not necessarily a single answer in practice situations. Consequently, the ability to practice in contexts of uncertainty and complexity is critical. Conducting difficult conversations with parents and carers is a reminder of the need to accept uncertainty and complexity as integral to relationships with clients. Research suggests that practitioners' confidence in conducting difficult conversations can be increased through interactive multiprofessional workshops.[77]

The pedagogical approach of narrative learning and an awareness of the victim, rescuer and persecutor roles in difficult conversations requires practitioners to reflect on their actions and hold themselves accountable for the impact these have on families and colleagues. Health visitors can then consider the extent to which an encounter was meaningful or helpful.

Whilst there is recognition within the literature of the importance of relationship – building with families[4,63] there is limited guidance on the micro-skills of how to build such a partnership.[64] Social workers participating in the 2008 Forrester study were observed to demonstrate a high level of confrontation and low level of listening when interacting with actors playing simulated clients. Core communication skills such as the use of open questions alongside empathy and reflection were rarely observed in the simulations. Roadblocks to listening interfered with engaging parents and working with resistance in situations where there were concerns about family welfare.[64] The answer may lie in Motivational Interviewing techniques, which aim to understand the nature of resistance and find ways of reducing it.[65–67]

Motivational interviewing is based on these assumptions:

- how we speak to people is likely to be just as important as what we say
- being listened to and understood is an important part of the process of change
- the person who has the problem is the person who has the answer to solving it
- people only change their behaviour when they feel ready – not when they are told to do so
- the solutions people find for themselves are the most enduring and effective.

There are four general principles of motivational interviewing:

- R – resist the urge to change the individual's course of action through didactic means
- U – understand it's the individual's reasons for change, not those of the practitioner, that will elicit a change in behaviour
- L – listening is important; the solutions lie within the individual, not the practitioner
- E – empower the individual to understand that they have the ability to change their behaviour.[66]

## THINKING SPACE

Ask yourself….
- What conversations do you find difficult?

Your responses may include, amongst other things, the following:

Asking clients (adults, young people and children) about their experience of domestic abuse/mental health/alcohol or substance use/poor hygiene/sexual health and relationships.

Addressing issues of conflict with colleagues – challenging attitudes/resistance to change.
- What is it exactly that is difficult about having these conversations?

Your responses may include, amongst other things, the following:

I don't feel I have the experience/skills/words/have not been trained/don't feel it's part of my role/not comfortable/too close for comfort/frightened.

Now read through the following section on 'Preparing for a difficult conversation'. Is this helpful?

## Preparing for a difficult conversation

Meaningful exchanges between health professionals and children and their families are characterised by a genuine interest toward the child and the family, demonstrating a sensitivity to all aspects of verbal and nonverbal communication.[68] Communication skills such as active listening, paraphrasing, summarising, reflecting and questioning are considered fundamental to the development of rapport and empathic therapeutic relationships.[69]

If possible, in advance of the conversation, the practitioner might give some thought into how they are feeling at that moment. This enables self-compassion and resilience and may give a sense of whether this is the right time to have the conversation. Additionally, the individual with whom the conversation is to take place may not be ready to speak. If the circumstances permit this can be acknowledged, and an agreement made to come back to it at another time. However, there are occasions when a conversation can't wait and is necessary, even though the person does not want it.

There are advantages to taking time to plan the conversation, including identifying any specific challenge and framing the conversation in such a way as to maintain honesty, yet ensuring the hearer feels respected throughout.

Acknowledging the difficulty of the conversation may be helpful, also that what is being said may or may not be difficult to hear. Silence can be as powerful as speech, so allowing space for the client to process and respond to what is being said can help individuals to appreciate they are being listened to and asked about their perspective.

The importance of nonverbal communication can't be over-estimated: appearing calm, speaking clearly and levelly, maintaining normal eye contact and careful positioning in relation to the client should be considered throughout the conversation (GMCUK 2016).[70]

## THINKING SPACE

Consider the following difficult conversations:

You are visiting the home of a young mother to complete the 6- to 8-week developmental assessment. The mother undresses the baby and you observe a fading bruise on the baby's thigh. How would you address this?

A mother comes to the Health Centre for some family planning advice. You observe a bruise on the mother's eye. She says her ex-partner hit her but the children (9 years, 5 years and 4 months) were not in the same room when this happened. How would you address this?

You are visiting the home of a family on your caseload. An 8-year-old boy answered the door saying his mother was out and he'd been left to care for his brothers, aged 2 years and 9 months old. After 15 minutes the mother returns, saying this is the first time she's ever left the children alone. How would you address this?

## The safeguarding supervision process

Safeguarding supervision takes place where known or suspected child protection concerns about children, young people and families are formally reviewed by a practitioner and supervisor, ensuring competent, accountable practice is maintained. It is a formal process which should be embedded within the governance structure of the organisation within which it takes place. A supervisory structure, pathway and contract which the organisation, supervisor and supervisee understand and adhere to reflects the seriousness of the activity, retaining a child focus at the heart of all supervisory discussions and actions. Effective practitioner supervision can play a critical role in ensuring a clear focus on a child's welfare and it should support practitioners to reflect critically on the impact of their decisions and actions on the child and their family (SG 2014, LSCB 2017).[40,77] Indeed, all staff working with children and families should be provided with appropriate supervision and support to safeguard their health and well-being (SG 2014, LSCB 2017).[40,77]

Morrison and Wonnecott[71] describe supervision as a complex activity, requiring practical and emotional intelligence on the part of the supervisor to support the confidence and competency of the supervisee. They identify key links in the supervision chain suggesting the supervisor should be able to demonstrate emotional competence and empathy, model accurate and effective assessment and partnership working in relation to the supervisee and their practice families. Child-focused planning and intervention should be a priority of the supervisory process and a clear supervision policy, held at organisational level, should underpin clarity and the security roles of both the supervisee and the supervisor.[71]

The purpose of supervision – a definition.

Supervision is the process by which one worker is given responsibility by the organisation to work with another worker(s) in order to meet certain organisational, professional and personal objectives which promote the best outcomes for service users. These functions are:

(i) Competent, accountable performance/practice – organisation
(ii) Continuing professional development – empowerment, knowledge and skills
(iii) Personal support – emotional containment
(iv) Engaging the individual with the organisation – mediation[72]

Morrison[72:205] describes a supervisory framework that stresses the importance of maintaining a balanced relationship between thinking, feeling and action in relation to safeguarding practice. He highlights the danger of becoming *stuck* at key points in the think, feel, act cycle. When stuck in reflection (feeling), the practitioners' own feelings dominate; their thinking is be suppressed and actions can be driven only by feelings. When stuck in analysing (thinking), the practitioner is dominated by thinking; their feelings are suppressed and their actions driven by rigid thinking. When stuck in action (doing), the practitioner is dominated by action; their thinking and feelings are suppressed. Finally, Morrison describes the practitioner being stuck in experience; being overwhelmed by their experiences, risking the practitioner shutting down and disconnecting from all feelings, thinking and action. The practitioner stuck in experience is in danger of *burn out.*

Botham[73] noted a lack of consensus about the supervision models and frameworks being used in practice, though her review highlighted the benefits for health visitors of supervision: these included, stress reduction, the provision of support and opportunities for personal learning and development, including enhanced critical thinking skills. Rooke[74] study supports this finding; health visitors discussed the importance of supervision providing personal support, a safe space to talk about feelings, especially fear, anger, sadness, repulsion or helplessness arising from safeguarding work.

Gilovich (1991) suggests that individuals are inclined to find alternative ways of interpreting or 'framing' what they encounter and are adept at finding a frame that is acceptable to them. These relatively subtle shifts of criteria and interpretation may produce significant errors of judgement. Critical reflection through supervision is known to strengthen analysis and professional challenge and provide some protection against these biases in assessments and decision-making.[71]

## Reflective supervision provides emotional containment and challenges any distortion in perception

Supervision should aim to be sensitive, constructive and challenging, demonstrating respect for supervisees and an acceptance of differing value bases where this is not discriminatory.

In line with the purpose of personal support, supervision should provide a safe space to talk about feelings, especially fear, anger, sadness, repulsion or helplessness arising from work. An exploration of any emotional blocks to engaging the family should be addressed. Mezirow[85] states that reflective feedback enables us to correct distortions in our beliefs and errors in problem-solving and explore any emotional blocks to engaging the family. The benefit of reflective supervision is that it allows us to learn from discussing our experiences with individuals who may raise alternatives, ask challenging questions and suggest alternative interpretations. Individual processes in reflective dialogue, which involve one teller and one listener, have the potential to explore experiences in depth (Mezirow, 1990).

Morrison[75:205] suggests the partnership of the supervisor and supervisee should reflect the positive modelling that is also, ideally, mirroring the desired behaviours of practitioners with families. An open, honest and respectful relationship should form the basis of both the supervisory relationship and the worker's relationship with the family and should empower the practitioner to challenge authoritatively and appropriately. Supervision aims to support the practitioners' professional development, intervening early to identify any additional training needs and support practice: for example, managing conflict, negotiating skills or improving time management.

Morrison[72:302–303] highlights the importance of the supervisory role within safeguarding supervision, asking how it is to be sustained, supported and developed. He stresses the importance of selecting supervisors who have the emotional and personal competencies to perform the role. He highlights the need for supervisors to be trained to carry out supervision and, crucially, receive ongoing developmental supervision themselves to maintain quality and focus.

## CONCLUSION

This chapter has focused on the attitudinal and relational approaches which enhance effective working with complex families; the core elements of the 'how' rather than the 'what'. The cultivation of emotions, values, and reflection in daily practice is seen at the heart of work with families. Understanding dynamics, the ability to build relationships and engage with people are skills that don't just apply to the health visitor's work with families, they also apply to working effectively within a team.

Practical aspects of family engagement and challenge within practice have been viewed through a pedagogical lens of narrative and discovery learning theory. The significance of dangerous dynamics, intuitive and IC and self-reflection in achieving unconscious competence has been explored. The view that competence depends on habits of mind, including attentiveness, critical curiosity, self-awareness has been promoted throughout this chapter. Safeguarding supervision unites and underpins all aspects of complex casework, fostering skilled, accountable practice, providing professional empowerment and emotional support. Additionally, the mediation role of supervision ensures the individual practitioner complies with NMC and organisational aims and standards.

### KEY LEARNING POINTS

- Development of the competency to recognise child maltreatment and take effective action to protect children.
- Challenge own beliefs and attitudes and have the inter-cultural competency to communicate with parents and carers about their perceived identity, personal and family history, their experience of being parented and their approaches to parenting.
- Be prepared with the skills to 'read' complex situations and dynamics and build strong relationships with children and their families.
- Improve work with non-engaging/non-compliant families, including the confidence to challenge disguised compliance.
- Have access to effective safeguarding supervision to support accountable, emotionally contained practice.

## REFERENCES

1. Keys, M. (2009). Determining the skills for Child Protection Practice: Emerging from the quagmire. *Child Abuse Review, 18,* 316–332. https://onlinelibrary.wiley.com/doi/pdf/10.1002/car.1089. Accessed 28 August 2020.
2. Brandon, M., Belderson, P., Warren, C., Howe, D., Gardener, R., Dodsworth, J., & Black, J. (2008). *Analysing child death and serious injury through abuse and neglect: What can we learn? A Biennial analysis of SCRs 2003 – 2005.* UEA.
3. Brandon, M., Bailey, S., & Belderson, P. (2011). *Building on the learning from Serious Case Reviews: A two-year analysis of child protection database notifications 2005–2007 & 2007–2009.* Department of Education.
4. Astbury, R., Shepherd, A., & Cheyne, H. (2016). Working in partnership: The application of shared decision-making to health visitor practice. *Journal of Clinical Nursing, 26*(1–2). https://onlinelibrary.wiley.com/doi/pdf/10.1111/jocn.13480. Accessed 28 August 2020. p221–222
5. Royal College Nursing. (2019). *Safeguarding children and young people: Roles and competencies for Healthcare staff.* (4th ed.)
6. Scottish Government. (2012). *National Risk Framework to support the assessment of children and young people.* https://www.gov.scot/publications/national-risk-framework-support-assessment-children-young-people/. Accessed 28 August 2020.
7. Pollice, G. (2003). *Teaching versus training.* http://www.ibm.com/developerworks/rational/library/3810.html. Accessed 26 August 2020.
8. Epstein, R. M., & Hundert, E. M. (2002). Defining and assessing professional competence. *Journal of American Medical Association, 287,* 226–235. Journal of American Medical Association
9. Sidebotham, P., Brandon, M., Powell, C., Solebo, C., Koistinen, J., & Ellis, C. (2008). *Learning from Serious Case Reviews: Report of a research study on the methods of learning lessons nationally from Serious Care Reviews.* Department of Education.

10. Ofsted. (2010). *Learning lessons from serious case reviews 2009–2010*. Sections 103–106.

11. Trevithick, P. (2011). Understanding defences and defensiveness in social work. *Journal of Social Work Practice, 25*(4), 389–412.

12. Mattinson, J. (1975). *The reflection process in casework supervision*. London: Tavistock.

13. Gigerenzer, G. (2002). *Reckoning with risk: Learning to live with uncertainty* (p. 228). London: Allen Lane.

14. Polanyi, M. (1967). *The tacit dimension*. London: Routledge & Kegan Ltd. 4, 18, 25.

15. Fonteyn, M. E., & Grobe, S. (1993). Expert nurses' clinical reasoning under uncertainty: Representation, structure, and process. *Proceedings of the Annual Symposium on Computer Applications in Medical Care*, 405–409.

16. Helm, D. (2010). *Making sense of child and family assessment: How to interpret children's needs* (pp. 187–188). London: Jessica Kingsley Publishers.

17. Saltiel, D. (2015). Observing front line decision making in child protection. *British Journal of Social Work*. doi:10. 1093/bjsw/bcv112.

18. Munro, E. (2011). *The Munro review of child protection: Final report. A child-centred system*. Department of Education, Sections 6.24 & 6.25: 90.

19. Care Inspectorate – (2019). *Learning from significant case reviews. March 2015 to April 2018.* https://www.careinspectorate.com/index.php/low-graphics/8-news/5063-learning-from-significant-case-reviews-march-2015-to-april-2018. Accessed 28 August 2020.

20. Cicchetti, D., & Valentino, K. (2006). An ecological transactional perspective on child maltreatment: Failure of the average expectable environment and its influence upon child development. In D. Cicchetti, & D. J. Cohen (Eds.), *Developmental psychopathology, second edition: risk, disorder, and adaptation (Vol. 3)*. New York: Wiley.

21. Department of Health, Department for Education and Employment, Home Office. (2000). *Framework for the assessment of children in need and their families*. London: The Stationery Office.

22. Scottish Government. (2016). *GIRFEC national practice model*. https://www.gov.scot/publications/girfec-national-practice-model/. Accessed 28 August 2020.

23. Laming Lord. (2003). *The Victoria Climbie inquiry: Report of the inquiry by Lord Laming*. Norwich: TSO.

24. World Health Organisation. (2020). Regional Office for Europe. https://www.euro.who.int/en/health-topics/health-emergencies/coronavirus-covid-19#:~:text=WHO%20announced%20COVID-19,on%2011%20March%202020. Accessed 3 September 2020.

25. PMO. (2020). *Prime Ministers statement on coronavirus (Covid-19): 23 March 2020.* https://www.gov.uk/government/speeches/pm-address-to-the-nation-on-coronavirus-23-march-2020. Accessed 3 September 2020.

26. Child Poverty Action Group. (2020). *Poverty in the pandemic: The impact of coronavirus on low-income families and children*. August 2020. CPAG wesite - https://cpag.org.uk/policy-and-campaigns/report/poverty-pandemic-impact-coronavirus-low-income-families-and-children. Accessed 11 September 2020

27. Corlett, A., Clarke, S., McCurdy, C., Rahman, F., & Whittaker, M. (2020). The Living Standards Audit 2019, Resolution Foundation. https://www.resolutionfoundation.org/app/uploads/2019/07/Living-Standards-Audit-2019.pdf. Accessed 26 December 2021.

28. Refuge. (2020). *COVID-19 Response*. www.refuge.org.uk/refuge-responds-to-covid-19. Accessed 30 March 2020.

29. Scottish Government. (2020). Children, young people and families COVID-19 evidence and intelligence report. https://www.gov.scot/binaries/content/documents/govscot/publications/research-and-analysis/2020/07/children-young-people-families-covid-19-evidence-intelligence-report2/documents/children-young-people-families-covid-19-evidence-intelligence-report/children-young-people-families-covid-19-evidence-intelligence-report/govscot%3Adocument/children-young-people-families-covid-19-evidence-intelligence-report.pdf. Accessed 5 September 2020.

30. NHS. (2020). *COVID-19 prioritisation within community health services*. www.england.nhs.uk/coronavirus/wpcontent/uploads/sites/52/2020/03/COVID-19-prioritisation-within-community-health-services-19-March-2020-version-1.1.pdf. Accessed 26 August 2020.

31. Royal College of Paediatrics and Child Health. (2020). *COVID-19 – Guiding principles for safeguarding partnerships during the pandemic*. https://www.rcpch.ac.uk/resources/covid-19-guiding-principles-safeguarding-partnerships-during-pandemic. Accessed 26 August 2020.

32. Cook, L. L. & Zschomler, D. (2020). *Child and family social work in the context of COVID-19: Practice issues and innovations*. Briefing Paper. Norwich: CRCF. http://www.uea.ac.uk/crcf.

33. Musimbe-Rix, S. (2021). Research: Domestic abuse evidence review. https://interventionsalliance.com/domestic-abuse-evidence-review/. Accessed 26 December 2021.

34. Lowes, L., & Prowse, M. (2001). Standing outside the interview process? The illusion of objectivity in phenomenological data generation. *International Journal of Nurse Studies, 38*(4), 471–480.

35. Deardorff, D. (2006). Identification and assessment of intercultural competence as a student outcome of inter-

nationalization. In M. Byram, & A. Feng (Eds.), *Living and studying abroad* (pp. 232–256). Clevedon: Multilingual Matters.

36. Bhopal, R. S. (2012). The quest for culturally sensitive health-care systems in Scotland: Insights for a multi-ethnic Europe. *Journal of Public Health, 34*(1), 5–11. https://academic.oup.com/jpubhealth/article/34/1/5/1555017.

37. Crichton, J., Paige, M., Papademetre, L., & Scarino, A. (2004). *Integrated resources for intercultural teaching and learning in the context of internationalization in higher education.* Research Centre for Languages and Cultures Education, School of International Studies, University of South Australia.

38. Deardorff, D. (2006). Identification and assessment of intercultural competence as a student outcome of internationalization, *Journal of International Education, Fall 2006, 10,* 241–266. https://doi.org/10.1177/1028315306287002

39. LeBaron, M., & Pillay, V. (2006). *Conflict across cultures: A unique experience of bridging differences.* Yarmouth, ME: Intercultural Press.

40. HM Government. (2018). *Working together to safeguard children: A guide to inter-agency working to safeguard and promote the welfare of children.* 2018, 28–29.

41. Scottish Government. (2005). *The Prohibition of Female Genital Mutilation (Scotland) Act.*

42. HM Government. (2016). *Multi-agency guidance on Female Genital Mutilation.* London: Stationary Office. https://www.gov.uk/government/uploads/system/uploads/attachment_data/file/512906/Multi_Agency_Statutory_Guidance_on_FGM__-_FINAL.pdf. Accessed 28 August 2020.

43. Karpman, S. (1968). *Fairy tales and script drama analysis.* http://www.karpmandramatriangle.com/pdf/DramaTriangle.pdf. Accessed 28 August 2020.

44. Bruner, J. (2002). *Making stories, law, literature, life.* Harvard Press. Cambridge Massachusetts. London England.

45. Goding, L. (2013). Intuition and health visiting practice. *British Journal of Community Health Nursing, 2*(4). https://www.magonlinelibrary.com/doi/abs/10.12968/bjch.1997.2.4.7310.

46. Ling, M. S., & Luker, K. A. (2000). Protecting children: Intuition and awareness in the work of health visitors. *Journal of Advanced Nursing, 32*(3), 572–579. https://onlinelibrary.wiley.com/doi/pdf/10.1046/j.1365-2648.2000.01520.x. Accessed 13 September 2020.

47. Littlechild, B. (2006). Men's use of violence and intimidation against family members and child protection workers. In C. Humphreys, & N. Stanley (Eds.), *Domestic violence and child protection* (pp. 208). London: Jessica Kingsley.

48. Department for Communities & Local Government. (2012). Working with troubled families: A guide to working practice. https://assets.publishing.service.gov.uk/government/uploads/system/uploads/attachment_data/file/66113/121214_Working_with_troubled_families_FINAL_v2.pdf. Accessed 3 September 2020.

49. Turnell, A., & Edwards, S. (1999). *Signs of safety: A safety and solution-oriented approach to child protection casework.* New York: WW Norton. https://www.signsofsafety.net/what-is-sofs/.

50. Dale, P., Davies, M., & Morrison, T. (1990). *Dangerous families: Assessment and treatment of child abuse.* Tavistock Pub, London.

51. Reder, P. Duncan, S & Grey, M., et al. (1993). *Beyond blame: Child abuse tragedies re-visited.* London: Routledge.

52. Care Inspectorate. (2016). *Significant Case Reviews in Scotland 2012 to 2015, Dundee.*

53. Sidebotham, P., Brandon, M., Bailey, S., Belderson, P., Dodsworth, J., Garstang, J., et al. (2016). *Pathways to harm, pathways to protection: A triennial analysis of serious case reviews 2011 to 2014.* London: Department of Education.

54. Kettle, M., & Jackson, S. (2017). Revisiting the rule of optimism. *The British Journal of Social Work, 47*(6), 1624–1640. https://doi.org/10.1093/bjsw/bcx090. Accessed 28 August 2020.

55. Egonsdotter, G. Bengtsson, S. Magnus, I & Borell, K. (2020). *Child protection and cultural awareness: Simulation-based learning, Journal of Ethnic & Cultural Diversity in Social Work,* 29:5, 362–376, DOI: 10.1080/15313204.2018.1493013.

56. Shemmings, D., Shemmings, Y., & Cook, A. (2012). *Gaining the trust of 'highly resistant' families: Insights from attachment theory and research Child and Family Social Work.* Wiley. Journal of Child & Family Social Work, 2012, 17, pp. 130–137.

57. Rawlings, A., Paliokosta, P., Maisey, D., Johnson, J., Capstick, J., & Jones, R. (2014). *Study to investigate the barriers to learning from serious case reviews and identify ways of overcoming these barriers* (pp. 7–9). DoE.

58. Sprague, J., & Stuart, D. (2000). *The speakers handbook.* Fort Worth, TX: Harcourt College Publishers.

59. Ambrose, S., Bridges, M., & Lovett, M. (2010). *How learning works: 7 research-based principles for smart learning.* Jossey-Bass. A Wiley Imprint. New York, USA.

60. Westcott, M. (1968). *Towards a contemporary psychology of intuition.* New York, NY: Rinehart & Winston, Holt.

61. Resnick, L. B. (1976). Task analysis in instructional design: Some cases from Mathematics. In D. Klahr (Ed.),

*Cognition and instruction* (pp. 51–80). Hillside, NJ: Erlbaum.

62. McGaghie, W., & Issenberg, S. B. (2010). Does simulation-based medical education with deliberate practice yield better results than traditional clinical education? A meta-analytic comparative review of the evidence. *Academic Medicine, 86*(6), 706–711.

63. Cowley, S., Whittaker, K., Malone, M., Donetto, S., Grigulis, A., & Maben, J. (2015). Why health visiting? Examining the public health benefits within a universal service; a narrative review of the literature. *International Journal of Nursing Studies. 52*(1), pp. 465–480.

64. Forrester, D., McCambridge, J., Waissbein, C., & Rollnick, S. (2008). How do child and family social workers talk to parents about child welfare concerns? *Child Abuse Review, 17*, 23–35. doi:10.1002/car.981. https://onlinelibrary.wiley.com/toc/10990852/2008/17/1.

65. Britt, E., Hudson, S., & Blampied, N. (2003). *Motivational interviewing in health settings: A review.* Elsevier. http://web.vu.lt/mf/r.viliuniene/files/2019/05/Motivational_Interviewing_Article.pdf. Accessed 28 August 2020. Christchurch, New Zealand

66. Rollnick, S., Miller, W., & Butler, C. (2008). *Motivational interviewing in healthcare: Helping patients change behaviour.* London and New York: Guildford Press.

67. Scott, G. (2010). Motivational interviewing 1: Background, key principles and application in healthcare. *Nursing Times, 106*(34), 21–22.

68. Hough, M. (2010), *Counselling skills and theory* (3rd ed.). UK: Hodder.

69. Roberts, J. F., Fenton, G., & Barnard, M. C. (2015). *Developing effective therapeutic relationships with children, young people and their families.* Manchester: University of Salford http://dx.doi.org/10.7748/ncyp.27.4.30.e5. Accessed 26 August 2020.

70. General Medical Council United Kingdom (2016). *Handling difficult conversations: Ten top tips.* https://gmcuk.wordpress.com/2016/05/13/handling-difficult-conversations-ten-top-tips/. Accessed 9 September 2020.

71. Morrison, T., & Wonnecott, J. (2010). *Supervision: Now or never. Reclaiming reflective supervision in social work.* In-Trac Training and Consultancy. https://www.in-trac.co.uk/supervision-now-or-never/. Accessed 26 August 2020.

72. Morrison, T. (2006). *Staff supervision in social care: Making a real difference for staff and service users.* Pavilion Publishing. ISBN 184196168X.

73. Botham, J. (2013). What constitutes safeguarding children supervision for health visitors and school nurses? *Community Practitioner, 86*(3), 28–34.

74. Rooke, J. (2015). Exploring the support mechanisms health visitors use in safeguarding and child protection practice. *Community Practitioner, 88*(10), 42–45.

75. Benner, P., & Tanner, C. (1987). How expert nurses use intuition. *American Journal of Nursing, 87*(1).

76. Benner, P., Tanner, C., & Chesla, C. (1992). From beginner to expert: Gaining a differentiated clinical world in critical care nursing. *Advances in Nursing Science, 14*(3).

77. Brighton, L., Selman, L., Gough, N., Nadicksbernd, J., Bristowe, K., Millington-Sanders, C., & Koffman, J. (2017). Difficult conversations: Evaluation of multi-professional training. *BMJ Journals: Supportive and Palliative Care, 8*(1). https://spcare.bmj.com/content/8/1/45. Accessed 28 August 2020.

78. Brandon, M. (2014). *Learning from serious case reviews about how to work with child neglect.* NSPCC. Slide 5. https://www.norfolklscb.org/wp-content/uploads/2015/04/Neglect-Learning-from-SCR%92s-%96-Marion-Brandon.pdf. Accessed 19 September 2020.

79. Cleaver, H., Unell, I., & Aldgate, J. (2011). *Children's needs – Parenting capacity. Child abuse: Parental mental illness, learning disability, substance misuse, and domestic violence* (2nd ed.). TSO. London.

80. Dingwall, R., Eeekelhaar, J., & Murray, T. (1983). The Protection of Children: State Intervention and Family Life, London: Blackwell.

81. Gilovich, T. (1991). *How we know what isn't so: The fallibility of human reason in everyday life* (p. 75). New York: The Free Press.

82. Hammersley, V., Donaghy, E., Parker, R., McNeilly, H., Atherton, H., Bikker, A., et al. (2020). Comparing the content and quality of video, telephone, and face-to-face consultations: A non-randomised, quasi-experimental, exploratory study in UK primary care. *British Journal of General Practice, 69*(686), e595–e604. https://doi.org/10.3399/bjgp19X704573. Accessed 3 September 2020.

83. London Safeguarding Children Board. (2017). *3. Supervision. London Child Protection Procedures.* (5th ed.). Sections 3 to 3.6.

84. London Safeguarding Children Board. (2017). *7. Managing work with families where there are obstacles and resistance in London child protection procedures.* (5th ed.). Sections 7.1.1 and 7.1.2. https://www.londoncp.co.uk/chapters/supervision.html. Accessed 28 August 2020.

85. Mezirow, J. (1990). *How critical reflection triggers transformative learning, in Fostering Critical Thinking in Adulthood* (p. 1). http://184.182.233.150/rid=1LW06D9V6-26428MK-1Z64/Mezirow's%20chapter,%20How%20Critical%20Refletion%20Triggers%20TL.pdf. Accessed 26 August 2020.

86. Refuge.org.uk. (2017). http://www.refuge.org.uk/get-help-now/what-is-domestic-violence/domestic-violence-the-facts/. Accessed 3 September 2020.

87. Safeguarding Board Northern Ireland. *Safeguarding Board highlights drop in referrals for children that may have experienced harm during COVID-19.* www.safeguardingni.org/safeguarding-board-highlights-drop-referrals-children-may-have-experienced-harm-during-covid-19. Accessed 7 May 2020.

88. Scottish Government. (2014). *The Children and Young People Scotland Act*, GIRFEC approach. UNCRC.

89. Scottish Government. (2014). *National guidance for child protection in Scotland.* https://www.gov.scot/publications/national-guidance-child-protection-scotland/pages/7/. Accessed 28 August 2020.

90. Sroufe, L. A., Egeland, B., Carlson, E. A., & Collins, W. A. (2007). *The development of the person: The Minnesota study of risk and adaptation from birth to adulthood* (p. 91). New York, London: Guildford Press.

91. West of Scotland Child Protection Consortium. (2016). *Practitioner portfolio: Working with resistance.* http://childprotectionnorthayrshire.info/cpc/professionals/non-engaging-families/. Accessed 9 September 2020.

92. Egonsdotter, G., Bengtsson, S., Israelsson, M., & Borell, K. (2020). Child protection and cultural awareness: Simulation-based learning. *Journal of Ethnic & Cultural Diversity in Social Work, 29*(5), 362–376.

93. Strengthening families, protecting children (SFPC) programme. https://www.gov.uk/guidance/strengthening-families-protecting-children-sfpc-programme#history. Accessed at 26 December 2021.

94. Dingwall, R. (2013). The Rule of Optimism—Thirty Years On, Thousand Oaks, Social Science Space. http://www.socialsciencespace.com/2013/09/the-rule-of-optimism-thirty-years-on/#. Accessed 26 December 2021.

# 13 PERINATAL MENTAL HEALTH

PATRICIA BURROWS ▪ MARY MALONE ▪ SHARIN BALDWIN

## CHAPTER CONTENTS

INTRODUCTION

OVERVIEW OF PERINATAL MENTAL HEALTH DISORDERS

RISK FACTORS FOR PERINATAL MENTAL HEALTH DISORDERS

IDENTIFICATION OF PERINATAL MENTAL HEALTH DISORDERS

POST-ADOPTION DEPRESSION

IMPACT OF MATERNAL ANTENATAL MENTAL HEALTH DISORDERS

IMPACT OF MATERNAL POSTNATAL MENTAL HEALTH DISORDERS

IMPACT OF PATERNAL MENTAL HEALTH DISORDERS

FINANCIAL IMPLICATION OF PERINATAL MENTAL HEALTH DISORDERS

IMPACT OF COVID-19 ON MATERNAL AND PATERNAL MENTAL HEALTH

INTERVENTIONS TO SUPPORT WOMEN AND THEIR FAMILIES

CONCLUSION

## LEARNING OUTCOMES

*To:*

- describe perinatal mental health and its associated perinatal health conditions
- understand the prevalence of perinatal mental health and its contributing factors
- understand the role of the health visitors in the assessment and identification of mental health disorders in mothers and fathers
- understand how depression may affect parents following adoption
- understand the impact of maternal and paternal mental health on pregnancy and the growth and development of infants and children
- understand the effectiveness of interventions to support women and their families

## INTRODUCTION

This chapter provides an overview of perinatal mental health and includes discussions of the risk factors, signs and symptoms parents may display and the impact of perinatal mental health problems on the whole family. It highlights the important role that health visitors play in identifying parental mental health problems and supporting them during this crucial period. Evidence on interventions to support parental mental health and well-being and the challenges associated with the current Covid-19 context are presented.

Before perinatal mental health can be explored, it is important to define the term 'perinatal' and clarify the period it covers. According to the World

Health Organisation (WHO) the perinatal period commences at 22 weeks of pregnancy and ends 7 days after birth.[1] The Collins English Dictionary describes it as

*'the period from about three months before to one month after birth'.*[2]

NHS England on the other hand refers to perinatal mental health (PMH) problems as those which occur during pregnancy or in the first year following the birth of a child.[3] In this chapter perinatal mental health will be used as an umbrella term that encompasses mental health problems, psychological distress and psychological well-being, from conception to one year after birth. It can include pre-existing mental health conditions as well as the onset of new ones and will focus, not only on treating and preventing mental health problems, but also the promotion of psychological well-being.

## OVERVIEW OF PERINATAL MENTAL HEALTH DISORDERS

Mental health disorders affecting expectant or new parents in the perinatal period covers a wide range of conditions, including depression, anxiety, eating disorders, drug and alcohol use disorders as well as severe mental illnesses such as psychosis, bipolar disorder and schizophrenia.[4] The phenomenology and risk factors for mental disorders in the perinatal period are largely similar to those for the disorders at other times, but the treatment may vary for women during pregnancy and breastfeeding. Another important factor for focusing on mental health problems in the perinatal period is that it requires a more urgent and effective response due to the impact it can have on the woman, her partner and their baby.

A list of definitions for a range of perinatal mental health conditions are presented in Box 13.1.

Anxiety and depression are the most common perinatal mental health disorders in both women and men, and for that reason the vast majority of research to date has focused on these conditions.

There are wide variations in the reported prevalence rates of depression in the perinatal period. In a review of the prevalence of maternal postnatal depression across different countries and cultures, Arifin and colleagues[7] reported the rate to range from 4.0% to 63.9%. They included a total of 124 research papers from more than 50 countries and although there were wide variations in the screening instruments and diagnostic tools used, the Edinburgh Postnatal Depression Scale (EPDS) was the most common instrument. Studies from Japan reported the lowest rates of maternal postnatal depression in this review and America the highest.

In recent systematic review and meta-analysis of 58 papers (N = 37,294 women), the incidence of postnatal depression among healthy mothers without a prior history of depression was reported as 12%, while the overall prevalence of depression was 17%.[8] Prevalence was similar regardless of the type of diagnostic tool used; however, there were statistical differences in the prevalence between different geographical regions, with the Middle East having the highest prevalence (26%) and Europe the lowest (8%).

While the widely cited prevalence rate for maternal postnatal depression is 10% to 15%, data from various studies suggest that depression during pregnancy may affect up to 20% of women[9] and 10% to 22% in the postnatal period.[10–13]

Similarly, there are wide variations in the reported prevalence rates of depression in fathers in the perinatal period. In an integrative review of 20 studies Goodman[14] reported depression in fathers (both first-time and subsequent) to range from 1.2% to 25.5% in the first year following the birth of their baby. Using data from the Avon Longitudinal Study of Parents and Children (ALSPAC), a

## BOX 13.1
### PERINATAL MENTAL HEALTH DISORDERS

**Depression:** Persistent and pervasive low mood of varying severity and duration. It can affect men and women in the antenatal and postnatal period. Symptoms include on-going feelings of sadness, despair, difficulty dealing with daily life, constant tiredness, lack of energy, sleep disruption, self-blame, appetite disruption, impaired concentration, hopelessness, loss of motivation, self-neglect and suicidal ideation.

**Anxiety disorders:** Anxiety disorders, including panic disorder, generalised anxiety disorder (GAD), obsessive-compulsive disorder (OCD) and post-traumatic stress disorder (PTSD) can occur on their own or can co-exist with depression. Anxiety may include excessive worries about a number of life domains along with various physical symptoms. The main symptoms of general anxiety include feeling edgy/restless/jumpy, apprehensive, nervous, experiencing fatigue, sleep disturbances, difficulty concentrating/focusing on things and stomach problems (nausea, diarrhoea).

- **Obsessive compulsive disorder** is a type of anxiety and a mental health condition in which a person has obsessive thoughts and compulsive behaviours. Women are at higher risk of OCD during the perinatal period and symptoms are more prevalent after delivery. Obsessions are unwanted unpleasant ideas and thoughts that are persistent and repetitive in nature. They are often related to the baby and can cause deep feelings of anxiety, disgust and unease. Compulsions may include repetitive behaviour that temporarily relieves the unpleasant feelings brought on by the obsessive thought (e.g. those related to cleaning, washing and checking).
- **Post-traumatic stress disorder** is a type of anxiety that can occur for the first time, reoccur or worsen during the perinatal period (Howard et al 2014). Some women and their partners will experience PTSD as a direct result of a difficult labour or traumatic delivery. It is therefore important to give the woman and men suspected of depression the opportunity to recount the birthing experience to rule out this condition when screening for depression. Symptoms include anxiety, panic attacks, flashbacks, depressive symptoms and fear of sexual intimacy.
- **Eating disorders:** Eating disorders are a persistent disturbance of eating that significantly impairs health or psychosocial functioning. Classified by DSM-5 as four broad categories: (i) anorexia nervosa, (ii) bulimia nervosa, (iii) binge eating disorder, and (iv) other specified feeding or eating disorders (OSFED). Symptoms may include menstrual dysfunction, fertility problems, intense fear of weight gain, severe emotional distress.[5] Women with a history of an eating disorder may be at increased risk of perinatal depression.[6]

**Postnatal psychosis (puerperal psychosis):** This is a severe mental illness, with acute onset of symptoms, characterised by psychotic depression, mania or atypical psychosis. Symptoms include rapidly changing mood, bizarre behaviour, lack of inhibition, hallucinations (distortion of the five senses), delusions, confusion, agitation and lack of insight. Immediate assessment and treatment, usually with antipsychotic medication in an inpatient setting by specialist mental health services, are required for postnatal psychosis, and treatment by specialist mental health services are required for puerperal psychosis.

Adapted from Baldwin, S., Walker, M., & Parker, R. (2019). *Institute of Health Visiting Good Practice Points for Health Visitors: Understanding mothers' mental health & well-being during their transition to motherhood.* London: IHV. Reproduced with permission.

---

large UK longitudinal cohort study, which included 8431 fathers, Ramchandani et al[15] reported the presence of depressive symptoms in 4% of fathers at 8 weeks after birth. However, a later meta-analysis of 43 studies reported depression in 10.4% of fathers between the first trimester of their partner's pregnancy and one year postpartum, with the peak time of 3 to 6 months postnatally, a rate similar to findings for postnatal women.[16] The most recent updated meta-analysis of studies published from January 1980 to November 2015, with a total of 74 studies providing data on 41,480 participants, reported prevalence rates of paternal depression as 8.4% from pregnancy through the first postpartum year.[17]

Although there are varying rates of depression reported in men and women in the perinatal period, it is nonetheless an important public health issue that health visitors need to focus on in order to provide the right level of support to parents and their children.

Anxiety disorders cover a range of conditions, including panic disorder, generalised anxiety disorder (GAD), obsessive-compulsive disorder (OCD) and post-traumatic stress disorder (PTSD). While they can occur on their own they often co-exist with depression. The prevalence rate of GAD in women is 8.5% to 0.5% during pregnancy and 4.4% to 10.8% postpartum (Misri et al 2015)[156], whereas for men it ranges between 4.1% to 16.0% during their partner's pregnancy and 2.4% to 18.0% during the 6- to 8-week postnatal period.[18] Women with a history of an eating disorder may be at increased risk of perinatal depression.[6] There is also a higher risk of OCD in pregnant and postnatal women than in nonpregnant women, while tokophobia is a type of anxiety disorder that relates to the pathological fear of childbirth, affecting 6% to 10% of pregnant women.[19] Complications of pregnancy and birth can be traumatic and lead to PTSD or other mental health problems in both women and men.

Other severe mental health illnesses, relating to women in the perinatal period, include bipolar disorders and psychosis.[20] Bipolar disorder is commonly known as manic depression. Although this may be a pre-existing condition in some women, childbirth can often trigger it or make it worse. Bipolar disorder is characterised by severe 'highs' (where the individual may display increased energy levels and the inability to relax) and severe 'lows' (feelings of low mood, sadness, despair and lack of motivation). Some symptoms of bipolar disorder may present as being similar to those of psychosis,[25]. Postpartum psychosis is a severe mental illness, that affects one to two in 1000 mothers. The onset is rapid, usually 3 days after birth, but it can take several weeks for it to be detected in some cases. While 50% of women who experience postnatal psychosis have no history of mental health problems, women with bipolar disorder are at increased risk of experiencing postnatal psychosis. The rate of postpartum psychosis is almost double in women who have bipolar disorder and a family history of postpartum psychosis, compared to that of women with bipolar without a family history of postpartum psychosis. There is currently limited knowledge on bipolar disorders and psychosis relating to men's perinatal mental health, therefore these are areas that would benefit from more research.

### A poem about antenatal depression

*I'm so tired*
*I feel like s\*\*t*
*My head's sore*
*I have loads of zits!*
*With trembling hands*
*I comb my hair*
*Comes out in lumps*
*But I don't care!*
*My diet's rubbish*
*My weight goes up and down*
*I've lost my appetite*
*My face is a permanent frown.*
*My stomach is churning*
*My heart beats so fast*
*My skin looks awful*
*How long will it last?*

*Written by Health visitors in London North West Healthcare Trust during their Perinatal Mental Health training session.*

In general, the postnatal period has historically been the focus of far greater research attention than the antenatal period, despite the fact that some studies have shown a decrease, rather than an increase, in depression and anxiety after childbirth.[21] A review by Norhayati et al[22] reported that antenatal depression and anxiety are significant risk factors for postnatal depression in both developed and developing countries. This highlights the importance of assessing parental mental health in the antenatal period so that the right support and interventions can be put in place to prevent or minimise the impact in the postnatal period.

## RISK FACTORS FOR PERINATAL MENTAL HEALTH DISORDERS

Many personal, biological, psychological, social and family issues may act as predisposing factors for perinatal mental health disorders. These include poverty, migration, extreme stress, exposure to violence (domestic, sexual and gender-based), emergency and conflict situations, natural disasters, trauma and low social support.[23] Pearlstein and colleagues[11] reported risk factors for postnatal depression in women to include a history of mental health problems, childhood abuse and neglect, domestic violence, interpersonal conflict, inadequate social support, alcohol or drug abuse, unplanned or unwanted pregnancy, and migration status. Whereas a family or personal history of bipolar disorder is reported to significantly increase the risk of developing postpartum psychosis.[24,25]

Many risk factors for anxiety and depression in men during the perinatal period are similar to those of women, such as unsupportive marital relationship, unplanned pregnancy[26–28]; history of depression, higher social deprivation; poor social and emotional support (Castle et al 2008),[163] having a partner with elevated depressive symptoms or depression, and poor relationship satisfaction.[30] In addition to this, young parental age, paternal unemployment, having a partner in a more prestigious occupation and low parental self-efficacy have also been reported to contribute to poor mental health in fathers.[31] Maternal depression is, however, the strongest predictor of paternal depression during the postpartum period.[14,30,32] Bereavement by miscarriage, stillbirth or neonatal death can lead to mental health problems in both parents.[33]

## IDENTIFICATION OF PERINATAL MENTAL HEALTH DISORDERS

As health visitors in the UK have the most extended period of contact with families, from pregnancy up to 5 years post birth, they are in an ideal position to assess parents' mental health and identify any risk of perinatal mental health disorders. The Healthy Child Programme (HCP) for England, which was originally published in 2009[34] and reviewed and updated in 2015[35] and 2021,[162] recognised the importance of this early intervention and the need for health professionals to work effectively with parents to ensure that their children have the best start in life.

In England, the routine five contacts undertaken by health visitors provide an opportunity to support new parents in their transition to parenthood, promote child development, improve child health outcomes and ensure that families at risk are identified at the earliest opportunity.[36] The first three of the five contacts are ideal for carrying out comprehensive and holistic assessments of the expectant/new mothers' and fathers' needs. The Department of Health for England stated that the 6- to 8-week health visitor visit 'is crucial for assessing the baby's growth and well-being alongside the health of the parent, particularly looking for signs of postnatal depression. It is a key time for discussing key public health messages, including breastfeeding, dental health, healthy start vitamins, immunisations, sensitive parenting and for supporting parents on specific issues such as sleep'.[37:17] The importance of assessing parental mental health during the perinatal period is also reflected in the Universal Health Visiting Pathway in Scotland.[38] This highlights opportunities to assess parental mental health throughout five of the eight home visits offered to all families between pregnancy and the first year after birth. Similarly, health visitor contacts in the antenatal period, and postnatally at 1 to 6 weeks and 6 months are emphasised as key time-points for assessing and supporting parental mental health in the Healthy Child Wales Programme,[39] and the Universal Child Health Promotion Programme in Northern Ireland.[40]

According to NICE,[4] the assessment and diagnosis of a suspected mental health problem in pregnancy and the postnatal period should include:

- History of any mental health problem, including in pregnancy or the postnatal period
- Physical well-being (including weight, smoking, nutrition and activity level) and history of any physical health problem
- Alcohol and drug misuse
- The woman's attitude towards the pregnancy, including denial of pregnancy
- The woman's experience of pregnancy and any problems experienced by her, the fetus or the baby
- The mother–baby relationship
- Any past or present treatment for a mental health problem, and response to any treatment
- Social networks and quality of interpersonal relationships
- Living conditions and social isolation
- Family history (first-degree relative) of mental health problems
- Domestic violence and abuse, sexual abuse, trauma or childhood maltreatment
- Housing, employment, economic and immigration status
- Responsibilities as a carer for other children and young people or other adults

For the most common perinatal mental illnesses, anxiety and depression, NICE[4] advocates the use of the Depression Identification Questions (previously referred to as the Whooley Questions) for depression, and the Generalised Anxiety Disorder 2-item (GAD-2) screening tool for GAD in women. It is important that when asking these questions, health visitors use their clinical skills such as observation, listening, paraphrasing and professional judgement to determine if the mother is at risk. Further assessment using an assessment tool such as the EPDS or Patient Health Questionnaire 9 (PHQ9) can then be used to support the findings. While the tool choice may vary and will be dependent on local organisational policies, the EPDS is the most commonly used depression identification tool by health visitors. This is because it was developed in primary care specifically for the use of health visitors with mothers. The EPDS is a self-report questionnaire consisting of 10 questions, widely recognised and used internationally, and its use is endorsed by NICE.[4] Moreover, it can be used in the antenatal and postnatal period and has also been validated for use with fathers,[41] another reason why it is cited as the tool of choice by health professional and researchers. It is also available and validated in 58 different languages, which may make it more acceptable to non-English speaking parents and to those from different cultural backgrounds.

The PHQ-9 is another self-report assessment tool used for depression and anxiety, which has been validated for use in primary care.[42] It is the nine-item depression scale of the patient health questionnaire. It is one of the most validated tools in mental health and can be a powerful tool to assist clinicians with diagnosing depression and monitoring treatment response.

It is important to remember that with any assessment tool it is possible to have false positive (suggests the presence of depression/anxiety, when in reality it is not present) and false negative (fails to suggest a presence of depression/anxiety, when in reality it is present) results. It is therefore essential that assessments and subsequent decisions are based on clinical assessment and judgement of the professional. Health visitors need to be trained in the use of recommended and validated assessment tools in order to carry out accurate assessments of mothers and fathers in the perinatal period.

## THINKING SPACE

- *Do you use any of these assessment tools with mothers and fathers?*
- *Were you aware that the Edinburgh Postnatal Depression Scale (EPDS) has been validated for use with fathers?*

*You can find out more from: Matthey, S., Barnett, B., Kavanagh. D. J., & Howie, P. J. (2001). Validation of the Edinburgh Postnatal Depression Scale for men, and comparison of item endorsement with their partners.* Journal of Affective Disorders, 64 (2–3), 175–184.

It is important for health visitors to be aware of the risk factors for perinatal mental health disorders, as well as the sign and symptoms, which may be different for men and women. For example, signs and symptoms for feelings of abandonment and powerlessness may be similarly reported in men and women who are depressed, whereas alcohol and substance abuse may more frequently manifest in men.[43] Another example relates to the different communication and coping styles between men and women. Men may be less likely to access health services, more reluctant to discuss their mental health symptoms or concerns due to wanting to put their partner's needs first, or even present with different mental health symptoms and needs (Baldwin et al 2018).[44-47,164] In their integrative review of paternal depression, Edward and colleagues[32] highlighted that men and women differed in their knowledge and beliefs about the symptoms and causes of postnatal depression. Many women perceived postnatal depression to be associated with the biological rather than psychosocial cause and therefore unique to women's pregnancy and birth. This could potentially exclude men in the consideration for depression by their partners, in the perinatal period. Using the same methods for assessing and managing men's and women's mental health needs may not be appropriate, given that there may be gender differences in the presentation of mental health problems. The different signs and symptoms displayed by men and women highlight some of the complexities around the mental health needs of parents during their transition to parenthood and emphasise the need for better understanding of these by health professionals.

To be able to effectively identify mental health problems, health visitors need to be aware of cultural issues relating to perinatal mental health. For example, it is common practice for many Asian women to live with their husband's family, which is often seen by health visitors as a source of additional support[48]; however, numerous studies have reported that this is often not the case. Increased difficulties, stress and conflict experienced by women living in extended family settings, especially where the mother-in-law is over intrusive and controlling, has been strongly linked to maternal depression and anxiety.[49-51]

It is also important to consider language difficulties associated with perinatal mental health. In many languages (such as Urdu, Thai and those spoken in Nigeria and Cambodia) there is no direct translation for the word 'depression'. Therefore, this word may be interpreted differently by parents speaking those languages. It is also important to use properly qualified interpreters for non-English speaking clients, rather than family members.[52] Having a good understanding of issues relating to stigma and mental health, and how this may influence parental help seeking behaviours is vital to the effective identification and management of perinatal mental health problems and the provision of culturally sensitive care.

## THINKING SPACE

- *Can you think of any societal or cultural factors preventing parents that you work with from discussing their mental health or seeking help in the perinatal period? How can you support these parents or enable them to get help?*
- *Do you offer information to parents in any languages other than English? Do you use interpreters to communicate with fathers who do not speak English?*

*Did you know that the Edinburgh Postnatal Depression Scale (EPDS) is available in 58 different languages? You can find out more from: Cox, J., Holden, J., & Henshaw, C. (2014). Perinatal mental health. The Edinburgh Postnatal Depression Scale (EPDS) Manual (2nd ed.). RCPsych Publications.*

*For more information on communication and cultural aspects relating to maternal mental health, please refer to the chapter 'Working with diverse communities' by Baldwin and Johnson in Luker et al.*[52]

Men's perinatal mental health has not been given the same level of priority as women's in the UK. Screening tools such as the EPDS, which is commonly used by health visitors in the UK, has been validated for use with men in the antenatal and postnatal period as mentioned earlier but NICE guidance[4:53] does not currently include fathers in the recommended routine assessment and management of perinatal mental health. Until recently NICE guidelines on antenatal and postnatal mental health[4] recommended routine assessment of women, but did not include any reference or recommendations for fathers or partners. In the updated guidelines published in 2018, it was acknowledged that

> *'the mental health needs of fathers/partners whose health and functioning will inevitably be affected by mental health problems in women, are also important and should be considered'.*[53:37]

This suggested that it is necessary for services to also consider the needs of fathers/partners, carers and other children in the family, with care also tailored to meet their needs, which could include the provision of specialist inpatient services, integration of specific mental health services and maternity services, and dedicated treatment programmes.[53] However, it fails to inform how these needs will be identified for fathers in the first place, with no recommendation for routine mental health assessment of fathers in the perinatal period.

A recent qualitative study of 21 first-time fathers in London reported that men wanted to be asked about their own mental health and well-being by health professionals and offered the same level of support as women.[152] Most fathers stated that they would be willing to speak to health professionals about their mental health and considered that it would be better to be given an opportunity to seek help, rather than dealing with it themselves. Interestingly, men stated that they would only feel able to disclose any mental health difficulties if they knew that the health professional assessment aimed to include their needs and not just those of their partner and baby.[152] This has implications for health visiting practice and the identification of perinatal mental health disorders in fathers. Health visitors therefore need to be adequately skilled to working with and identifying depressive symptoms in fathers as well as mothers and take more of a family/parent focused approach, rather than focusing primarily on the woman and child.

THINKING SPACE

- *Do you assess the mental health of expectant mothers and fathers at routine antenatal appointments?*
- *Do you assess fathers' mental health and well-being during all your contacts?*
- *Do you provide parents with any information about perinatal mental health?*

*iHV Tips on 'Understanding your mental health and emotional well-being during pregnancy and after the birth of your baby (mothers & fathers') are freely available from: /*

## POST-ADOPTION DEPRESSION

While this chapter has mainly focused on mental health disorders in the perinatal period, it is important to highlight that adoptive parents can also suffer symptoms of depression in the early placement period and at significant other times after an adoption, which is referred to as post-adoption depression.[54] Depression suffered by adoptive parents were previously not regarded as being the same as postnatal depression, which was thought to result from the hormonal changes relating to pregnancy and birth. Research studies however suggest comparable levels of depressive symptoms between adoptive and birth mothers, with no significant difference in the incidence of depression between the two groups.[55,56] Post-adoption depression can affect mothers as well as fathers, and therefore can also affect same-sex couples. It is important to be mindful that the likely cause of depression following adoption is the stress rather than the adoption itself.[56] Symptoms include depressed mood, decreased interest or pleasure in tasks, significant weight gain, difficulty sleeping and excessive sleeping, feeling agitated, fatigue, excessive guilt and shame, and indecisiveness.[57] Adoptive parents may experience increased levels of stresses that are unique to the adoption process, in addition to the stressors associated with changes to lifestyle, relationships, sleep deprivation and financial pressures that biological parents may experience. These include unexpected expectations of the new role, feelings of grief and loss regarding own fertility, feeling of guilt for the birth parents, high/unrealistic expectations of the child, gaps in knowledge about the child's background, parenting a traumatised child, difficulty in forming an attachment with the child, and acceptance by family, friends and society. Health visitors can play an important role in supporting adoptive parents by being proactive and getting involved in the pre-adoption period, where possible.

Assessing mental health (using the same methods as biological parents), providing reassurance post-placement, supporting them with attachment issues and connecting them with other community/support networks are all important steps in addressing the mental health needs and promoting mental well-being of adoptive parents.

THINKING SPACE

- *Do you assess the mental health needs of adoptive parents?*
- *Do you know where you can find more information to support adoptive parents? You can find more information on PAD here: /*

## IMPACT OF MATERNAL ANTENATAL MENTAL HEALTH DISORDERS

There is a plethora of literature that reveal the negative impact of antenatal depression and anxiety on the developing fetus and child.[58–60] Stein et al,[61] in their review of the evidence on the association of depression and anxiety and the impact on the fetus and the child, report that antenatal depression is associated with increased risk of premature delivery and low birthweight, this risk being reported as higher in lower-income countries. This is similarly echoed by Dadi et al (2020) in a systematic review of reviews examining antenatal depression and adverse birth outcomes that confirms antenatal depression increases the risk of preterm birth and low birth weight. Antenatal depression is not however associated with pre-eclampsia, Apgar scores or admission to neonatal intensive units.[61]

It is well established that antenatal depression is associated with an increased risk for child emotional and behavioural problems.[62–64] O'Connor et al[65] in the ALSPAC study demonstrated a significant association between antenatal anxiety and children's behavioural problems at age 4 years, specifically hyperactivity and inattention in boys and behavioural problems in both boys and girls. Noteworthy in this study is that the association between antenatal anxiety and behavioural and emotional development was independent of antenatal, obstetric and socio-demographic factors. Stein et al[61] additionally support this reporting from their review the association between antenatal depression and behavioural difficulties in children including attention deficit hyperactivity disorder, oppositional defiant disorder and conduct disorder.

Some explanations are put forward in the literature to explain the mechanisms central to the association between antenatal depression and anxiety on child growth and development.[61] Glover et al[66] explain that stress experienced by the mother directly affects the development of the hypothalamic pituitary adrenal (HPA) axis in the fetus.[67,68] This can result in stimulation of high cortisol production and release that can restrict flow of nutrients and oxygen to the fetus resulting in poor growth.[66,69,70] It has been proposed that antenatal depression may also affect the maternal immune system function via glucocorticoid hormone imbalance that may increase susceptibility to various microbial infections.[71,72] Dadi et al[153] in their review conclude that depressed mothers may be more likely to smoke and drink while being less likely to attend medical care and have poor appetite all of which can lead to malnourishment and impact on fetal development.

Weinstock[73] and Clarke et al[74] allude to animal studies that demonstrate maternal antenatal stress, resulting in behavioural disturbances in their offspring and providing evidence that antenatal stress leads to maladaptive cognitive and behavioural changes in rodent offspring. However, such findings are uncertain in human beings between antenatal depression or anxiety indicating that it is a more complex mechanism.[66] O'Connor et al[65] suggest in the findings from their longitudinal study that the correlation between antenatal anxiety and behavioural and emotional problems in boys and girls at 4 years of age is consistent with the notion that early life experiences can influence how an individual responds to later experiences.

Pearson et al[75] use the term maternal programming to explain that antenatal depression and anxiety may cause neurocognitive changes in the mother, resulting in reduced maternal responsiveness towards infants which therefore affects development of prenatal maternal–fetal bonding. McNamara et al[76] further suggest that the experience of mental health difficulties antenatally may impair a mother's ability to form a close bond with her unborn baby through lack of emotional resources, beliefs about poor suitability and competence as a parent, a lack of maternal role identity and negative attitudes towards caregiving.

Although there is an increased focus on the impact of a woman's psychological well-being during pregnancy and the development of prenatal maternal fetal bonding and maternal–fetal attachment (MFA), the impact of antenatal anxiety on maternal–fetal bonding is still not fully understood. It has been determined earlier in this chapter that the antenatal period can be associated with an increase in distress and anxiety.[77] The terms antenatal attachment and MFA are used interchangeably in the literature when exploring the impact of antenatal anxiety and depression on the relationship between the pregnant woman and her developing fetus.[153] Doan and Zimerman[78] ascertain that antenatal attachment represents a bond between a parent and a fetus characterised by the cognitive, emotional, and mental capacities needed to conceptualise another human being. Cranley[79] initially described MFA as the emotional bond between a mother and her unborn child during pregnancy. Subsequent authors have proposed and acknowledged that MFA and antenatal attachment signify the thoughts, behaviours, emotions and attitudes expectant mothers have in relation to their unborn baby and pregnancy.[79–82] It is proposed that such negative outcomes in childhood may be affected by the quality of the relationship between the pregnant woman and her developing baby with subsequent difficulty in postpartum bonding.[83–86]

Studies that have examined the impact of antenatal attachment report negative consequences on early childhood development. These include: behavioural and conduct difficulties, negative socioemotional regulations and cognitive development (Kingston & Tough, 2012).[87, 88] Cildir et al[88] investigated the association between antenatal attachment and child development, socioemotional behavioural problems, and competence in early childhood. Their study results demonstrate that antenatal attachment was shown to be even a stronger predictor of development than was worsening maternal depression in early childhood.

Rollè et al,[89] in their systematic review of 41 studies looking at the association between antenatal attachment and perinatal depression, report that antenatal depressive symptoms were found to be negatively associated with antenatal attachment. In addition, lower levels of antenatal attachment were related to higher postnatal depressive symptoms. McNamara et al[76] further sought to determine, in their systematic review, whether there was a relationship between maternal mental health and MFA and postpartum bonding. Findings confer that depression was associated with lower MFA and postpartum bonding in the majority of studies reviewed. McNamara and colleagues[76] conclude that these findings are supportive of the claim that maternal mood negatively impacts on a mother's ability to bond with her baby, both during pregnancy and in the early postpartum period. The authors from both studies do caution regarding interpretation of the findings as a number of the included studies varied in quality and scope.

## IMPACT OF MATERNAL POSTNATAL MENTAL HEALTH DISORDERS

The negative impact that postnatal depression can have on parenting and subsequent developmental outcomes in children is well documented.[61,90] This encompasses insecure attachment, emotional regulation, behavioural difficulties and poor cognitive development.[91–94]

The importance of attachment in a child's psychological, cognitive and social development is well established.[95,96] This is explored in depth in Chapter 14, Infant and Child Mental Health. The literature outlines that the symptoms of postnatal depression influence the mother's ability to respond to their environment, consequently affecting their parenting capabilities.[97] This, therefore, affects the mother's ability to respond sensitively to their infant, which can include a range of parenting patterns such as disengagement and withdrawal, missing of infant cues, poor responsiveness and intrusiveness during stressful situations and insufficient parental warmth.[76,92, 97–100] It has been reported that infants of depressed mothers at 9 months of age have lower social engagement, fewer mature regulatory behaviours and more negative emotionality, and higher cortisol reactivity.[101,102]

Barnes and Theule,[103] in a meta-analysis of 42 studies to determine the relationship between maternal depression and infant attachment security, report that there is a significant relationship between maternal depression and infant attachment. Infants of mothers with depression were nearly twice as likely to have a nonsecure attachment than were infants of healthy mothers. Śliwerski et al,[104] in their systematic review, investigated the influence of maternal depression on the relationship between mother and child, and on child attachment security, measured up to 24 months after birth. Their findings demonstrate that a history of major depressive disorders was found to affect child attachment style only when depression coexists with another mental disorder, or when it appears prior to the antenatal period.

Postnatal depression has been demonstrated to impact a range of cognitive learning outcomes in early childhood, achievement of developmental milestones and long-term academic achievement.[61,105–107] Impaired cognitive development is affected by the inability of the parent to focus attention on the infant's signals and provide adequate stimulation, supporting their engagement with their surrounding environment.[61,109] This in turn can contribute toward the infant's ability to control attention and effectively process information which is predictive of the intellectual capacity of the child.[61,92,108,109] The ALSPAC study (mentioned previously in this chapter) investigated the association between maternal and paternal depression and anxiety in the perinatal period, executive function at age eight, and academic achievement at the end of compulsory school at age 16.[109] The results demonstrate significant association between postnatal depression and academic achievement. Adolescents of postnatally depressed mothers were 1.5 times more likely than adolescents of nondepressed mothers to fail to achieve a 'pass' grade in maths.[109] Netsi et al[94] in their observational study of 9848 women with varying levels of postnatal depression and their children, found that children of women with persistent and severe depression were at an increased risk of behavioural problems by age 3.5 years, as well as lower mathematics grades and depression during adolescence.

It is clear from the evidence that factors such as low socioeconomic status, absence of social support (including partner support) and persistence of parental disorder increase the child's risk of an adverse outcome.[61,110] Conversely, when disorders occur in the absence of social adversity, and if they are of short duration, the risks to the child are generally low.[61] Children of mothers with higher socioeconomic status, education, or more optimal parenting behaviours have been found less likely to suffer from the adverse effects of maternal postnatal depression.[110] Nonetheless, despite adversity many children in such situations develop normally and remain healthy, showing resilience of parental care and child development.

## IMPACT OF PATERNAL MENTAL HEALTH DISORDERS

Research in recent years has started to focus on the implication of paternal mental health on children's development. These studies specifically look at the interaction and quality of the paternal-child interaction and the longer-term impact on child development.

Sethna et al[111] investigated the link between paternal depression and father–infant interactions at 3 months postpartum. The results demonstrate that paternal depression is associated with more withdrawn parental behaviour, with less verbal and behavioural stimulation during interactions with their young infants. McElwain and Volling[112] similarly report that depressed paternal mood was directly related to less intrusiveness for fathers in the free-play session with their 12-month-old. Davis et al[113] additionally report that depressed fathers (compared to nondepressed fathers) are less likely to engage in reading to their 1 year-old infants. Paulson et al[114] similarly report that paternal depressive symptoms result in decreased parent-to-child reading and relatively reduced child expressive language at age two.

This evidence of the impact of paternal depression on father–infant/child interaction does imply that such interactions may affect children's development.[115–119] Ramchandani et al[117] identified that disengaged interactions of fathers with their infants at 3 months postpartum predicted behavioural problems in children. In an earlier ALSPAC study by Ramchandani and colleagues[15] the presence of symptoms of severe self-reported postnatal depression in fathers (assessed using the EPDS) was associated with emotional and behavioural problems in their children at around 3 years of age, particularly in boys. Kvalevaag et al[116] similarly in their large Norwegian population study reported an association between symptoms of paternal antenatal depression and poor socioemotional and behavioural development of children at age 36 months.

Ramchandani et al[155] further report an increased risk of psychiatric, behavioural, and conduct disorders in children aged 7 years if their fathers had been depressed in the antenatal and postnatal periods. More recently, Gutierrez-Galve et al[120] using the ALSPAC data of over 3000 families in Bristol, identified a link between postnatal depression in men, as assessed using the EPDS, and an increased risk of depression in their teenage daughters at age 18.

## THINKING SPACE

- *What is your experience of the impact of maternal and paternal perinatal mental health disorders on the infant and family?*
- *Is this different for mothers and fathers?*

## FINANCIAL IMPLICATION OF PERINATAL MENTAL HEALTH DISORDERS

The maternal Mental Health Alliance commissioned an independent report on the economic and social impact of maternal mental health problems in the perinatal period including during pregnancy and the first year after childbirth for the UK.[121] The report demonstrates that the cost of perinatal mental health problems is exceptionally high, carrying a total long-term cost to society of up to £8.1 billion for each 1 year cohort of births in the UK.[121] The significance of this cost is further illustrated where a single case of perinatal depression is estimated at around £74,000. Nearly three-quarters (£51,000) of this cost relates to adverse impacts on the child rather than the mother (£23,000).

While the total cost of paternal perinatal mental health problems is currently unknown, it is likely to be considerable. In a UK study of 192 fathers recruited from two postnatal wards in southern England, Edoka and colleagues[122] estimated healthcare costs of paternal depression in the postnatal period, using data collection on self-reported resource use over the first postnatal year. Three groups of fathers were identified: fathers with depression (n = 31), fathers at high risk of developing depression (n = 67) and fathers without depression (n = 94). Mean father–child dyad costs were calculated based on health service resource-use by the father and child, as reported by the fathers, and was estimated at £1103.51, £1075.06 and £945.03 (2008 prices) in these three groups. After controlling for potential confounding factors, including father's age, academic qualifications, ethnicity, employment status, whether the father had other children, child's gender, child's birth weight and a diagnosis of postnatal depression in the child's mother, paternal depression was associated with significantly higher community care costs (mean cost difference of £132), mainly due to increased contacts with general practitioners (GPs) and psychologists between those with and without depression. While this study only estimated costs from a healthcare system perspective and did not consider other sectors of the economy, it nevertheless provides useful preliminary insights into the healthcare costs associated with paternal depression during the postnatal period.

## IMPACT OF COVID-19 ON MATERNAL AND PATERNAL MENTAL HEALTH

It is important to consider the impact of the Covid-19 pandemic on the mental health of mothers and their partners. Best Beginnings, Home Start and the Parent–Infant Foundation[126] reveal key findings from a joint online Covid-19 survey (Babies in Lockdown). The Babies in Lockdown report captures the experiences from a diverse group of expectant and new parents during the critical first months and years of their babies' development. More than half of the parents (61%) shared significant concerns about their mental health with a quarter (24%) of pregnant respondents citing mental health as a main concern said they would like help with this, rising to almost a third (32%) of those with a baby. Two-thirds (68%) of parents said their ability to cope with their pregnancy or baby had been impacted by Covid-19.

It has been suggested that there may be some quite serious long-term effects on the mental health of wider populations, with consequences of the lockdown involving symptoms similar to PTSD.[123] Saccone et al,[124] in their cross-sectional study of 100 pregnant women from Italy, found a moderate-to-severe psychological impact of the Covid-19 pandemic and highlighted the need for intervention to improve the mental health of this population. Davenport et al.[125] aimed to assess the influence of the Covid-19 pandemic and subsequent physical distancing/isolation measures on the mental health and physical activity of pregnant and postpartum women. The survey identified a substantial increase in the likelihood of maternal depression and anxiety during the Covid-19 pandemic with the number of women experiencing moderate to high anxiety symptoms increasing from 29% to 72%. The following findings from the 'Babies in Lockdown' survey[126] illustrate the enormous negative impact that Covid-19 has had on parents:

- Over half of parents (68%) reported that they found their ability to cope with their pregnancy or baby had been impacted as a result of Covid-19.
- Over half (68%) of the parents felt the changes brought about by Covid-19 were affecting their unborn baby, baby or young child.
- A third (34%) of respondents believed that their baby's interaction with them had changed during the lockdown period.
- A quarter (25%) of parents reported concern about their relationship with their baby, and one-third (35%) of these wanted to get help with this.

Conti and Dow,[127] in their survey investigating the impact of Covid-19 on the health visiting services in England, report that in some areas of England at least half of skilled health visitors were redeployed. This also included the redeployment of some health visitors from perinatal mental health and parent–infant teams into other health services in the initial period of the lockdown, therefore affecting the provision of services for pregnant women and their partners.

A combination of factors resulting from Covid-19 appear to directly affect maternal and paternal mental health. These include worry about infection, direct effects of the virus on the fetus or on an infant, visitor restrictions, social isolation, financial strain.[128] The number of calls to the UK national domestic abuse helpline for reported cases of domestic violence increased by 25%.[129] Symptoms of perinatal depression, anxiety, and PTSD are significantly associated with having experienced domestic violence.[130] In addition, the impact of no visitors in the postpartum period, or of no partner being permitted during Caesarean sections during Covid-19, may be anxiety-provoking for some with reduced social support in the postpartum period.[128,131]

## THINKING SPACE

■ *Consider the provision of health visitor services during Covid-19 and how this has impacted the emotional well-being of pregnant women and their partners.*

## INTERVENTIONS TO SUPPORT WOMEN AND THEIR FAMILIES

Just as perinatal mental health problems range from severe, for example perinatal psychosis and bipolar disorder, to less severe, for example mild to moderate depression and anxiety disorder, so too do the therapeutic interventions available. Identifying appropriate and effective interventions to help women with all forms of perinatal mental health problems is important because, as the previous section shows, the consequences of poor mental health are considerable. This section identifies the range of interventions available starting with those which are essential for women with more severe perinatal mental health conditions.

Severe psychiatric disorder is a major cause of maternal morbidity (UK Confidential Enquiry into Maternal Deaths, CEMD)[132] and all forms of disorder carry consequences for the mother, the infant and the whole family. Women with severe mental health disorders will often have experienced mental ill health before pregnancy and risks of recurrence are high. Assessment of mental and psychological well-being should be offered to all women at the antenatal contact but it is especially important for women who have been unwell in the past. As well as assessment at the antenatal contact, the new birth contact is also an important assessment point and should include a discussion of the mother's birth experience and the mother's views on her relationship with her new baby. Assessment should be followed by development of a comprehensive plan. Oates et al draws attention to health care professionals' tendency to underestimate the risk of recurrent mental ill health for all women and especially those from affluent and well-educated backgrounds and she highlights the risks this poses for perinatal mental health.[159]

## THINKING SPACE

■ *What are the most important learning points here?*

*Health professionals (midwives, health visitors, GPS and obstetricians) need to be confident in the importance of early contact and assessment of women in the antenatal period. For those women who have experienced mental ill health in the past the risk of recurrence is high. Health professionals need to be able to assess accurately in early pregnancy and communicate in an open and transparent manner with women and with each other about the risks of recurrence.*

Medication is the most usual intervention for women with severe mental health disorder with tricyclic or selective serotonin reuptake inhibitors (SSRIs) being the drugs of choice. Thompson and Thomson[133] found that tricyclic and other related antidepressants reduced anxiety and improved sleep in women with postnatal depression; Hollyman et al found that Amitryptaline, a tricyclic antidepressant, was an effective treatment for major depression in perinatal women.[157] The possibility of neonatal withdrawal or of infant serotonin overdose for the infants of mothers taking SSRIs in the third trimester of their pregnancy have been investigated with no evidence found to support this or of foetal abnormalities.[134,158]

Women may also be worried about the effects of medication on breastfeeding. Wisner et al[135] found that there were some adverse effects on the infants of women taking either Doxepin or Fluoxetine during breastfeeding, but they found no adverse effects on the infants of women taking other antidepressants. In breastfeeding infants over 10 weeks there was no evidence of accumulating drug serum levels.[135]

Hanley[158] points out that women may be reluctant to take medication in the perinatal period. Health professionals need to help the woman balance the benefits of taking medication against the possible consequences of not doing so. Intense feelings of depression, anxiety and low mood can, if they remain untreated, lead to lack of self-esteem, poor personal care, dietary deficiency, self-medication with alcohol or illicit drugs, and even self-harm. Helping women make the right decision for themselves and their families through articulating the risks and benefits of different decision pathways is an important part of perinatal health care and one which requires both knowledge of the alternative interventions and their potential consequences, and excellent communication skills from the practitioner.

### Case study 13.1

Mary is a 32-year-old woman who has just had her second baby. Mary meets her health visitor for a virtual new birth visit. She tells the health visitor that she did feel rather low after the birth of her first baby, Teddy, who is now 2 years old. Mary said she took medication at that time but she was worried all the time that it wasn't the right thing

to do. She felt she had failed because she needed medication and she was worried all the time that the medication might have an effect on the baby whom she breastfed. Now, with the new baby, Phoebe, Mary feels low again. Living at the time of the virus has made her feel worse she feels. Mary is constantly worried for the baby, for herself and has feelings of impending doom. She doesn't want to take medication again but she feels worse every day and she's noticed that she is crying a lot, sleeping very little and doesn't want to talk with her partner, Ed, whom she knows is worried that she is getting poorly again.

**What should the health visitor do?**

Assess Mary's mental, psychosocial and physical health by listening to Mary and observing Mary, her children and what she can see of their physical environment. Review Mary's records to assess the severity of her previous ill health. The health visitor should help Mary to consider the different options open to her by offering information on medication and on other therapies and interventions described below. The health visitor can also help Mary to understand the possible implications of choosing to take medication or choosing not to do so. The health visitor should suggest that Mary makes an appointment to see her GP and the health visitor should see Mary and her family for a face-to-face contact and re-assessment within 2 weeks of this contact.

Women with severe mental health disorders have also been shown to benefit from interventions combining medication and person-centred therapies. In their Cochrane Review, Bledsoe and Grote[136] undertook a meta-analysis of the available literature and identified large effect sizes when medication is combined with cognitive behavioural therapy (CBT) and interpersonal therapy (IPT). Evidence of effectiveness for medication alone in women with mild depression is less robust.[137,138]

In CBT[165] a therapist helps a woman identify symptoms she may be experiencing – such as panic, anxiety, low self-esteem and lack of confidence – and to challenge the meaning of these in her understanding of her situation. Appleby et al[139] found that CBT delivered by UK Health Visitors, focusing on maternal thoughts on childcare, engaging with others and accessing help from others, could be as effective as medication for women with major postnatal depression. Danger of relapse at the end of the 6-week treatment period treatment was the major worry for these women.

The best-known person-centred intervention in the UK is based upon the Rogerian concepts of unconditional positive regard and the development of positive self-regard[140] and takes the form of 'listening visits'. The relationship between mother and counsellor is the basis of this intervention as each share thoughts and perceptions on what the mother is experiencing. No advice is given but the counsellor helps the mother to explore the option open to her. Listening visits usually last for about an hour, are offered in sets of four or six sessions and take place within the woman's own home. Evidence suggests that their success depends on the health visitor's training in delivery of the therapeutic approach and on the availability of a referral pathway for those women who do not respond, or who need more than the allocated amount of contact.[141]

Shakespeare et al[141] and Slade et al[142] found that the relationship between the mother and the counsellor, both before and during the intervention, was pivotal to its success and determined the extent to which women accessed it. They also found that, when there was a good relationship with the health visitor, women enjoyed the visits but attributed their recovery to other interventions. Morrell et al[143] found that interventions led by health visitors trained in either CBT or other person-centred approaches, such as unconditional positive regard and listening visits, brought maternal benefit over usual care at both 6 and 12 months post intervention.

IPT is a form of time-limited psychotherapy focusing on the four areas of grief, interpersonal disputes, role transitions and interpersonal deficits and has been adopted for use in both the antenatal and postnatal periods. Spinelli et al[144] in an RCT identified that IPT in combination with a parenting education programme was equally effective in a three-centre bi-lingual trial (English and Spanish) of white, African, American and Hispanic women. Sockol et al[159] in a meta-analysis of 27 studies found that interventions including IPT were more effective than usual care and interventions with a CBT component.

Delivering interpersonal interventions within groups has also attracted attention for the positive effects it can offer. As Hanley (2009) points out, gathering women together in groups musters peer support and generates cohesiveness. Some women, however, may find groups difficult and have problems which they feel need individual attention. Group interventions take numerous forms, each of which has different foci and may work better for different women and their families. Scope et al (2013)[166] reviewed seven studies comparing group CBT to usual care and found evidence of effectiveness, albeit small, and diminishing over time. Honey et al[160] found psychoeducational groups work to be more effective than normal primary care in intervening with post-natal women experiencing mental distress, and in Australia Morgan[145] found that a group for postnatal women and their partners, which offered an intervention drawing on psychotherapeutic and CBT models, increased both women and men's self-esteem and decreased their levels of distress.

## THINKING SPACE

*On reflection, what are the main messages from the evidence on effectiveness of person-centred therapies as interventions to improve the mental well-being of women in the perinatal period?*

Answers:
- *They focus on the psychosocial context of the woman's whole experience*
- *They focus on the woman talking and others listening to the woman as she does so*
- *They promote egalitarian and therapeutic relationships rather than hierarchical and advice-giving and -receiving relationships*
- *They are based on trust and mutual positive regard*
- *They can be used and they work well when used with other interventions and they need to be part of an assessment and referral framework in order to have the most effect.*

As well as the interventions identified above by Hanley (2009)[158] there are also a number of other activities for which there is a more limited evidence base but which may enhance maternal well-being in the perinatal period. Baby massage helps to promote maternal and infant interactions and to promote feelings of maternal closeness to the new baby[146] and are viewed as fostering better interactions between the mother–infant dyad. Fujita et al[147] found that baby massage helped to improve maternal mood. Oren et al[148] found that 'light therapy' – exposing pregnant women to a bright light (10,000 lux) for 60 minutes during the first ten minutes of wakening over a 3- to 5-week period – could be effective. However, they failed to identify the optimum treatment duration and so need to do further investigation. In a similar way, the effectiveness alone as a treatment for perinatal mental health problems is supported by a sparse literature; however, Manber et al[149] argue that it may be effective when combined with other conventional treatments. Armstrong and Edwards[150] found that pram-walking mothers had better mental health and improved fitness levels when compared with a non-pram-walking comparison group.

In recent years there has been an increase in mindfulness-based interventions to improve mental health and well-being. Mindfulness works on the principle that becoming more aware of the present moment can help us enjoy the world around us more and understand ourselves better. A systematic review of 17 studies of mindfulness-based interventions in the perinatal period reported significant reductions in depression, anxiety and stress, and significant increases in mindfulness skills post-intervention, each with small- to medium-sized effects; qualitative data suggests that participants viewed mindfulness interventions positively.[151] While there is insufficient evidence from high quality research on which to base recommendations about the effectiveness of mindfulness to promote perinatal mental health, mindfulness is recommended by the National Institute for Health and Care Excellence (NICE) as a way to prevent depression in people who have had three or more bouts of depression in the past.[167] Therefore, it would be useful for health visitors to be aware of mindfulness-based interventions that parents could access in their local communities or via online platforms. For more information visit https://www.nhs.uk/conditions/stress-anxiety-depression/mindfulness/.

### Case study 13.2

Helen is a health visitor working during Covid. Helen knows that many of the perinatal families on her caseload are experiencing low mood which is being made worse by the crisis. In the past Helen has used groups as a way of fostering cohesiveness and helping families make friendships which affirm their parenting skills and help to improve mood. Helen is in virtual contact with the families.

**What can Helen do in the current situation?**

Helen can run online baby massage classes; for parents this will help to enhance mood and support positive connections with the new baby and for

Helen it will also offer the opportunity to engage with families frequently for assessment of health needs and intervention where necessary. Helen can also encourage families to organise themselves into pram-walking groups, which can meet in a safe socially distanced manner out of doors and get the benefit of social contact, affirming conversations and connections with other families. In this way the proven benefits for perinatal mental health of talking, listening, connecting and affirming each other as parents can be achieved safely.

In summary, there are numerous and different interventions available to support good mental health in the perinatal environment. Identifying the level of need and the wishes of the family are essential to identifying the right intervention for the family and all depend for success on assessment and re-assessment of current and previous mental health and well-being and a supportive network for referral and support to facilitate the most appropriate intervention for the individual family.

## THINKING SPACE

- *Do you have any policies/guidelines in your organisation that address the needs of fathers/ adoptive parents?*
- *Do you have any information resources designed for fathers or that are written to meet the needs of both parents?*
  *If not, is this something you could develop within your team/service?*

Working with parents with mental health disorders can be challenging and it is important for health visitors to ensure that they look after their own mental health and well-being. Building compassionate resilience can help with this, which allows individuals to cope positively with adversity.[168] Self-compassion is a key to resilience and learning how to maintain this resilience even in

challenging situations can help maintain personal positive mental well-being. Health professionals who are compassionate, encourage greater disclosure by patients about their concerns, symptoms and behaviour, and are ultimately more effective at delivering care (Larson & Yao)[161]. Refer to Chapter 3, Professional practice and practitioner well-being.

## THINKING SPACE

- *What steps do you take to maintain your own mental well-being?*
- *Have you heard of mindfulness? Do you incorporate mindfulness in your everyday practice?*
  *You may find these resources helpful: https:// www.nhs.uk/conditions/stress-anxiety-depression/ mindfulness/*
  *https://www.nhs.uk/conditions/stress-anxiety-depression/*

## CONCLUSION

This chapter has provided an overview of perinatal mental health disorders that encompass mental health problems, psychological distress and psychological well-being from conception to 1 year after birth. The prevalence, predisposing factors and impact of maternal and paternal perinatal mental health disorders have been described. The role of the health visitor in the assessment and identification of women and their partners at risk of developing perinatal mental health disorders is at the centre of universal health visiting service provision across the four nations of the UK. There are numerous and different interventions available to support the range of perinatal disorders that requires the health visitor to have the knowledge and skills to ascertain the level of need and wishes of the family so that the most appropriate referral, support and intervention is identified for the woman, her partner and family.

## KEY LEARNING POINTS

- Mental health disorders affecting expectant or new parents in the perinatal period covers a wide range of conditions, including depression, anxiety, eating disorders, drug and alcohol use disorders as well as severe mental illnesses such as psychosis, bipolar disorder and schizophrenia.
- There are wide variations in the reported prevalence rates of maternal depression in the perinatal period. The prevalence of maternal postnatal depression across different countries and cultures can range from 4.0% to 63.9%.
- The prevalence rates of depression in fathers in the perinatal period varies from 1.2% to 25.5% in the first year following the birth of their baby.
- A wide range of factors predispose towards the development of perinatal mental health disorders and include: personal, biological, psychological, social and family issues.
- Maternal and paternal mental health disorders have a negative impact on parenting and subsequent developmental outcomes in children. This encompasses insecure attachment, emotional regulation, behavioural difficulties and poor cognitive development.
- Health visitors within the UK are in a unique position to assess parents' mental health and identify any risk of perinatal mental health disorders.
- The range of assessment tools that can be used by the health visitor include:
  - Depression Identification Questions (Whooley questions) for depression
  - Generalised Anxiety Disorder 2-item (GAD-2) screening tool for generalised anxiety disorders
  - Edinburgh Postnatal Depression Scale (EPDS) or Patient Health Questionnaire 9 (PHQ9)
- It is essential that health visitors use their clinical skills, such as observation, listening, paraphrasing and professional judgement, to determine if the mother is at risk of developing a perinatal mental health disorder.
- Identifying appropriate and effective interventions to help women with all forms of perinatal mental health disorders is important. The range of therapeutic interventions will depend on the severity of the perinatal mental health disorder.

## FURTHER RESOURCES

Action on Postpartum Psychosis (APP). www.app-network.org/.

Baldwin, S., & Kelly, T. (2014). *A guide to postnatal depression in fathers (wheel)*. UK: KMMD. http://www.development-wheels.com/PND.htm.

iHV. *Good practice points for health visitors*. https://ihv.org.uk/for-health-visitors/resources/good-practice-points/.
Working with birth trauma
Understanding fathers' mental health & well-being
Understanding mothers' mental health & well-being
Postnatal psychosis
Traumatic events – Supporting families

Maternal Mental Health Alliance. www.maternalmentalhealthalliance.org/.

Mind. www.mind.org.uk/.

NCT: www.nct.org.uk/.

NHS. www.nhs.uk/.

PANDAS. Pre and postnatal depression advice and support. www.pandasfoundation.org.uk/.

*Post-adoption depression factsheet*. https://www.nhs.uk/Livewell/adoption-and-fostering/Documents/Adoption%20UK%20Factsheet%2014%20-%20Post-adoption%20depression%20June%202013.pdf.

RCGP. *Perinatal mental health toolkit*. https://www.rcgp.org.uk/clinical-and-research/resources/toolkits/perinatal-mental-health-toolkit.aspx.

The Fatherhood Institute. *Ten top tips for attracting fathers to programmes*. http://www.fatherhoodinstitute.org/wp-content/uploads/2014/11/Ten-top-tips-for-attracting-fathers-to-programmes.pdf.

*The perinatal mental health care pathways*. https://www.england.nhs.uk/publication/the-perinatal-mental-health-care-pathways/

Tommy's. *Pregnancy and post-birth well-being plan.* https://www.tommys.org/pregnancy-information/calculators-tools-resources/wellbeing-plan/pregnancy-and-post-birth-wellbeing-plan

## REFERENCES

1. WHO (1992). World Health Organisation. ICD-10: International statistical classification of diseases and health related problems. Geneva: WHO.
2. Collins English Dictionary. Copyright © HarperCollins Publishers. https://www.collinsdictionary.com/dictionary/english/perinatal.
3. NHS England. (2020). *Perinatal mental health.* https://www.england.nhs.uk/mental-health/perinatal/ Accessed 25 October 2020.
4. National Institute for Health and Care Excellence. (NICE). (2014). *Clinical guideline [CG192]: Antenatal and postnatal mental health: Clinical management and service guidance.* (Updated 2015). https://www.nice.org.uk/guidance/cg192. Accessed January 2020.
5. Bye, A., Walker, M., Mackintosh, N., Sandall, J., & Easter, A. (2018). Supporting women with eating disorders during pregnancy and the postnatal period. *Journal of Health Visiting, 6*(5), 224–228.
6. Bulik, C. M., Von Holle, A., Siega-Riz, A. M., et al. (2009). Birth outcomes in women with eating disorders in the Norwegian Mother and Child cohort study (MoBa). *International Journal of Eating Disorders, 42*(1), 9–18. doi:10.1002/eat.2057.
7. Arifin, S. R. M., Cheyne, H., & Maxwell, M. (2018). Review of the prevalence of postnatal depression across cultures. *AIMS Public Health, 5*(3), 260–295. doi:10.3934/publichealth.2018.3.260.
8. Shorey, S., Chee, C. Y. I., Ng, E. D., Chan, Y. H., Tam, W. W. S., & Chong, Y. S. (2018). Prevalence and incidence of postpartum depression among healthy mothers: A systematic review and meta-analysis. *Journal of Psychiatric Research, 104*, 235–248. doi:10.1016/j.jpsychires.2018.08.001.
9. Lorenzo, L., Byers, B., & Einarson, A. (2011). Antidepressant use in pregnancy. *Expert Opinion on Drug Safety, 10*(6), 883–889.
10. Gjerdingen, D., Fontaine, D., Scott, C., McGovern, P., Center, B., & Miner, M. (2009). Predictors of mothers' postpartum body dissatisfaction. *Women Health, 49*(6), 491–504.
11. Pearlstein, T., Howard, M., Salisbury, A., & Zlotnick, C. (2009). Postpartum depression. *American Journal of Obstetrics and Gynecology, 200*(4), 357–356.
12. Goodman, J. H., & Santangelo, G. (2011). Group treatment for postpartum depression: A systematic review.

*Database of Abstracts of Reviews of Effects (DARE): Quality-assessed Reviews.*
13. Liberto, T. L. (2012). Screening for depression and help-seeking in postpartum women during well-baby pediatric visits: An integrated review. *Journal of Pediatric Health Care, 26*(2), 109–117.
14. Goodman, J. H. (2004). Paternal postpartum depression, its relationship to maternal postpartum depression, and implications for family health. *Journal of Advanced Nursing, 45*(1), 26–35.
15. Ramchandani, P., Stein, A., Evans, J., & O'Connor, T. G. (2005). Paternal depression in the postnatal period and child development: A prospective population study. *Lancet, 365*, 2201–2205.
16. Paulson, J. F., & Bazemore, S. D. (2010). Prenatal and postpartum depression in fathers and its association with maternal depression: A meta-analysis. *The Journal of the American Medical Association, 303*(19), 1961–1969.
17. Cameron, E. E., Sedov, I. D., & Tomfohr-Madsen, L. M. (2016). Prevalence of paternal depression in pregnancy and the postpartum: An updated meta-analysis. *Journal of Affective Disorders, 206*, 189–203.
18. Leach, L. S., Poyser, C., Cooklin, A. R., & Giallo, R. (2016). Prevalence and course of anxiety disorders (and symptom levels) in men across the perinatal period: A systematic review. *Journal of Affective Disorders, 190*, 675–686.
19. Saisto, T., & Halmesmaki, E. (2003). Fear of childbirth: A neglected dilemma. *Acta obstetricia et gynecologica Scandinavica, 82*(3), 201–208.
20. Jones, I., Chandra, P. S., Dazzan, P., & Howard, L. M. (2014). Bipolar disorder, affective psychosis, and schizophrenia in pregnancy and the postpartum period. *Lancet, 384*, 1789–1799.
21. Heron, J., O'Connor, T. G., Evans, J., Golding, J., & Glover, V. (2004). The course of anxiety and depression through pregnancy and the postpartum in a community sample. *Journal of Affective Disorders, 80*, 65–73.
22. Norhayati, M. N., Nik Hazlina, N. H., Asrenee, A. R., & Wan Emilin, W. M. A. (2015). Magnitude and risk factors for postpartum symptoms: A literature review. *Journal of Affective Disorders, 175*, 34–52. doi:10.1016/j.jad.2014.12.041.
23. PHE (2019) Guidance 4. *Perinatal Mental Health.* https://www.gov.uk/government/publications/better-mental-health-jsna-toolkit/4-perinatal-mental-health#fn:5.
24. Howard, L. M., Molyneauxm, E., Dennis, C.-L., Rochat, T., Stein, A., & Milgrom, J. (2014). Non-psychotic mental disorders in the perinatal period. *The Lancet, 384*(9956), 1775–1788.

25. Jones, I., & Craddock, N. (2001). Familiarity of the *Puerperal Trigger in Bipolar Disorder: Results of a Family Study. American Journal of Psychiatry, 158*(6), 913–917.

26. Bradley, R., & Slade, P. (2011). A review of mental health problems in fathers following the birth of a child. *Journal of Reproductive and Infant Psychology, 29*(1), 19–42. doi:10.1080/02646838.2010.513047.

27. Schumacher, M., Zubaran, C., & White, G. (2008). Bringing birth-related paternal depression to the fore. *Women Birth, 21*(2), 65–70. doi:10.1016/j.wombi.2008.03.008.

28. Ballard, C., & Davies, R. (1996). Postnatal depression in fathers. *International Review of Psychiatry, 8*(1), 65–71.

29. Boyce, P., Condon, J., Bartona, J., & Corkindale, C. (2007). First-time fathers' study: Psychological distress in expectant fathers during pregnancy. *Australian & New Zealand Journal of Psychiatry, 41*, 718–725.

30. Wee, K. Y., Skouteris, H., Pier, C., Richardson, B., & Milgrom, J. (2011). Correlates of ante- and post-natal depression in fathers: A systematic review. *Journal of Affective Disorders, 130*(3), 358–377.

31. Giallo, R., D'Esposito, F., Cooklin, A., Mensah, F., Lucas, N., Wade, C., & Nicholson, J. M. (2013). Psychosocial risk factors associated with fathers' mental health in the postnatal period: Results from a population-based study. *Social Psychiatry and Psychiatric Epidemiology, 48*(4), 563–573.

32. Edward, K., Castle, D., Mills, C., Davis, L., & Casey, J. (2015). An integrative review of paternal depression. *American Journal of Men's Health, 9*(1), 26–34.

33. Royal College of GPs. (2016). *Position statement about Perinatal Mental Health.* https://www.rcgp.org.uk/policy/rcgp-policy-areas/perinatal-mental-health.aspx.

34. Department of Health. (2009). *The Healthy Child Programme – Pregnancy and the first five years of life.* London: DH.

35. Public Health England. (2015). *Rapid review to update evidence for the healthy child programme 0-5.* London: PHE. https://www.gov.uk/government/publications/healthy-child-programme-rapid-review-to-update-evidence.

36. Public Health England. (2018). *Best start in life and beyond: Improving public health outcomes for children, young people and families. Guidance to support the commissioning of the Healthy Child Programme 0–19: Health visiting and school nursing services.* London: PHE. https://www.gov.uk/government/publications/healthy-child-programme-0-to-19-health-visitor-and-school-nurse-commissioning.

37. Department of Health. (2015). *Universal Health Visitor Reviews: Advice for local authorities in delivery of the mandated universal health visitor reviews from 1 October 2015.* https://assets.publishing.service.gov.uk/government/uploads/system/uploads/attachment_data/file/464880/Universal_health_visitor_reviews_toolkit.pdf.

38. Scottish Government. (2015). Universal *Health Visiting Pathway* in Scotland: Pre-birth to pre-school. https://www.gov.scot/publications/universal-health-visiting-pathway-scotland-pre-birth-pre-school/.

39. NHS Wales. (2016). *An overview of the Healthy Child Wales Programme.* https://gov.wales/healthy-child-wales-programme-0

40. Department of Health, Social Services and Public Safety. (2010). *Healthy child, healthy future: A framework for the Universal Child Health Promotion Programme in Northern Ireland – Pregnancy to 19 years.* https://www.health-ni.gov.uk/publications/healthy-child-healthy-future.

41. Matthey, S., Barnett, B., Kavanagh, D. J., & Howie, P. (2001). Validation of the Edinburgh postnatal depression scale for men, and comparison of item endorsement with their partners. *Journal of Affective Disorders, 64*(2–3), 175–184.

42. Cameron, I. M., Crawford, J. R., Lawton, K., et al. (2008). Psychometric comparison of PHQ-9 and HADS for measuring depression severity in primary care. *British Journal of General Practice, 58*(546), 32–36. doi:10.3399/bjgp08X263794.

43. Madsen, S. A. (2011). Between autonomy and attachment: Psychotherapy for men with postnatal depression. In C. Blazina, & D. S. Shen-Miller (Eds.), *An international psychology of men: Theoretical advances, cases studies, and clinical innovations. Volume 7 of The Routledge Series on counseling and psychotherapy with boys and men* (pp. 315–340). New York: Routledge.

44. Morgan, M., Matthey, S., Barnett, B., & Richardson, C. (1997). A group programme for postnatally distressed women and their partners. *Journal of Advanced Nursing, 26*, 913–920.

45. Meighan, M., Davis, M. W., Thomas, S. P., & Droppleman, P. G. (1999). Living with postpartum depression: The father's experience. *The American Journal of Maternal Child Nursing, 24*(4), 202–208.

46. Robertson, S., Bagnall, A., & Walker, M. (2015). Evidence for a gender-based approach to mental health program: Identifying the key considerations associated with 'being male': An Evidence Check rapid review brokered by the Sax Institute (www.saxinstitute.org.au) for the Movember Foundation.

47. Darwin, Z., Galdas, P., Hinchliff, S., Littlewood, E., McMillan, D., McGowan, L., & Gilbody, S. (2017).

Fathers' views and experiences of their own mental health during pregnancy and the first postnatal year: A qualitative interview study of men participating in the UK Born and Bred in Yorkshire (BaBY) cohort. *BMC Pregnancy and Childbirth, 17*(1), 45.

48. Baldwin, S., & Griffiths, P. (2009). Do specialist community public health nurses assess risk factors for depression, suicide, and self-harm among South Asian mothers living in London? *Public Health Nursing, 26*(3), 277–289.

49. Cooper, J., Husain, N., Webb, R., Waheed, W., Kapur, N., Guthrie, E., et al. (2006). Self-harm in the UK: Differences between South Asians and Whites in rates, characteristics, provision of services and repetition. *Social Psychiatry and Psychiatric Epidemiology, 41*(10), 782–788.

50. Oates, M. R., Cox, J. L., Neema, S., Asten, P., Glangeaud-Freudenthal, N., Figueiredo, B., et al. (2004). Postnatal depression across countries and cultures: A qualitative study. *British Journal of Psychiatry, 184*(46), s10–s16.

51. Sonuga-Barke, E. J. S., & Mistry, M. (2000). The effect of extended family living on the mental health of three generations within two Asian communities. *British Journal of Clinical Psychology, 39*(2), 129–141. https://doi.org/10.1348/014466500163167.

52. Baldwin, S., Johnson, M. R. D. (2016). Working in Diverse Communities. In: Luker, K.A., McHugh, G.A., Bryar, R.N., (Eds) *Health Visiting: Preparation for Practice.* 220-251. Chichester UK: Wiley-Blackwell.

53. National Institute for Health and Care Excellence. (NICE). (2018). Antenatal and Postnatal Mental Health: Clinical Management and Service Guidance: Updated edition. National Clinical Guideline Number 192. NICE: The British Psychological Society and The Royal College of Psychiatrists. https://www.ncbi.nlm.nih.gov/books/NBK338568/.

54. Adoption UK. (2013). *Post-adoption depression, Factsheet 14.* https://www.nhs.uk/Livewell/adoption-and-fostering/Documents/Adoption%20UK%20Factsheet%20 14%20-%20Post-adoption%20depression%20June%20 2013.pdf.

55. Mott, S. L., Schiller, C. E., Richards, J. G., O'Hara, M. W., & Stuart, S. (2011). Depression and anxiety among postpartum and adoptive mothers. *Archives of Women's Mental Health, 14*(4), 335–343.

56. Senecky, Y., Agassi, H., Inbar, D., Horesh, N., Diamond, G., Bergman, Y. S., et al. (2009). Post-adoption depression among adoptive mothers. *Journal of Affective Disorders, 15*, 62–68.

57. Foli, K. J. (2009). Depression in adoptive parents: A model of understanding through grounded theory. *Western Journal of Nursing Research, 32*(3), 379–400.

58. Blackmore, E. R., Gustafsson, H., Gilchrist, M., Wyman, C., & O'Connor, T. G. (2016). Pregnancy-related anxiety: Evidence of distinct clinical significance from a pro-spective longitudinal study. *Journal of Affective Disorders, 197,* 251–258.

59. Koelewijn JM, Sluijs AM, Vrijkotte TGM. (2017). Possible relationship between general and pregnancy-related anxiety during the first half of pregnancy and the birth process: A prospective cohort study. BMJ Open. May 9;7(5):e013413. doi: 10.1136/bmjopen-2016-013413. PMID: 28490549; PMCID: PMC5623367.

60. Korja, R., Nolvi, S., Grant, K. A., & McMahon, C. (2017). The relations between maternal prenatal anxiety or stress and child's early negative reactivity or self-regulation: A systematic review. *Child Psychiatry and Human Development, 48*, 1–19.

61. Stein, A., Pearson, R. M., Goodman, S. H., Rapa, E., Rahman, A., McCallum, M., et al. (2014). Effects of perinatal mental disorders on the fetus and child. *Lancet., 384*(9956), 1800–1819. doi:10.1016/S0140-6736(14)61277-0. Epub 2014 Nov 14. PMID: 25455250.

62. Gerardin, P., Wendland, J., Bodeau, N., et al. (2011). Depression during pregnancy: Is the developmental impact earlier in boys? A prospective case-control study. *Journal of Clinical Psychiatry, 72*, 378–387.

63. Velders, F. P., Dieleman, G., Henrichs, J., et al. (2011). Prenatal and postnatal psychological symptoms of parents and family functioning: The impact on child emotional and behavioural problems. *European Child Adolesc Psychiatry, 20*(7), 341–350. doi:10.1007/s00787-011-0178-0. Epub 2011 Apr 27. PMID: 21523465; PMCID: PMC3135831.

64. Leis, J. A., Heron, J., Stuart, E. A., & Mendelson, T. (2013). Associations between maternal mental health and child emotional and behavioural problems: Does prenatal mental health matter? *J Abnorm Child Psychol, 42*, 161–171.

65. O'Connor, T. G., Heron, J., Golding, J., Beveridge, M., & Glover, V. (2002). Maternal antenatal anxiety and children's behavioural/emotional problems at 4 years. Report from the Avon Longitudinal Study of Parents and Children. *British Journal of Psychiatry, 180,* 502–508. doi:10.1192/bjp.180.6.502. PMID: 12042228.

66. Glover, V., O'Connor, T. G., & O'Donnell, K. (2010). Prenatal stress and the programming of the HPA axis. *Neuroscience and Biobehavioral Review, 35*, 17–22.

67. Henry, C., Kabbaj, M., Simon, H., et al. (1994). Prenatal stress increases the hypothalamic–pituitary–adrenal axis response in young and adult rats. *Journal of Neuroendocrinology, 6*, 341–345.

68. Schneider, M., & Moore, C. F. (2000). Effect of prenatal stress on development: A nonhuman primate model. In C. Nelson (Ed.), *Minnesota Symposium on Child Psychology* (pp. 201–243). New Jersey: Erlbaum.

69. Van den Bergh, B. R., Mulder, E. J., Mennes, M., & Glover, V. (2005). Antenatal maternal anxiety and stress and the neurobehavioural development of the fetus and child: Links and possible mechanisms. A review. *Neuroscience and Biobehavioral Review, 29*(2), 237–258.

70. O'Donnell, K., O'Connor, T. G., & Glover, V. (2009). Prenatal stress and neurodevelopment of the child: Focus on the HPA axis and role of the placenta. *Developmental Neuroscience, 31*(4), 285–292.

71. Reynolds, R. M. (2013). Glucocorticoid excess and the developmental origins of disease: Two decades of testing the hypothesis – 2012 Curt Richter award winner. *Psycho Neuroendocrinology, 38*(1), 1–11.

72. Couret, D., Prunier, A., Mounier, A. M., Thomas, F., Oswald, I. P., & Merlot, E. (2009). Comparative effects of a prenatal stress occurring during early or late gestation on pig immune response. *Physiology & Behavior, 98*(4), 498–504.

73. Weinstock, M. (1997). Does prenatal stress impair coping and regulation of hypothalamic–pituitary–adrenal axis? *Neuroscience and Biobehavioral Review, 21*, 1–10.

74. Clarke, A. S., Wittwer, D. J., Abbott, D. H., et al. (1994). Long-term effects of prenatal stress on HPA axis activity in juvenile Rhesus monkeys. *Developmental Psychobiology, 27*, 257–269.

75. Pearson, R. M., Melotti, R., Heron, J., et al. (2012). Disruption to the development of maternal responsiveness? The impact of prenatal depression on mother–infant interactions. *Infant Behavior and Development, 35*, 613–626.

76. McNamara, J., Townsend, M. L., & Herbert, J. S. (2019). A systemic review of maternal well-being and its relationship with maternal fetal attachment and early postpartum bonding. *PLoS One, 14*(7), e0220032. https://doi.org/10.1371/journal. Pone.0220032.

77. Göbela, A., Lydia Stuhrmanna, Y., Harderb, S., Schulte-Markworta, M., & Susanne Mudra, S. (2018). The association between maternal–fetal bonding and prenatal anxiety: An explanatory analysis and systematic review. *Journal of Affective Disorders, 15*(239), 313–327.

78. Doan, H. M., & Zimerman, A. (2003). Conceptualizing Prenatal Attachment: Toward a Multidimensional View. *Journal of Prenatal & Perinatal Psychology & Health, 18*, 109–129. https://www.researchgate.net/publication/310671845_Conceptualizing_prenatal_attachment_Toward_a_multidimensional_view. Accessed 20 August 2019.

79. Cranley, M. S. (1981). Development of a tool for the measurement of maternal attachment during pregnancy. *Nursing Research, 30*(5), 281–284.

80. Muller, M. E. (1992). A critical review of prenatal attachment research. *Scholarly Inquiry for Nursing Practice, 6*(1), 5–22.

81. Brandon, A. R., Pitts, S., Denton, W. H., Stringer, C. A., & Evans, H. M. (2009). A history of the theory of prenatal attachment. *Journal of Prenatal and Perinatal Psychology and Health, 23*(4), 201–222.

82. Van den Bergh, B., & Simons, A. (2009). A review of scales to measure the mother–foetus relationship. *Journal of Reproductive and Infant Psychology, 27*(2), 114–126.

83. Figueiredo, B., & Costa, R. (2009). Mother's stress, mood and emotional involvement with the infant: Three months before and three months after childbirth. *Archives of Women's Mental Health, 12*(3), 143–153.

84. Ohoka, H., Koide, T., Goto, S., Murase, S., Kanai, A., Masuda, T., et al. (2014). Effects of maternal depressive symptomatology during pregnancy and the postpartum period on infant–mother attachment. *Psychiatry and Clinical Neurosciences, 68*(8), 631–639. doi:10.1111/pcn.12171.

85. O'Hara, M., Okada, T., Kubota, C., Nakamura, Y., Shiino, T., Aleksic, B., et al. (2017). Relationship between maternal depression and bonding failure: A prospective cohort study of pregnant women. *Psychiatry and Clinical Neurosciences, 71*(10), 733–741. doi:10.1111/pcn.12541.

86. Doster, A., Wallwiener, S., Müller, M., Matthies, L. M., Plewniok, K., Feller, S., et al. (2018). Reliability and validity of the German version of the Maternal–Fetal Attachment Scale. *Archives of Gynecology and Obstetrics, 297*, 1157–1167.

87. Branjerdporn, G., Meredith, P., Strong, J., & Garcia, J. (2017). Associations between maternal–foetal attachment and infant developmental outcomes: A systematic review. *Journal of Maternal and Child Health, 21*, 540–553. doi:10.1007/s10995-016-2138-2.

88. Cildir, D. A., Ozbek, A., Topuzoglu, A., Orcin, E., & Janbakhishov, C. E. (2019). Association of prenatal attachment and early childhood emotional, behavioral, and developmental characteristics: A longitudinal study. *Infant Mental Health 41*(4), 517–529. doi:10.1002/imhj.21822.

89. Rollè, L., Giordano, M., Santoniccolo, F., & Trombetta, T. (2020). Prenatal attachment and perinatal depression: A systematic review. *International Journal of Environmental Research and Public Health, 17*(8), 2644. doi:10.3390/ijerph17082644.PMID: 32290590.

90. Pearson, R. M., Evans, J., Kounali, D., et al. (2013). Maternal depression during pregnancy and the postnatal period: Risks and possible mechanisms for off spring depression at age 18 years. *JAMA Psychiatry, 70*, 1312–1319.

91. Deave, T., Heron, J., Evans, J., & Emond, A. (2008). The impact of maternal depression in pregnancy on early child development. *International Journal of Obstetrics and Gynaecology, 115*(8), 1043–1051.

92. Murray, L., Halligan, S. L., & Cooper, P. (2010). Effects of postnatal depression on mother–infant interactions, and child development. In J. G. Bremner, & T. D. Wachs (Eds.), *Handbook of infant development* (2nd ed.). Malden, UK: Wiley-Blackwell.

93. Murray, L., Arteche, A., Fearon, P., Halligan, S., Goodyer, I., & Cooper, P. (2011). Maternal postnatal depression and the development of depression in off spring up to 16 years of age. *Journal of the American Academy of Child and Adolescent Psychiatry, 50*, 460–470.

94. Netsi, E., Pearson, R. M., Murray, L., Cooper, P., Craske, M. G., & Stein, A. (2018). Association of persistent and severe postnatal depression with child outcomes. *JAMA Psychiatry, 75*(3), 247–253.

95. Bowlby, J. (1982). Attachment and loss: Retrospect and prospect. *American Journal of Orthopsychiatry, 52*(4), 664–678. https://doi.org/10.1111/j.1939-0025.1982.tb01456.x. PMID: 7148988 31.

96. Ainsworth, M. S. (1979). Infant–mother attachment. *American Psychologist, 34*(10), 932–937. https://doi.org/10.1037/0003-066X.34.10.932.

97. Stein A, Craske MG, Lehtonen A, Harvey A, Savage-McGlynn E, Davies B, Goodwin J, Murray L, Cortina-Borja M, Counsell N. (2012). Maternal cognitions and mother-infant interaction in postnatal depression and generalized anxiety disorder. *J Abnorm Psychol. 121*(4), 795–809. doi: 10.1037/a0026847. Epub 2012 Jan 30. PMID: 22288906; PMCID: PMC3506203.

98. Field, T. (2010). Postpartum depression effects on early interactions, parenting, and safety practices: A review. *Infant Behavior and Development, 33*, 1–6.

99. Everett, W., Susan, M., Dominique, T., Judith, C., & Leah, A. (2000). Attachment security in infancy and early adulthood: A twenty-year longitudinal study. *Child Development, 71*(3), 684–689.

100. Antonucci, T. C., Akiyama, H., & Takahashi, K. (2004). Attachment and close relationships across the life span. *Attachment and Human Development, 6*(4), 353–370. doi:10.1080/1461673042000303136. PMID:15764124.

101. Alhusen, J. L., Gross, D., Hayat, M. J., Rose, L., & Sharps, P. (2012). The role of mental health on maternal–fetal attach-mentin low-income women. *Journal of Obstetric, Gynecologic, and Neonatal Nursing, 41*(6), e71–e81. https://doi.org/10.1111/j.1552-6909.2012.01385.x. PMID:22788921.

102. Robinson, M., Oddy, W. H., Jianghong, L., Kendall, G. E., de Klerk, N. H., Silburn, S. R., et al. (2008). Pre- and post-natal influences on preschool mental health: A large-scale cohort study. *Journal of Child Psychology and Psychiatry, 49*(10), 1118–1128. https://doi.org/10.1111/j.1469-7610.2008.01955.x. PMID: 19017026.

103. Barnes, J., & Theule, J. (2019). Maternal depression and infant attachment security: A meta-analysis. *Infant Mental Health Journal. 40*(6), 817–834.

104. Śliwerski, A., Kossakowska, K., Jarecka, K., Świtalska, J., & Bielawska-Batorowicz, E. (2020). The effect of maternal depression on infant attachment: A systematic review. *International Journal of Environmental Research and Public Health, 17*(8), 2675. doi:10.3390/ijerph17082675. PMID: 32295106; PMCID: PMC7216154.

105. Quevedo, L. A., Silva, R. A., Godoy, R., et al. (2012). The impact of maternal postpartum depression on the language development of children at 12 months. *Child Care Health Development, 38*, 420–424.

106. Sutter-Dallay, A. L., Murray, L., Dequae-Merchadou, L., Glatigny-Dallay, E., Bourgeois, M. L., & Verdoux, H. (2011). A prospective longitudinal study of the impact of early postnatal vs chronic maternal depressive symptoms on child development. *European Psychiatrists, 26*, 484–489.

107. Kaplan, P. S., Danko, C. M., Diaz, A., & Kalinka, C. J. (2011). An associative learning deficit in 1-year-old infants of depressed mothers: Role of depression duration. *Infant Behavior and Development, 34*(1), 35–44.

108. Stanley, C., Murray, L., & Stein, A. (2004). The effect of postnatal depression on mother infant interaction, in fant response to the still-face perturbation, and performance on an instrumental learning task. *Development and Psychopathology, 16*, 1–18.

109. Pearson, R. M., Bornstein, M., Cordero, M., Scerif, G., Mahedy, L., Evans, J., Abioye, A., & Stein, A. (2016). Maternal perinatal mental health and offspring academic achievement at age 16: The mediating role of childhood executive function. *Journal of Child Psychology and Psychiatry, 57*(4), 491–501. https://acamh.onlinelibrary.wiley.com/doi/pdf/10.1111/jcpp.12483.

110. Takács, L., Kandrnal, V., Kaňková, Š., et al. (2020). The effects of pre- and post-partum depression on child behavior and psychological development from birth to pre-school age: A protocol for a systematic review and meta-analysis. *Systematic Review, 9*(146), 1–7. https://doi.org/10.1186/s13643-019-1267-2.

111. Sethna, V., Murray, L., Netsi, E., Psychogiou, L., & Ramchandani, P. G. (2015). Paternal depression in the postnatal period and early father–infant interactions. *Parenting Science and Practice*, 15(1), 1–8. 1529-5192.

112. McElwain, N., & Volling, B. L. (1999). Depressed mood and marital conflict: Relations to maternal and paternal intrusiveness with one-year-old infants. *Journal of Applied Developmental Psychology*, 20(1), 63–83. https://www.sciencedirect.com/science/article/abs/pii/S0193397399800045.

113. Davis, R. N., Davis, M. M., Freed, G. L., & Clark, S. J. (2011). Fathers' depression related to positive and negative parenting behaviors with 1-year-old children. *Pediatrics*, 127(4), 612–618.

114. Paulson, J. F., Keefe, H. A., & Leiferman, J. A. (2009). Early parental depression and child language development. *Journal of Child Psychology and Psychiatry*, 50, 254–262.

115. Paulson, J. F., Dauber, S., & Leifermann, J. C. (2006). Individual and combined effects of postpartum depression in mothers and fathers on parenting behaviour. *Pediatrics*, 118, 659–668.

116. Kvalevaag, A. L., Ramchandani, P. G., Hove, O., Assmus, J., Eberhard-Gran, M., & Biringer, E. (2013). Paternal mental health and socioemotional and behavioral development in their children. *Pediatrics*, 131, e463–469.

117. Ramchandani, P. G., Domoney, J., Sethna, V., Vlachos, H., & Murray, L. (2013). Do early father–infant interactions predict the onset of externalising behaviours in young children? Findings from a longitudinal cohort study. *The Journal of Child Psychology and Psychiatry*, 54(1), 56–64.

118. Sweeney, S., & MacBeth, A. (2016). The effects of paternal depression on child and adolescent outcomes: A systematic review. *Journal of Affective Disorders*, 205, 44–59. doi:10.1016/j.jad.2016.05.073. Epub 2016 Jun 24. PMID: 27414953.

119. Gentile, S., & Fusco, M. L. (2017). Untreated perinatal paternal depression: effects on offspring. *Psychiatry Research*, 252, 325–332.

120. Gutierrez-Galve, L., Stein, A., Hanington, L., Heron, J., Lewis, G., O'Farrelly, C., & Ramchandani, P. G. (2019). Association of *maternal and paternal depression in the postnatal period with offspring depression at age 18 years*. *JAMA Psychiatry*, 76(3), 290–296.

121. Bauer, A., Parsonage, M., Knapp, M., Iemmi, V., & Adelaja, B. (2014). *Costs of perinatal mental health problems*. London: Centre for Mental Health and London School of Economics Health. https://www.centreformental-health.org.uk/costs-of-perinatal-mh-problems.

122. Edoka, I. P., Petrou, S., & Ramchandani, P. G. (2011). Healthcare costs of paternal depression in the postnatal period. *Journal of Affective Disorders*, 133, 356–360.

123. World Economic Forum. (2020). Lockdown is the world's biggest psychological experiment – and we will pay the price. https://www.weforum.org/agenda/2020/04/this-is-the-psychological-side-of-the-covid-19-pandemic-that-were-ignoring/. Accessed October 10, 2020.

124. Saccone, G., Florio, A., Aiello, F., Venturella, R., De Angelis, M. C., Locci, M., et al. (2020). Psychological impact of Covid-19 in pregnant women. *American Journal of Obstetrics and Gynecology*, doi:10.1016/j.ajog.2020.05.003. [Epub ahead of print].

125. Davenport, M. H., Meyer, S., Meah, V. L., Strynadka, M. C., & Khurana, R. (2020). Moms Are Not OK: Covid-19 and Maternal Mental Health. *Frontiers in Global Women's Health*, 1(1). https://www.frontiersin.org/articles/10.3389/fgwh.2020.00001/full.

126. Babies in Lockdown: Listening to parents to build back better. (2020). Best Beginnings, Home-Start UK, and the Parent–Infant Foundation. UK. https://babiesin-lockdown.files.wordpress.com/2020/08/babies_in_lockdown_executive_summary.pdf.

127. Conti, G., & Dow, A. (2020). *The Impact of Covid-19 on Health Visitor in England-first Results*. London: UCL. https://discovery.ucl.ac.uk/id/eprint/10106430/8/Conti_Dow_The%20impacts%20of%20COVID-19%20on%20Health%20Visiting%20in%20England%20250920.pdf.

128. O'Connor, K., Wrigley, M., Jennings, R., Hill, M., & Niazi, A. (2021). Mental health impacts of COVID-19 in Ireland and the need for a secondary care mental health service response. *Irish journal of psychological medicine*, 38(2), 99–107. https://doi.org/10.1017/ipm.2020.64

129. Refuge. (2021). Press release-A year of lockdown: Refuge releases new figures showing dramatic increase in activity across its specialist domestic abuse services (online). https://www.refuge.org.uk/a-year-of-lockdown/. Accessed 15 September 2021).

130. Howard, L.M., Oram, S., Galley, H., Trevillion, K., Feder, G. (2013). Domestic violence and perinatal mental disorders: A systematic review and meta-analysis. *PLoS Med*. 10(5):e1001452. doi:10.1371/journal.pmed.1001452. Epub 2013 May 28. PMID: 23723741; PMCID: PMC3665851.

131. Bick, D., Cheyne, H., Chang, Y. S., & Fisher, J. (2020). Maternal postnatal health during the Covid-19 pandemic: Vigilance is needed. *Midwifery*, 88, 102781. https://doi.org/10.1016/j.midw.2020.102781.

132. MBRRACE-UK. (2019). In M. Knight, K. Bunch, D. Tuffnell, J. Shakespeare, R. Kotnis, S. Kenyon, & J. J.

Kurinczuk (Eds.), *Saving lives, improving mothers' care – Lessons learned to inform maternity care from the UK and Ireland confidential enquiries into maternal deaths and morbidity 2015-2017*. Oxford: National Perinatal Epidemiology Unit, University of Oxford.

133. Thompson, C., & Thomson, C. M. (1989). The prescribing of antidepressants in general practice. 11: A placebo controlled trial of low dose dothiepin. *Human Psychopharmacology, 4*, 191–204.

134. Bonari, L., Bennett, H., Einarso, A., & Koren, G. (2004). Risks of untreated depression in pregnancy. *Can Family Physician, 50*, 37–29.

135. Wisner, K., James, P., & Findling, R. L. (1997). Antidepressant treatment during breastfeeding. *Obstetrical and Gynaecological Survey, 62*(4), 223–224.

136. Bledsoe, S.E., Grote, N.K. (2006). Treating depression during pregnancy and the postpartum: A preliminary meta-analysis. In: Database of Abstracts of Reviews of Effects (DARE): Quality-assessed Reviews [Internet]. York (UK): Centre for Reviews and Dissemination (UK); 1995-. Available from: https://www.ncbi.nlm.nih.gov/books/NBK73095/.

137. Elkin, I., Shea, M. T., Watkins, J. L., et al. (1989). General effectiveness of treatments. *Archives of General Psychiatry, 46*, 971–982.

138. National Institute for Health and Care Excellence. (NICE). (2004). *Depression: Management of depression in primary and secondary care. Clinical practice guideline No 23.* London: NICE.

139. Appleby, L., Warner, R., Whitton, A., & Faragher, B. (1997). A controlled study of fluoxetine and cognitive behavioural counselling in the treatment of postnatal depression. *British Medical Journal, 314*(7085), 932–936. 29.

140. Rogers, C. (1957). The necessary and sufficient conditions of therapeutic personality change. *Journal of Consulting Psychology, 21*(2), 95–103.

141. Shakespeare, J., Blake, F., & Garcia, J. (2006). How do women with postnatal depression experience listening visits in primary care? A qualitative interview study. *Journal of Reproductive and Infant Psychology, 24*, 149–162.

142. Slade, P., Morrell, C. J., Rigby, A., et al. (2010). Postnatal women's experiences of management of depressive symptoms: a qualitative study. *British Journal of General Practice, 60*, e440–e448.

143. Morrell, J., Slade, P., Warner, R., et al. (2009). Clinical effectiveness of health visitor training in psychologically informed approaches for depression in postnatal women: Pragmatic cluster randomised trial in primary care. *British Medical Journal, 338*, a3045.

144. Spinelli, M., G Endicott, J., Leo, A. C., et al. (2013). A controlled clinical treatment trial of interpersonal psychotherapy for depressed pregnant women at 3 New York City sites. *Journal of Clinical Psychiatry, 74*, 393–399.

145. Morgan, M. (1997). A group programme for postnatally depressed women and their partners. *Journal of Advanced Nursing, 26*(5), 913–920.

146. Higgins, M., St James Roberts, I., & Glover, V. (2007). Post-natal depression and mother and infant outcomes after infant massage. *Journal of Affective Disorder, 15*, 189–92.

147. Fujita, M., Endoh, Y., Saimon, N., & Yagaguchi, S. (2006). Effects of massaging babies on mothers: A pilot study on the changes in mood states and salivary cortisol level. *Complementary Therapies in Clinical Practice, 12*(3), 181–185.

148. Oren, D., Wisner, K., Spinelli, M., et al. (2002). An open trial of morning light therapy for treatment of antepartum depression. *American Journal of Psychiatry, 159*, 666–669.

149. Manber, R., Allen, J. J., & Morris, M. M. (2002). Alternative treatments for depression: Empirical support and relevance to women. *Journal of Clinical Psychiatry, 63*, 628–640.

150. Armstrong, K., & Edwards, H. (2004). The effectiveness of a pram-walking exercise programme in reducing depressive symptomology for post-natal women. *International Journal of Nursing Practice, 10*(4), 177–194.

151. Lever, T. B., Cavanagh, K., & Strauss, C. (2016). The effectiveness of mindfulness based interventions in the perinatal period: A systematic review and meta-analysis. *PLoS One., 11*(5), e0155720. doi:10.1371/journal.pone.0155720. PMID: 27182732; PMCID: PMC4868288.

152. Baldwin, S., Walker, M., & Parker, R. (2019). *Institute of Health Visiting Good Practice Points for Health Visitors. Understanding Mothers' Mental Health & Well-Being During their Transition to Motherhood.* London: iHV.

153. Dadi, A. F., Miller, E. R., & Mwanri, L. (2020). Postnatal depression and its association with adverse infant health outcomes in low- and middle-income countries: A systematic review and meta-analysis. *BMC Pregnancy Childbirth, 20*(1), 416.

154. NSPCC. (2020). Mental health risks for new and pregnant mothers during coronavirus. https://www.nspcc.org.uk/about-us/news-opinion/2020/mental-health-risks-new-pregnant-mothers-cornavirus/. Accessed 10 October 2020.

155. Ramchandani, P. G., O'Connor, T. G., Evans, J., Heron, J., Murray, L., & Stein, A. (2008). The effects of pre- and post-natal depression in fathers: a natural experiment

comparing the effects of exposure to depression on offspring. *Journal of Child Psychology and Psychiatry, and Allied Sisciplines, 49*(10), 1069–1078. https://doi.org/10.1111/j.1469-7610.2008.02000.x.

156. Misri, S., Abizadeh, J., Sanders, S., & Swift, E. (2015). Perinatal generalized anxiety disorder: Assessment and treatment. Journal of women's health, 24(9), 762–770.

157. Hollyman, J.A., Freeling, P. & Paykel, E.S. (1998). Double-blind placebo-controlled trial of amitriptyline among depressed patients in general practice. *Journal of the Royal Collage of General Practitioners, 38,* 393–397.

158. Hanley, J. (2009). Perinatal Mental Health, John Wiley and Sons. West Sussex.

159. Sockol, LE. (2018). A systematic review and meta-analysis of interpersonal psychotherapy for perinatal women. *J Affect Disord.* May;232:316–328.

160. Honey, KL, Bennett, P, Morgan, M. (2002). A brief psycho-educational group intervention for post natal depression. *B J Clin, Psych.* 41(4), 405–9.

161. Larson, EB, Yao, X. (2005). Clinical empathy as emotional labor in the patient-physician relationship. *JAMA.* 293(9), 1100–6. doi: 10.1001/jama.293.9.1100. PMID: 15741532.

162. PHE (2021). Guidance, Health visiting and school nursing service delivery model, updated 2021. https://www.gov.uk/government/publications/commissioning-of-public-health-services-for-children/health-visiting-and-school-nursing-service-delivery-model.

163. Castle H, Slade P, et al (2008). Attitudes to emotional expression, social support and postnatal adjustment in new parents. Journal of Reproductive and Infant Psychology, 26(3), 180-194, DOI: 10.1080/02646830701691319.

164. Baldwin, S., Malone, M., Sandall, J., Bick, D. (2018). Mental health and wellbeing during the transition to fatherhood: a systematic review of first time fathers' experiences. JBI Database System Rev Implement Rep. 16(11), 2118-2191. doi: 10.11124/JBISRIR-2017-003773. PMID: 30289768; PMCID: PMC6259734.

165. Beck, A. (1970). Cognitive therapy: Nature and relation to behavior therapy. Behavior Therapy, 1(2), 184-200. https://www.sciencedirect.com/science/article/pii/S0005789470800302?via%3Dihub#aep-article-footnote-id1.

166. Scope, A., Leaviss, J., Kaltenthaler, E. et al. (2013). Is group cognitive behaviour therapy for postnatal depression evidence-based practice? A systematic review. BMC Psychiatry 13, 321. https://doi.org/10.1186/1471-244X-13-321.

167. NICE (2009). Depression in adults: recognition and management. Clinical Guideline. https://www.nice.org.uk/guidance/cg90.

168. Institute of Health Visiting (2015). Developing Resilience with Compassion: A Health Visiting Framework, Managers Document.

# 14

# EMOTIONAL AND MENTAL HEALTH WELL-BEING AND DEVELOPMENT OF INFANTS AND CHILDREN

KIRSTEN COULL ▪ AMANDA HOLLAND

## CHAPTER CONTENTS

INTRODUCTION

INFANT AND CHILD MENTAL HEALTH IN CONTEXT

BRAIN ARCHITECTURE – AN OVERVIEW

THE 'EXPERIENCE-DEPENDENT' BRAIN

IMPACT OF NEGLECT ON BRAIN ARCHITECTURE

PARENT–INFANT INTERACTION

SERVE AND RETURN INTERACTIONS

RUPTURE AND REPAIR

THEORIES OF EMOTIONAL DEVELOPMENT

PARENTAL REPRESENTATIONS

RISK FACTORS THAT IMPACT ON INFANT AND CHILD EMOTIONAL AND MENTAL HEALTH, WELL-BEING AND DEVELOPMENT

THE IMPACT OF PARENTAL MENTAL HEALTH DIFFICULTIES ON INFANT AND CHILD EMOTIONAL MENTAL HEALTH AND WELL-BEING

THE IMPACT OF DOMESTIC VIOLENCE AND ABUSE ON INFANT AND CHILD EMOTIONAL MENTAL HEALTH AND WELL-BEING

THE IMPACT OF SUBSTANCE ABUSE OR MISUSE ON INFANT AND CHILD EMOTIONAL MENTAL HEALTH AND WELL-BEING

SUMMARY

RELATIONSHIP-BASED THERAPEUTIC INTERVENTIONS

PROGRAMMES THAT PROMOTE ATTACHMENT AND PARENTAL SENSITIVITY

PROGRAMMES INVOLVING LIVE DEMONSTRATIONS

MEDIA-BASED METHODS

BABY MASSAGE

PROGRAMMES THAT PROMOTE EMOTIONAL, SOCIAL AND BEHAVIOURAL DEVELOPMENT

PROFESSIONAL ROLES IN SUPPORTING POSITIVE ATTACHMENTS

CONTAINMENT

PROVIDING THE EXPERIENCE OF A SAFE, NURTURING RELATIONSHIP

OBSERVING, DESCRIBING AND BEING CURIOUS

UNDERSTANDING CHILD DEVELOPMENT AND APPROPRIATE EXPECTATIONS

HARNESSING A SENSE OF WONDER

MODELLING, IN PARTICULAR PLAY

FACILITATING APPROPRIATE SUPPORT FOR CAREGIVERS INDIVIDUALLY AND, WHERE APPROPRIATE, AS A COUPLE

CONCLUSION

## LEARNING OUTCOMES

*To:*

- gain an understanding of early brain architecture and the impact of infant experiences on their developing brain.
- gain a recognition of the importance of sensitive, attuned interactions for positive infant development, and the potential impact of their absence.

- gain an understanding of key risk factors that impact infant and child emotional mental health and well-being.
- gain awareness of evidence-based therapeutic interventions to promote attachment and parental sensitivity.
- gain an awareness of potential professional roles in supporting the development of positive mental health.

## INTRODUCTION

The human baby is born more helpless than any other species on the earth and is dependent on its parents for far longer. They will have the genetic blueprints inherited from their parents and wider family; however the intricacies of how their brain architecture develops and their understanding of themselves, their world and those around them will be shaped by the experiences they have, even before they are born.

Over the course of this chapter we will explore what is meant by infant mental health (IMH) and why it has such an impact on the trajectory of the developing child. We will outline the core aspects of infant brain development and discuss those elements which are essential for optimal growth and progress towards individual potential. With this in mind, consideration will be given to the challenges that can arise to impact healthy infant and child mental health and well-being, how we recognise these, and how best they can be supported within the health visitor role.

Throughout the chapter we largely refer to 'parent' which, unless otherwise specified, refers to the primary caregiver whether they be mother, father or any other biological or non-biological significant person in the child's life. As we will

go on to explore, infant development takes place within a rich medley of influencing factors, with all of those around the infant having a role to play in their unfolding trajectory.

## INFANT AND CHILD MENTAL HEALTH IN CONTEXT

IMH refers to the positive growth of emotional, social and cognitive development across the early months and years of life. It describes the process of optimal brain development resulting from interactions between the inherent structure of the infant brain, and the life experiences which shape the connections therein. Responsive and nurturing interactions with a consistent caregiver form the foundations for positive IMH.[1]

Evidence highlights that the experiences that an infant has through the period of rapid growth and development over the first 3 years of their life, and in particular the first 1001 days, will have the most profound impact upon the child's ongoing developmental trajectory through to adolescence and adulthood[2]. Given this recognition, it is perhaps intuitive that optimising this period as an opportunity for significant growth should be a key priority.

The majority of children will receive the sensitive and nurturing care that they need to develop strong and healthy brain connections as a foundation for ongoing positive mental health. Babies do not need to be, nor should they be, bombarded by stimuli at all times. Rather, they require predictable, attuned interactions with a primary caregiver and a network of support around that caregiver, to facilitate what Winnicott[3] labelled 'good enough' parenting for optimal development. In some circumstances however, for a multitude of reasons which we shall explore across this chapter, factors impact on this pathway which affect the developing brain and subsequent well-being.

Early mental health difficulties can manifest in a range of presentations and, by the pre-school years, are largely classified as oppositional defiant and conduct disorders, attention deficit hyperactivity disorders, anxiety disorders and depressive disorders.[4] Prevalence rates vary significantly, partly due to difficulties in defining what constitutes mental health difficulties in the early years.[5] Within the UK, a recent study by the Department of Health and Social Care in England,[6] using rigorous application of diagnostic criteria with a large sample, found prevalence of 5.5% (1 in 18) preschool (2- to 4-year-old) children with at least one 'mental disorder' (according to ICD-10 diagnostic criteria). Overall prevalence within this age range was slightly higher in boys compared with girls (6.8% compared with 4.2%) with behavioural disorders constituting the highest prevalence of difficulties (2.5% prevalence).

Although there are wide variations in prevalence estimates, it has been demonstrated repeatedly that intervention for any difficulties highlighted during this critical period, and indeed across the pre-school years of a child's life, will elicit the highest rewards for the child, their family and their wider society.[7]

## BRAIN ARCHITECTURE – AN OVERVIEW

In order to appreciate the critical nature of the first months and years upon a child's future trajectory, it is important to understand the architecture of the developing brain in the foetus and infant.

Cells which will go on to form the brain begin to develop within 3 weeks of conception,[8] with recognisable brain structures in place at just 7 weeks' gestation. The brainstem is the first area to develop, situated at the top of the newly formed spinal cord. As one of the most primitive areas of the brain, this controls basic, essential functions such as temperature, heart rate and blood pressure. The midbrain follows next, controlling appetite and sleep, with the limbic system, our seat of emotion and impulse, following. The final brain structure to develop in utero is the cerebral cortex, reaching basic functionality at full gestation, although as the centre of rational, conscious thought as well as planning and logic, the cortex continues to develop across the first years of life and beyond. Indeed, the neocortex, or frontal lobes, the seat of our executive function – our 'air traffic control system' – is not fully mature until late adolescence.[9]

Given the rapid development of fundamental brain structures across gestation, the foetal brain is highly sensitive to any disruption to this process caused by factors such as maternal stress and the intake of alcohol and toxins, including smoking. Clear links have been demonstrated between prenatal anxiety and depression and later emotional and behavioural outcomes[10] and exposure to toxins during pregnancy, from nicotine through to cocaine, amphetamines, opiates and Ecstasy, can lead to multiple serious physical and mental health outcomes including stillbirth, prematurity, low birth weight and long-term neurological damage.[11] Alcohol use during pregnancy has been shown to have as much, if not more, impact as illicit substances, and although the prevalence of alcohol-related developmental difficulties has largely been thought to be underrepresented, one recent UK study suggested that 6% to 17% of children within the (regional, population-based) study showed signs of prenatal alcohol exposure.[12] Foetal alcohol spectrum disorder (FASD) encompasses a range of diagnoses linked to prenatal alcohol exposure, the effects of which impact to varying degrees across physical, emotional, cognitive and social domains.

By the time an infant reaches full gestation, the structural template for their brain development is largely in place. They will have over 100 billion neurons, but the vast majority of connections between these will not be formed until after they are born and begin to interact with the world around them. The networks that these neurons make will depend on the unique experiences of each individual infant.

## THE 'EXPERIENCE-DEPENDENT' BRAIN

When an infant experiences any form of stimulus, electrical signals are fired along the neurons in the brain to carry information to the relevant area. Neurons which are used regularly form pathways, with each neuron connected to the next by a synapse. Those pathways which are used repeatedly are reinforced by the body of the neuron, the axon, becoming myelinated. The process of myelination is when the axon is coated in a fatty sheath, called 'myelin'. This increases the signal transmission along the neural pathway by up to 100 times the unmyelinated speed.[13] Therefore, pathways which are used most frequently become more strongly wired within the infant brain, whether these be in response to positive, protective stimuli but also if they are in response to adverse stimuli. This process is often recalled by the phrase 'those neurons that fire together, wire together' (coined by Shatz in 1992 to describe the

work of Donald Hebb, who recognised that it is the process of one neuron repeatedly causing an outcome in another which underpins this pathway of neural transmission.[14])

The creation of these synapses, synaptogenesis, increases steadily from 24 weeks' gestation through the early years of life, with maximum synapses present at 5 years of age and then plateauing across the primary school years.[13] During infancy, the distribution of these synapses is not uniform. Indeed, specific areas of the brain will reach peak synaptic density at different stages of development, which relates to particularly sensitive periods, or 'windows of opportunity' for the consolidation of specific learning.[15] For example, maximum synaptogenesis occurs in the visual cortex between 4 and 8 months of age, with the peak in the prefrontal cortex at approximately 15 months.[16] Recognition of these sensitive periods allows an understanding of how the infant's experiences at different stages of development might impact on the architecture of their still-evolving brain structure and the functions arising.

Alongside the creation of new synapses and the consolidation of repeatedly used neural pathways, the converse is also true. Those neurons with less stimulation and fewer connections will be 'pruned' in order to make way for new learning. Synaptic pruning is particularly prolific during adolescence, when the brain undertakes the greatest period of growth and change after infancy.[17]

This neuroplasticity of the brain changing in structure and function as a result of experience, is present across the lifespan, and forms the foundation for adaptation, for example, following traumatic brain injury.[15] This capacity is at its peak for infants through pre- and post-natal periods and the 'use it or lose it' principle that describes plasticity becomes particularly pertinent when we consider the impact for those infants and children who do not receive the consistent, nurturing, responsive care that promotes the development of healthy brain connections.

## IMPACT OF NEGLECT ON BRAIN ARCHITECTURE

It is essential to recognise that the absence of fundamental human connection can have as much detrimental impact as the presence of perhaps more easily recognised harmful experiences. Lack of appropriate stimulation and sensitive care can elicit physiological changes to the developing brain structure which can lead to lifelong difficulties in health, learning and behaviour.[18] Extreme neglect has been demonstrated to impact on brain structure and function, increasing the risk of difficulties with attention and cognition, and altering stress response systems which can affect ongoing resilience and children's emotional resources to face any adversity. We will explore later in this chapter the impact of stress on infant and child mental health, within which neglect can be considered. However, first we must address what we mean by positive interactions and protective human connections.

### THINKING SPACE

- Neural pathways which are used repeatedly become hardwired – 'those neurons that fire together, wire together'.
- Pathways or connections which are not used are pruned away to make space for others – **'use it or lose it'.**
- The human brain has capacity for plasticity, which means shaping the brain according to experiences. This capacity is optimal during infancy and early childhood.

## PARENT–INFANT INTERACTION

Given our understanding of infant brain development, it is clear that in order to lay down the crucial pathways for optimal IMH, an infant needs to experience a predictable, consistent, warm and nurturing relationship with at least one caregiver. To facilitate this, infants are born with an innate

predisposition for social interaction. Since Harlow's work with primates in 1960s, which identified a predisposition for comfort over food,[19] there is widespread recognition that babies need more than simply their basic physical needs met in order to develop fully into healthy, functioning children and adults. In order to facilitate this, even prior to their birth, infants have the inherent capacity and drive for seeking social cues and responding to these.

## SERVE AND RETURN INTERACTIONS

'Serve and return interactions' form the basis of the reciprocal, responsive interactions that shape infant brain development. They describe the caregiver's capacity to appropriately interpret their infant or child's cues and to respond in a sensitive and timely manner.[9] This give-and-take dance of communication, or indeed the 'musicality' of the dialogue between parent and child,[20] is relevant to all interactions across childhood and beyond, but is particularly important over the early period in which the caregiver's responses will set a template for future interactions and relationships.

Parental contingent responsiveness is the process by which the parent is able to interpret the cues of the infant and attune their behavioural responses accordingly with a positive response that nurtures development. These responses might be in facial expression alongside tone of voice and even touch. Beebe and Lachman[21] highlighted the importance of this responsiveness falling within 'mid-range contingency' in which parents are able to balance their own emotional regulation as well as being able to support the infant's emotional regulation. Provision of this attuned response for the infant has been shown to have positive impact on their relationship with their parent.[22] However, a parent's capacity to provide attuned responsiveness can be influenced by a number of factors, as we will go on to explore.

## RUPTURE AND REPAIR

It is important to recognise that, although consistency and predictability of response form a core foundation of parent–infant interactions, it is unrealistic to expect any parent to maintain the same level of responsiveness regardless of demands in their internal and external environments. Consequently, there are moments when their responses will not be as nurturing or sensitive as usual. When these 'ruptures' take place, they provide an essential learning process for the developing infant. If the parent is able to recognise these departures from their customary responsive care, and 'repair' the interaction by reconnecting with their child's cues and responding in an attuned way, this cycle is likely to reinforce the secure nature of the relationship. It also allows the child to develop resilience in recognising that they can experience and survive these periods of rupture, secure in the knowledge that a safe base will continue to exist for them to return to an emotional equilibrium.[23]

There may be periods in which the rhythm of interaction is interrupted or inconsistent, due to a host of potential reasons which we shall go on to explore. The 'still face paradigm' was an experiment designed initially by Tronick, which requests a parent to interact animatedly with their baby and then to disengage, giving the baby a blank expression or 'still' face. The experiment demonstrates the almost immediate emotional dysregulation of infants when the anticipated interaction is removed, with the infant trying to reengage the parent and becoming increasingly distressed in their unsuccessful attempts.[24] Although this is often linked to potential disruption to sensitive interactions due to parental mental health difficulties, there is also a growing awareness of the potential impact of parental distraction and disengagement due to the use of technology,[25] which has become a societal norm across many cultures over recent years.

## THEORIES OF EMOTIONAL DEVELOPMENT

### Ecological systems theory

In order to consider those factors which influence the interactions and connections that an infant will make, we can refer briefly to Bronfenbrenner's Ecological Systems Theory. Bronfenbrenner described that there are five layers of ecological systems around a child. From the micro system, which encompasses the direct environment of family and friends, through wider social and cultural contexts, the theory highlights that all systems will interact with each other, as well as with the child, to exert influence across all areas of development.[26] The construct allows consideration of the breadth of influencers upon the infant as well as recognition of the scope for intervention when difficulties arise.

### Attachment theory

Attachment theory differs in that it places the core influential relationship of the infant on the primary caregiver. Infants are born with the neural pathways in place to recognise their own mother's voice and to be comforted by the scent of her breast milk,[27] which are inherent biological features to support the early development of a relationship between parent and child. Bonding is the emotional connection between parent and child. In some instances, this may develop shortly after birth, with some mothers describing the process of 'falling in love' with their baby as something which happened without conscious thought. For other mothers, this process may take longer, particularly if there are factors which impact, such as a traumatic birth or a mother's own experience of being parented (which we shall go on to explore further).

Although often used interchangeably, bonding is inherently different to attachment. Bonding is a process that a parent undertakes in connecting with their baby; however, attachment is a mechanism which the infant develops in response to their interactions with their caregivers and the caregiving environment.

Attachment theory emerged from the seminal work of John Bowlby and Mary Ainsworth in the 1960s, in understanding children's distress when separated from their main caregiver. Attachment theory describes the deep and enduring emotional connection between child and caregiver and is essentially a survival mechanism, designed to equip the child with the tools necessary to navigate the emotional environment within which they are raised.

Attachment patterns will also form a basis for how the child will go on to experience their sense of self and other relationships. The patterns of interaction with their primary caregiver, and the responses that they come to anticipate across a range of emotional circumstances, will determine the template upon which the child will map their future interactions. These form the underpinnings of 'internal working models' which allow the child to recognise, interpret and respond to the behavioural patterns of those around them.[28]

Attachment classifications were developed by Ainsworth as a result of observations of infant behaviours in the Strange Situation task.[29] These classifications are still in use today and form a basis for our understanding of how attachment might present in practice. The core aspects of how attachment patterns might arise and manifest are outlined in Table 14.1, but it is essential

### TABLE 14.1
### Attachment categorisations

| Attachment style | Caregiver response | Infant/child behaviour | Possible internal working models for infant/child |
|---|---|---|---|
| Secure attachment | Sensitive, responsive, consistent, attuned, reliable. For example, prompt comforting when child is distressed, warm interested response to infant's wish to communicate or play | Able to regulate emotions, seek help from others when distressed, adaptable to changing circumstances and able to explore the world | Feels worthy of attention and can depend on others for comfort if needed. Feels confident to explore the world around them and knows that distress can be survived. |
| Insecure (avoidant) | Connected enough to protect the infant; minimises the importance of attachment issues; can be dismissive of infant's attachment cues; insensitive to infant's signals and emotional needs. Distant, irritated, anxious | Shows little distress on separation and minimal joy when reunited with caregiver; avoidance of emotional intimacy and defensive focus on exploration. Does not seek out physical contact. Indiscriminate about who they interact with. | Does not expect or depend on comfort from others to regulate emotions. World feels safer if depend on self. |
| Insecure (ambivalent/resistant) | Inconsistent or unpredictable emotional availability and responses to infant's emotional needs. For example, at times overprotective or overstimulating and at other times rejecting or ignoring. | Overly engaged with attachment figure and may feel too anxious about caregiver's emotional availability to freely explore the environment. | Can never be sure if needs will be met. Self-worth dependent on reassurance from others but hard to trust positive regard. |
| Disorganised insecure attachment | Unresponsive, intrusive, hostile or violent. These parents may have experienced trauma themselves. | Chaotic and confusing behaviour; e.g., hypervigilant, freeze or fear when parent appears. | Sense of self and world constantly changing and overwhelming. No opportunity to lay down models of interaction. |

Holland & Coull, 2020 Adapted from[29,32]

to recognise that, although classifications can be helpful in understanding patterns of relationships and behaviour, there is not an inevitable, causal relationship between insecure or disorganised attachment and later psychopathology. It is recognised that early attachment difficulties, and the internal working models that might arise from them, can heighten the risk of later emergence of mental and even physical health difficulties.[30] However, there are many other factors which will interact to determine the ultimate developmental trajectory.[31]

## PARENTAL REPRESENTATIONS

A parent's own experience of being parented and their own attachment patterns will have significant impact on how they perceive their child and on the interactions they initiate. Parents develop mental representations of their baby before and during pregnancy, which can go on to impact on their interactions and relationship with their infant. Representations link closely with a parent's capacity to mentalise – to be able to think about their own internal state as well as their baby's emotional mental state – which is a core foundation for the development of attuned interactions and a secure relationship. Multiple factors will impact on mentalisation capacity, including parental mental well-being, the support network around them and their own representations of being a parent. Parents who have unresolved traumas from their own childhood are likely to find it more difficult to mentalise for themselves and their child. This can impact the interactions they engage in with their child, a process that has been described as 'ghosts in the nursery'.[33] The converse of this however, 'angels in the nursery',[34] describes the transmission of resilience and nurture, arising from parental experience of one positive attachment relationship in childhood, even in the context of other traumas.

### Case study 14.1: Ghosts and angels in the nursery

Sarah is mother to 3-month-old Eliza. Eliza is a thriving, engaging baby and the health visitor has been delighted to observe the attuned and sensitive interactions between Sarah and Eliza which characterise their developing relationship.

Sarah has spoken of her own childhood being fraught and unpredictable. Sarah's mother had significant mental health difficulties, which meant that she was not present, emotionally or physically, for long periods of time. Sarah's parents had a very volatile relationship and although her father was largely absent, Sarah remembers him as an intimidating man who was verbally aggressive towards her as well as her mother.

Sarah has spoken to her health visitor about wanting to do things differently from her parents and her wish to give Eliza the best start she can. She relayed her fears, in the first weeks of Eliza's life, that she too would become unwell and let down Eliza as she herself felt let down by her parents.

Sarah has described her maternal grandmother as her 'rock', as she stepped in to take care of Sarah during those periods when her mother was unable to. The health visitor observed Sarah singing a lullaby to Eliza, and the warmth of the shared gaze between mother and infant. When she described this interaction to Sarah, Sarah recalled that her grandmother used to sing the same lullaby to her, and it still helps her to feel safe and calm. Her face lit up with the recognition that it had the same effect on Eliza.

Despite the 'ghosts' of Sarah's early history trying to gain presence in her new motherhood, Sarah's resilience, harboured from the sensitive care and safe base she received from her grandmother, is allowing her to write a fresh pathway for her and her infant daughter.

The capacity to mentalise is linked with 'high reflective function', which describes a parent's ability to communicate to their baby that they recognise that they might have a different mental state to themselves.[35] This is closely related to 'mind-mindedness', which is a parent's capacity to interpret what their baby is thinking and feeling.[36] Also related is 'parental sensitivity', which requires the parent to see the infant as a separate entity with different emotional experiences, and to 'read' the cues that the infant portrays.[37] If we consider these abilities in the context of parent–infant interaction, it is intuitive to infer that those parents with high reflective function, mind-mindedness and sensitivity will be best placed to accurately interpret their infant's cues and to respond appropriately in helping their infant manage the emotions they are relaying. Unsurprisingly therefore, these constructs have been shown to have clear links with positive attachment and further positive developmental outcomes.[36]

## RISK FACTORS THAT IMPACT ON INFANT AND CHILD EMOTIONAL AND MENTAL HEALTH, WELL-BEING AND DEVELOPMENT

As we have explored over preceding pages, the human brain adapts and develops, for better or for worse, according to the quality of its environment of human relationships and experiences. The building blocks for healthy emotional development are dependent on secure, loving, sensitive and responsive relationships from conception.

We shall go on to discuss those parental factors which can impact significantly upon a child's developmental pathway. However, it is important to acknowledge first that by the very nature of being grounded in a two-way transactional process, the infant will also influence the relationship. Human infants are born with an innate temperament, the nature of which will interact with their parent's temperament to elicit patterns of responses. In addition, factors such as prematurity and chronic child health conditions can have a substantial impact upon parental representations and the developing parent–child relationship.

Human ethology assumes that parenting behaviours are pre-programmed and ready to develop when conditions elicit them. However, not all parenting behaviour patterns manifest automatically but are learnt through experiences, examples or education.[32] Indeed, not all parents are able to respond and engage positively with their child due to complex factors such as poor parental mental health, substance misuse and domestic violence or dysfunctional family relationships. As a result, infants can experience disruption that interferes with the development of secure relationships, thereby resulting in an increased risk of poor attachment and negative long-term physical and psychological outcomes. These factors are known as adverse childhood experiences (ACEs) and increase the risk of child abuse and neglect.[38]

Frequent, excessive or prolonged adversity experienced in utero and the first 3 years of life can seriously damage the developing brain, resulting in short and long-term disturbances in cognitive and emotional outcomes, including behavioural problems.[39] Evidence from the National Scientific Council on the Developing Child[40] indicates how adverse experiences trigger various levels of stress as the body's stress responses of 'fight or flight' deal with the threat (see Table 14.2). This results in physiological reactions, including increased heart rate, a rise in blood pressure and elevated levels of stress hormones. This can be short-lived, as in the case of 'positive' stress, where a child may experience stress as a result of receiving a vaccine injection, or longer-lasting 'tolerable' stress triggered by a frightening accident or the loss of a loved one. The body's responses to the effects of stress can be tolerated and over time return to normal when buffered by a caring, sensitive and responsive adult who can support the child with learning how to cope and adapt to stressful situations. Experience of certain amounts of stress is normal and essential for healthy child development, as they learn the skills needed to manage stress and develop resilience.[41] In the absence of

### TABLE 14.2
### Three categories of stress[40]

| Type of stress | Examples |
| --- | --- |
| **Positive stress**<br>Results from early childhood experiences causing short-lived minor physiological changes including increased heart rate and mild changes in hormone levels. With sensitive, responsive caregiving, children learn how to manage and overcome stress. | ■ receiving an immunisation<br>■ meeting new people<br>■ first day with a new carer<br>■ coping with adult set routines and boundaries<br>■ experiencing frustrations<br>■ mastering separation |
| **Tolerable stress**<br>More intense stress as a result of more severe longer-lasting difficulties. Activates the body's alert systems to greater degree. When stress is buffered by a supportive adult relationship, children learn to adapt, and the body's alert systems recover. Can become positive stress and benefit child development if a caring adult is consistently available to support and buffer the effects of stress. Where adult support is lacking tolerable stress can become toxic stress and negatively impact health and development. | ■ a frightening accident<br>■ natural disasters<br>■ family separation or divorce<br>■ the loss of a loved one<br>■ an act of terrorism |
| **Toxic stress**<br>Results from intense, frequent and/or prolonged adverse experiences over weeks, months or years. Can disrupt the development of brain architecture and other organ systems, increase the risk for stress-related disease and cognitive impairment, well into the adult years. | ■ maltreatment<br>■ physical abuse<br>■ sexual abuse<br>■ emotional abuse<br>■ chronic neglect<br>■ exposure to domestic violence<br>■ caregiver substance abuse<br>■ caregiver mental health illness<br>■ burdens of family economic hardship |

a protective adult buffer, stress management responses can become strong and prolonged, with persistent elevations of stress hormones and key brain chemicals resulting in toxic stress and alterations in the developing brain. Toxic stress can lead to cognitive and emotional difficulties, and in the longer-term can affect the immune and metabolic systems, causing mental health problems, such as depression and anxiety, and stress-related chronic diseases, such as heart disease, hypertension and diabetes.

## THE IMPACT OF PARENTAL MENTAL HEALTH DIFFICULTIES ON INFANT AND CHILD EMOTIONAL MENTAL HEALTH AND WELL-BEING

The perinatal period describes the period of time between pregnancy, childbirth and the first year after the birth. At least 1 in every 10 postnatal women are affected by mental health disorders, and at least 13% experience depression and anxiety in the perinatal period.[42] There is a correlation between maternal and paternal postnatal depression with 1 in 10 men experiencing anxiety and depression following the birth of their baby.[43] Fathers are known to experience anxiety and depression during the transition to fatherhood[44] with between 4% and 25% of new fathers reporting an experience of postpartum (the period up to 6 weeks following child birth) depression, although the prevalence may be underreported due to difficulties in recognising postpartum depression in men. A recent review found between 5% and 15% of men were affected by anxiety disorder in the postnatal period.[45]

During the perinatal period infant brain growth is at its greatest and healthy development is reliant on loving, attuned, responsive parenting, yet some parents, affected by poor mental health, may less likely be emotionally available, responsive to infant cues, or engage in attuned, timely and consistent interactions. Extended periods of disrupted interactions can create barriers to the development of secure infant attachments, and in severe cases increase the risk of toxic stress.[46]

Research indicates the potential implications of poor parental mental health on the emotional health and well-being of children. Stein et al.[47] conducted a review of evidence exploring the impact of anxiety and depression on the foetus and child. The review indicated a correlation between antenatal depression and premature delivery (<37 weeks' gestation). Prematurity can be a major factor of behavioural dysregulation and can result in feeding difficulties, irregular sleeping problems and unpredictable crying behaviour. Problems in infancy can worsen and continue into the preschool years and beyond, impacting on regulation difficulties in the long term.[48] Some research suggests an association between stress and depression in pregnancy and increased risk of a disorganised pattern of attachment,[47] neurodevelopmental problems including anxiety and depression, attention deficit hyperactivity disorder and autism spectrum disorder.[49,50]

Beyond the perinatal period, parental mental health continues to impact upon the developing child. Preschool children whose parents have a diagnosed mental health difficulty are almost three times more likely to themselves have diagnosable mental health difficulties than those whose parents do not have poor mental health.[6] The mechanisms of this association are a complex interplay of familial, social and environmental factors, with short and long-term impact across domains of child development.[51]

## THE IMPACT OF DOMESTIC VIOLENCE AND ABUSE ON INFANT AND CHILD EMOTIONAL MENTAL HEALTH AND WELL-BEING

Domestic violence and abuse or intermate partner violence (IPV) include acts of physical, sexual, emotional, psychological and controlling behaviours by those who are or have been intimate partners or family members.[52] IPV occurs in heterosexual and same-sex relationships and is perpetrated by both men and women, but women are more likely to be victims of IPV perpetrated by men.[53] A recent survey indicated that an estimated 1.3 million (7.9%) of women and girls aged over 16 and 695,000 (4.2%) of men and boys aged over 16 years were victims of IPV.[54] Evidence indicates substantially higher rates of IPV during the perinatal period and the risks increase where mental health problems[55] and substance misuse[56] co-occur. The consequences of IPV against women are significant, resulting in physical, emotional and psychological problems with increased risk of suicide and death.[52] During pregnancy IPV can result in increased risk of miscarriage, stillbirth, premature birth, low birth weight, physical malformation and mental health problems.

Victims of IPV may experience physical abuse and mental health problems, such as anxiety and depression. This can impact on parental regulation, responsiveness and sensitivity towards their child and cause disruptions in the development of a positive parent–infant relationship. The perinatal period is a time when a woman's normative maternal representations about her child and self as a mother develop. Caregiving systems designed to facilitate protective and nurturing parenting develop at this time, however this does not develop equally in all women. In the case of domestic violence, for example, this can result in women feeling helpless to protect their child or themselves from danger, thereby increasing the risk of adverse childhood outcomes, abuse and neglect. Children who witness domestic violence in the home are not only exposed to an increased risk of physical abuse themselves from 'being caught in the crossfire' or perhaps trying to prevent the violence, but also experience high levels of emotional stress from seeing and hearing violence, and may live in constant fear.

Children experience chronic toxic stress as a result of exposure to IPV. Under-fives are especially vulnerable to adversity, due to the plasticity of their developing brain. In the absence of a reliable non-violent caregiving buffer, the architecture of the developing brain can become seriously damaged resulting in short- and long-term disturbances in cognitive, emotional and behavioural outcomes. As a consequence, children can experience anxiety, depression, delays in achieving developmental milestones, and poor performance at school.[57] Evidence indicates an association between exposure to IPV against the mother, perpetrated by the male partner, and female experience of IPV later in life.[58,59]

## THE IMPACT OF SUBSTANCE ABUSE OR MISUSE ON INFANT AND CHILD EMOTIONAL MENTAL HEALTH AND WELL-BEING

Substance abuse or misuse refers to the continued misuse of harmful or hazardous psychoactive substances, including alcohol and illicit drugs. Dependency on substances can result in behavioural, cognitive, and physiological problems due to regular continued use, difficulties in controlling its use, increased tolerance, symptoms of withdrawal and placing priority on drug use rather than other activities and obligations.[60] People use substances for many reasons; for example, to relax, for pleasure or a way of coping with problems, such as their own traumatic childhood, although it does not make the problem go away. Parents who use alcohol or drugs in moderation are not necessarily a risk to their children, however, when the use of substances becomes the prime focus of a parent's attention as in substance misuse and addiction, it can affect parenting awareness and capacity to care for their child and act responsively to their emotional and physical needs. They may be unavailable, unpredictable, inconsistent, lacking in the capacity to provide a safe, loving and nurturing environment needed for healthy child development. With no available, reliable carer to buffer the effects, this can lead to chronic stress causing permanent changes to the developing brain, and impact on long-term neurological and physical development.[61]

Parental substance misuse is strongly associated with ACEs, placing children at increased risk of physical and emotional abuse or neglect. The use of substances such as alcohol – and illicit drugs such as cannabis, crack, cocaine, amphetamines, opiates and ecstasy – during pregnancy can lead to multiple serious physical and mental health outcomes, including stillbirth, prematurity, low birth weight, and long-term neurological damage and physical malformations.[11] Parental substance misuse in the postnatal period can adversely affect the parent–child relationship due to the impact on parenting capacity and problems that can co-occur with substance dependency, such as mental health problems, domestic violence, poverty, and chaotic and unpredictable environments.[62] The impact of substance misuse on children can vary according to their developmental age, personality, health and relationships within the household, and the trauma experienced can stretch beyond childhood into adulthood.

## SUMMARY

The importance of positive parent–infant/child relationships in promoting healthy child development in the early years has been discussed. Complex issues, such as perinatal mental health problems, IPV and substance misuse, can result in ACEs and increase the risk of abuse and neglect. Chronic stress resulting from ACEs can negatively impact on emotional, psychological and physiological development of infants and children and accelerate stress related disease.

Health visitors, because of their unique role of home visiting, work closely with families, implementing the principles of health visiting, building therapeutic relationships and working in partnership. Using expert communication skills health visitors identify health needs, stimulate awareness of health needs and can facilitate health-enhancing activities to support parents in building positive secure relationships with their infants and children. Where any risk of harm is suspected or identified local safeguarding procedures must be followed. The following section of this chapter focuses on interventions aimed at improving infant/child attachment and the parent–infant/child relationship from conception to the age of five.

## RELATIONSHIP-BASED THERAPEUTIC INTERVENTIONS

There are many relationship-based therapeutic programmes available that focus on prevention and early intervention to encourage positive parenting and child interaction. Below you will find a brief discussion of some universal and targeted programmes. These have been presented as: (1) programmes that promote attachment and parental sensitivity, and (2) programmes that promote emotional, social and behaviour development.[63] The list is not exhaustive and there will likely be some crossover. For more information see the Early Intervention Foundation (EIF) website https://www.eif.org.uk/report/the-best-start-at-home and the NHS Education for Scotland Early Intervention Framework for Children and Young People's Mental Health and Mental Wellbeing http://earlyinterventionframework.nhs.scot/.

## PROGRAMMES THAT PROMOTE ATTACHMENT AND PARENTAL SENSITIVITY

### Group-based programmes

The EIF highlights the family foundations programme (FFP) as an evidence-based group psycho-educational programme that provides education, training and support to parents to build their confidence and transition to parenthood. The aim is to promote secure attachments as parents gain insight about their own emotional needs and the needs of their new baby. Right from the Start (RFTS) is another group-based intervention that focuses on enhancing attunement between parents and infants whereby parents recognise and respond appropriately to infant cues. RFTS uses videos of parent–infant interaction to stimulate discussion and shared learning. The FFP is provided during the perinatal period and RFTS commences during the postnatal stage and both are typically delivered during 2-hour sessions over 8 to 9 weeks. Qualified professionals such as health visitors and midwives deliver the FFP; however RFTS is delivered by a specialist with a background in education psychology, early childhood education and experience in education and intervention with families of infants at risk.

### Home-visiting programmes

The Family Nurse Partnership (FNP) is an intensive evidence-based early childhood home visiting-based programme for vulnerable first-time mothers under the age of 19 years (or up to 25 years in Scotland if further vulnerability factors are present). Structured home visits commence antenatally and continue until the child reaches the age of two. The programme is aimed at improving pregnancy outcomes, child health and development, parental physical and mental health, parenting skills and social networks. It is delivered by specially trained family nurses who build therapeutic relationships with the family, working in a strength-based approach to meet the needs of parents and infants. The programme is underpinned by the theories of attachment, ecology and self-efficacy. American-based research suggests the programme has a positive impact on a wide range of parenting and child outcomes, including improved prenatal health behaviours, birth outcomes, sensitive childcare, and reduced child injuries, abuse and neglect.[64] UK research is following up findings of an RCT of FNP in England in 2015 and a recent Scottish study on the value of FNP concluded that FNP in Scotland impacts consistently, showing improvements across domains of parent and child health and well-being.[65]

Minding the Baby is a home-visiting programme aimed at first-time mothers, between the ages of 14 and 25 years, from the third trimester until the child reaches 2 years of age. It focuses on improving reflective functioning of mothers experiencing problems during the perinatal period for example, child protection issues, depression, substance misuse, homelessness, poverty and violent relationships. It focusses on the construct of mentalisation,[66] which involves holding the child in mind through parental reflective functioning. This aids in understanding the child's thoughts and feelings and behaviours as mental states. The programme is delivered for an hour a week by a qualified nurse and social worker who provide guidance on child development, parenting skills and crisis intervention. Evidence indicates that the programme is effective in promoting secure infant attachment to mothers by the age of 1.[67]

## PROGRAMMES INVOLVING LIVE DEMONSTRATIONS

The Newborn Behavioural Observation (NBO) Scale is an evidence-based observation of infant behavioural responses and development in partnership with parents. It involves demonstration of infant perceptual and interactive capabilities by a trained practitioner such as a health visitor or midwife. The aim is to enable parents to gain an understanding of their infant's abilities, strengths and challenges and to formulate caregiving strategies to meet the needs of the baby. It is delivered in the home from birth to 3 months of age and can be used with babies from 35 weeks' gestation and developmentally delayed babies. Evidence suggests that the NBO enables parents to learn about their new babies and become sensitive to their needs, thereby supporting the development of a positive parent–infant relationship.[68] (See Case study 14.2: Implementing the NBO.)

Evidence-based video feedback techniques to promote positive parenting have been found to positively impact on parental sensitivity and secure attachment. Video-feedback Intervention to Promote Positive Parenting, Circle of Security and Attachment and Bio-Behavioural Catch-Up (ABC) programmes are highlighted by the EIF report as home-based interventions targeting children at risk of maltreatment. These techniques aim to help parents understand their infant's or child's capabilities with a view of enabling parents to recognise cues and respond in an attuned and timely way to their child. The programmes are delivered by health visitors, midwives or social workers who video tape 10 minutes of interaction between the parents and infant/child, then subsequently returning to examine video recordings with the parent pointing out examples of positive parenting. The duration of the programmes varies from 10 1-hour sessions to 20 weekly 75-minute sessions.[63]

## MEDIA-BASED METHODS

Media-based methods have been developed to provide good evidence-based information to parents during the first few years of their child's life. They include information about the communication strategies of babies and help parents in understanding and recognising appropriate, timely responses to encourage and promote the development of positive relationships and healthy child development. Media-based methods include providing information related to the child's age through a newsletter or resource packs and/or books and DVDs/videos. The EIF highlight the Baby Express newsletter and the Social Baby DVD as evidence-based media information sources shown to positively improve parental sensitivity and attachment security.

The Baby Buddy app, created by Best Beginnings,[69] is an evidence-based pregnancy and parenting app that is now available via the NHS Apps Library. The app aims to provide support to parents during and after pregnancy; it monitors physical health and aims to empower parents and build confidence in parenting. An evaluation survey of the first 46,000 downloads of the app indicated that users learnt more about their pregnancy and felt closer to their baby.[70]

## BABY MASSAGE

Over the last 30 years, baby massage has become widely implemented throughout Western cultures to support parental sensitivity and promote bonding and attachment. Touch plays an essential role in forming early parent–child relationships. The types of touch facilitated through massage helps parents to express and develop emotional connections and increases awareness of their baby's cues.[71] Babies may find massage too stimulating in the early weeks, so it is recommended from 6 weeks onwards. Trained practitioners with various qualifications, such as health visitors and nursery nurses, have been trained to teach baby massage in the home, it is also delivered in small groups involving weekly classes of 1 hour over 4 to 6 weeks.

There is not yet robust evidence to support the use of baby massage with low-risk families and the available evidence supporting its use in promoting maternal sensitivity has been criticised due to significant problems in evaluation design.[72] A lack of high-quality evidence does not mean baby massage is not beneficial; indeed, many parents and babies enjoy the experience. However, further research is recommended.

### Case study 14.2: Implementing the NBO

As a Flying Start health visitor practising in Wales, I visited the home of a Polish couple to undertake a pre-arranged routine primary birth visit. Mother Ava, and father Stephan, both understood and spoke some English and declined an interpreter. Baby Anna was the couple's first child, she was 10 days of age, healthy, breast-feeding well and gaining weight. As part of the primary birth visit, I gained consent to perform Brazelton's Newborn Behavioural Observation (NBO). This involved 18 neurobehavioural observations of Anna in partnership with her parents and included observing her capacity to habituate to external light and sound stimuli, quality of motor tone and activity level, capacity for self-regulation, responses to stress, visual and auditory and social interactive capacities. As the NBO involves the need to elicit stimuli through hands-on manoeuvres (and the use of NBO equipment, that is a red ball, bell, rattle and a small torch), I have always found it a perfect way to observe and demonstrate an infant's uniquenesses, challenges and communications techniques in partnership with parents where English is not a first language.

On arrival at the home Anna was in her mother's arms in a drowsy, semi-alert state. Her mother said she had been sleeping. Together, with Anna's father sat nearby, we observed Anna move smoothly into a quiet alert state. This suggested Anna was able to transition smoothly through behavioural states, regulating her emotions, which I highlighted as a strength when explaining this to her parents. Anna was in a perfect state of alertness to perform some of the NBO. Performing an NBO can take anything between 5 minutes to an hour, depending on the infant's behaviour, the parents' needs, my goals for the session and the nature of my relationship with the parents. This was the first time I had met the family and I found performing the NBO enhanced my relationship with the parents as they put their trust in me as they watched me gently handle Anna, while praising her and them as parents, sharing in their sense of pride.

The NBO created a good opportunity to role-model handling and gentle safe stimulation as together we observed her behavioural preferences and vulnerabilities. Anna's parents were engaged in the experience and able to tell me some her of likes and dislikes while I performed manoeuvres. This demonstrated to me how much they already knew about their baby and that they were beginning to understand her communication signals and her needs. Together with her parents we observed how she was able to fix on and follow my face and a red ball (visual capacity), and turn to the sound of a rattle and her mother's voice (auditory capacity). Both parents seemed overjoyed to see their baby's responses. They said the word 'normal' with huge smiles on their faces, while looking at their baby adoringly. It was a joyous moment for me to observe how they interacted with Anna, showing such pride in her.

I performed manoeuvres to observe Anna's muscle tone and reflexes and while I did this I was able to talk about different aspects of Anna's development. I talked about protecting Anna's head, as I performed the pull-to-sit manoeuvre to observe shoulder and neck tone, and I promoted tummy time and safe sleeping as I placed Anna on her stomach to elicit the crawling response. Her crawling response was very strong and her parents were amazed on observing it. Anna was calm and seemed content to be handled throughout the observation; however, I explained to her parents that should she cry at any point we would stop the observation so her parents could sooth her if needed. Had this happened it would have facilitated an opportunity to observe how her parents soothed her and whether Anna was able sooth herself. When performing the NBO I always take the baby as I find them and a crying baby is a perfect opportunity to discuss crying, types of cries and soothing techniques and to observe how parents respond to their crying baby. As a health visitor it is a good time to show empathy, discuss support networks and very sensitively highlight the risks of shaking a baby.

After approximately 15 minutes Anna became actively alert and began rooting. Her father said she needed to feed. It was wonderful to see how Stephan and Ava were already attuned to Anna's feeding cues. As Anna fed from her mother's breast, Ava was happy for me to observe her feeding. Ava told me she was happy with breast-feeding and enjoying the experience. I was able to assess attachment and positioning and pointed out how well Ava had positioned Anna and how well she had attached to the breast, sucking strongly.

During the visit I had completed many aspects of the NBO, in partnership with the parents. Together we observed Anna's strengths and challenges and I gave anticipatory guidance while performing manoeuvres and role-modelling. I was able to observe how the parent–infant relationship was developing positively as Ava and Stephan already knew so much about their baby and responded to her communication signals and needs. I also felt that we had begun to develop a therapeutic relationship as they put their trust in me to handle Anna and we talked openly about her development, health and safety.

## PROGRAMMES THAT PROMOTE EMOTIONAL, SOCIAL AND BEHAVIOURAL DEVELOPMENT

### Group-based programmes

The Solihull Approach parenting group is a universal group parenting programme, based on the Solihull Approach, which integrates psychotherapy and behavioural concepts aimed at supporting parents with their child's social, emotional and behavioural development.[73] The Solihull Approach incorporates three concepts of containment, reciprocity and behaviour management. Containment is where a person contains their perturbed feelings and communicates their emotions in a way that restores their capacity to think without feeling overwhelmed. Reciprocity refers to the parent's ability to appropriately interpret their infant's cues and respond sensitively, engaging in the serve and return dance of interaction. Behaviour management refers to the parent's ability to harness these aspects in supporting their child's behaviour. The aim of the programme is for parents to develop the ability to contain their infant's or child's emotions through reciprocity and develop positive parenting strategies, while feeling supported by the professional.[74]

The suite of parenting groups have relevant programmes both antenatally and postnatally and include online resources. The groups are typically delivered over 2-hour sessions and run over 10 weeks. The groups are mostly led by educational psychologists, psychologists or professionals with a BA/Masters degree. The effectiveness of the Solihull group is supported by formative evidence; however, RCT trials are currently underway.

Mellow Parenting is a programme targeting parents who are hard to reach, experiencing child protection concerns, family violence, mental health difficulties and poverty. The programme helps parents to reflect on their own experiences and it uses videos and direct work with parents and children to explore problems. It focuses on building parental strengths and aims to improve parental understanding of their infant/child and improve interaction, communication and play. The programme is delivered by trained practitioners and offered from the antenatal period up to the age of five. Delivery consists of 14 5-hour weekly sessions in groups of six parents in a community setting. Research indicates positive effects in mother–child interaction, maternal well-being and child development and behaviour, with sustained effects and some further improvement 1 year on.[75]

## PROFESSIONAL ROLES IN SUPPORTING POSITIVE ATTACHMENTS

As has become evident over preceding pages, the sensitive, responsive care of a consistent caregiver is a core factor in supporting an infant or young child towards optimal brain development and a positive mental health trajectory. For many parents, however, providing this care can be challenging, for the variety of reasons which we have explored. As a professional working closely with a young family, health visitors are in a position to support this caregiver–child relationship and scaffold caregiver recognition of their role in shaping their child's emotional well-being.

## CONTAINMENT

Containment is the process by which an individual receives and understands the emotional communication of another, without being overwhelmed by it, and communicates this back to the other person. This process can restore the capacity to think in an individual previously overwhelmed[73].

A core facet of an infant's development of emotional regulation capacity is the experience of having their emotions recognised, acknowledged and tolerated by a caregiver. This is also true for adults, and particularly pertinent for those who are emotionally overwhelmed. If a professional is able to listen, empathise and acknowledge the emotions that a caregiver is trying to manage, without trying to minimise or jump in to solutions, they can support the caregiver to feel less overwhelmed and more emotionally available to providing their child with the support to manage their sense of distress.

In order for professionals to be able to provide containment to their clients, they themselves need to have the emotional space to help process difficult feelings. Appropriate supervision and self-care are essential components of being able to provide containment to others.

## PROVIDING THE EXPERIENCE OF A SAFE, NURTURING RELATIONSHIP

Many caregivers will have had little or no experience themselves of being held within the unconditional positive regard of a nurturing caregiver.

They may have never experienced what a safe base looks or feels like and their own attachment patterns and templates for relationships might make it very difficult for them to develop or sustain relationships with others. Health visitors have an opportunity to demonstrate to caregivers what this can look like in practice. They can model the maintenance of appropriate boundaries, the dance of serve and return interactions and the stability of a professional relationship even in the face of challenges. The impact of this investment by their health visitor upon a caregiver's sense of worth cannot be overestimated.

## OBSERVING, DESCRIBING AND BEING CURIOUS

One of the most powerful tools that professionals can use with caregivers and infants is simply observing the patterns of interactions which take place across family relationships. Being able to describe how an infant might gaze at their caregiver and expressing curiosity about their internal world can open the caregiver's mind to the possibility that their child seeks their response and might have thoughts and feelings separate to themselves.

## UNDERSTANDING CHILD DEVELOPMENT AND APPROPRIATE EXPECTATIONS

In order to appropriately interpret and respond to a child's cues, a caregiver must have a sense of what they might expect with regard to their child's developmental pathway. If a caregiver's expectations of their child's responses are set either too high or too low, it will be more challenging for them to pitch their interactions at a level that is appropriate to fully engage with their child.

Being able to lend insight into child development can support caregivers to set their expectations of their child at a realistic level and allow them to more successfully engage with their child in ways that their child can respond to, paving the way for serve and return interactions.

## HARNESSING A SENSE OF WONDER

Closely linked to observing and scaffolding expectations lies the capacity for a professional to be able to voice the wonder of the developing infant or child. For many caregivers, particularly those overwhelmed with the tasks upon them, or those who are caught in the difficult representations of their own experiences of being parented, it may feel like little joy is present in their caregiving role. If a trusted professional is able to marvel at their child and reinforce their parental role in creating this developing human, this can have potential to allow caregivers to also recognise the wonder that might exist alongside the very real challenges of parenting.

## MODELLING, IN PARTICULAR PLAY

Play is known to be one of the most beneficial ways of harnessing shared enjoyment between parent and child. There will be many caregivers however, particularly those who themselves have not experienced positive parental relationships, who might not know how to play with their child, how to share enjoyment of a book or toy with an infant or what responding to an infant's cues might look like in practice. By involving the infant or child, along with other children in the family, in contacts with the caregiver, a sense of how this might look and feel can develop for the caregiver within the safe environment of a professional relationship.

## FACILITATING APPROPRIATE SUPPORT FOR CAREGIVERS INDIVIDUALLY AND, WHERE APPROPRIATE, AS A COUPLE

Parenting is challenging for all caregivers, for a host of different reasons and at different stages for both caregiver and child. Appropriate support is essential, the extent of which cannot fall within the realm of one professional alone, and a comprehensive assessment of what supports might be necessary and accessible for a family can ensure that caregivers are facilitated to engage with the most appropriate networks to lend them what they need to fulfil their parenting capacity.

In addition to appropriate supports for caregiver and child, both individually and as a dyad, consideration must also be given where relevant, to the relationship between the parental couple. Evidence is growing to support the concept that the parental relationship is a key factor in the development and maintenance of a child's emotional well-being,[76] and the professional role of being able to observe this relationship and explore its facets as well as identifying appropriate supports, can form an important aspect of involvement.

## THINKING SPACE

What networks or resources local to you might be available to link in with families to specifically support them in scaffolding positive interactions between caregiver and their children?

## CONCLUSION

This chapter has explored what is meant by IMH and why it has such impact on the trajectory of the developing child. We have presented an overview of brain architecture and considered core aspects of infant brain development and how these are impacted by experiences, for better or for worse.

Theories of emotional development help us gain an understanding of the important role parents and carers play in nurturing infant and child mental health and well-being. Evidence indicates how risk factors such as poor parental mental health, domestic abuse and substance misuse can interfere with the development of positive parent–infant/child relationships, and in severe cases result in ACEs, neglect and abuse. The role of the health visitor is key to early identification of risk factors that can impact on infant/child mental health and well-being. To support health visitor practice, relationship-based therapeutic intervention programmes, aimed at promoting bonding and attachment, and emotional, social and behavioural development are discussed. Through implementing the principles of health visiting, using expert communication skills, and knowledge gained from reading this chapter, health visitors can support parents with understanding their child's mental health development and through partnership working facilitate health enhancing activities.

### KEY LEARNING POINTS

- Positive infant and child mental health is highly influenced by the experiences of the infant in utero and across their earliest years.
- Infant humans are born with the capacity to make positive, resilient brain connections, and to do so they need to be provided with sensitive and nurturing interactions and care.
- The absence of attuned care, or the presence of a range of key potential risk factors in the infant's environment, can impact on the developing brain structure and on the child's ongoing developmental trajectory.
- There are a range of evidence-based therapeutic interventions which can be engaged with families to promote attachment and parental sensitivity to support positive mental health development.

■ The health visitor is in a position to be able to support positive infant and child mental health through their awareness of infant brain development and their roles in supporting positive relationships within the family.

## FURTHER RESOURCES

Centre on the Developing Child. https://developingchild.harvard.edu/

Association of Infant Mental Health. https://aimh.org.uk/

https://www.nhsinform.scot/ready-steady-baby

https://www.bbc.co.uk/tiny-happy-people

https://www.eif.org.uk/report/the-best-start-at-home

## REFERENCES

1. https://aimh.uk/why-infant-mental-health
2. https://parentinfantfoundation.org.uk/1001days
3. Winnicott, D. (1953). Transitional objects and transitional phenomena. *International Journal of Psychoanalysis, 34,* 89–97.
4. Egger, H. L., & Angold, A. (2006). Common emotional and behavioral disorders in preschool children: Presentation, nosology, and epidemiology. *J Child Psychol Psychiatry, 47*(3–4), 313–337.
5. Dougherty, L. R., Leppert, K. A., Merwin, S. M., et al. (2015). Advances and Directions in Preschool Mental Health Research. *Child Development Perspectives, 9*(1), 14–19.
6. Department of Health and Social Care in England. (2017). Mental health of children and young people in England.
7. https://heckmanequation.org/resource/invest-in-early-childhood-development-reduce-deficits-strengthen-the-economy/.
8. Konkel, L. (2018). The brain before birth: Using fMRI to explore the secrets of fetal neurodevelopment. *Environmental Health Perspectives, 126*(11), 112001.
9. Center on the Developing Child at Harvard University. (2011). *Building the Brain's 'Air Traffic Control' system: How early experiences shape the development of executive function*: Working Paper No. 11.
10. Glover, V. (2014). Maternal depression, anxiety and stress during pregnancy and child outcome; what needs to be done. *Best Practice Research in Clinical Obstetrics & Gynaecology, 28*(1), 25–350.
11. Ross, E. J., Graham, D. L., Money, K. M., & Stanwood, G. D. (2015). Developmental consequences of fetal exposure to drugs: What we know and what we still must learn. *Neuropsychopharmacology, 40*(1), 61–87.
12. McQuire, C., Mukherjee, R., Hurt, L., et al. (2019). Screening prevalence of fetal alcohol spectrum disorders in a region of the United Kingdom: A population-based birth-cohort study. *Prev Med, 118,* 344–351.
13. Linderkamp, O., Janus, L., Linder, R., & Skoruppa, D. B. (2009). Time table of normal foetal brain development. *International Journal of Prenatal and Perinatal Psychology and Medicine, 21,* 4–16.
14. Keysers, C., Gazzola, V. (2014). Hebbian learning and predictive mirror neurons for actions, sensations and emotions. *Philosophical Transactions of the Royal Society of London. Series B, Biological Sciences, 369*(1644), 20130175.
15. Ismail, F. Y., Fatemi, A., & Johnston, M. V. (2017). Cerebral plasticity: Windows of opportunity in the developing brain. *European Journal of Paediatric Neurology, 21*(1), 23–48.
16. Tierney, A., & Nelson, C., III. (2009) Brain development and the role of experience in the early years. *Zero Three,* 30(2): 9–13.
17. Blakemore, S. J., & Choudhury, S. (2006). Development of the adolescent brain: Implications for executive function and social cognition. *Journal of Child Psychology and Psychiatry, 47,* 296–312.
18. National Scientific Council on Developing Child. (2012). The science of neglect: The persistent absence of responsive care disrupts the developing brain. Working Paper 12. http://www.developingchild.harvard.edu.
19. Harlow, H. F., Dodsworth, R. O., & Harlow, M. K. (1965). Total social isolation in monkeys. *Proceedings of the National Academy of Sciences of the United States of America.*
20. Malloch, S. N. (1999). Mothers and infants and communicative musicality. *Musicae Scientiae, 3,* 29–57.
21. Beebe, B., & Lachmann, F. (2014). Relational perspectives book series. The origins of attachment: Infant research and adult treatment.
22. Beebe, B., Jaffe, J., Markese, S., et al. (2010). The origins of 12-month attachment: A microanalysis of 4-month mother–infant interaction. *Attachment & Human Development, 12,* 3–141.
23. Tronick, E. (1989). Emotions and Emotional Communication in Infants. *The American Psychologist, 44,* 112–119.
24. Tronick, E., Adamson, L., Als, H., & Brazelton, T. (1975). Infant emotions in normal and perturbated interactions. *Paper presented at the biennial meeting of the Society for Research in Child Development, Denver, CO.*
25. McDaniel, B. T. (2019). Parent distraction with phones, reasons for use, and impacts on parenting and child outcomes: A review of the emerging research. *Human Behaviour & Emerging Technology, 1,* 72–78r.

26. Bronfenbrenner, U. (1979). *The ecology of human development*. Harvard University Press.

27. Nishitani, S., Miyamura, T., Tagawa, M., Sumi, M., et al. (2008). The calming effect of a maternal breast milk odor on the human newborn infant. *Neuroscience Research, 63*, 66–71.

28. Bowlby, J. (1979). *The making and breaking of affectional bonds*. London, UK: Tavistock.

29. Ainsworth, M. S., Blehar, M., Waters, E., & Wall, S. (1978). *Patterns of Attachment: A Psychological Study of the Strange Situation*. Hillsdale, NJ: Erlbaum.

30. Mikulincer, M., & Shaver, P. R. (2012). An attachment perspective on psychopathology. *World Psychiatry, 11*(1), 11–15.

31. Sroufe, L. A. (2005). Attachment and development: A prospective, longitudinal study from birth to adulthood. *Attachment & Human Development, 7*, 349–367.

32. Bowlby, J. (1988). *A secure base*. USA: Routledge.

33. Fraiberg, S., Adelson, E., & Shapiro, V. (1975). Ghosts in the nursery: A psychoanalytic approach to the problems of impaired infant–mother relationships. *Journal of American Academy of Child Psychiatry, 14*(3), 387–421.

34. Lieberman, A. F., Padrón, E., Van Horn, P., & Harris, W. W. (2005). Angels in the nursery: The intergenerational transmission of benevolent parental influences. *Infant Mental Health Journal, 26*, 504–520.

35. Fonagy, P., Steele, M., Steele, H., et al. (1991). The capacity for understanding mental states: The reflective self in parent and child and its significance for security of attachment. *Infant Mental Health Journal, Infant Mental Health Journal, 12*, 201–218.

36. Meins, E., Fernyhough, C., Wainwright, R., Das Gupta, M., et al. (2002). Maternal mind-mindedness and attachment security as predictors of theory of mind understanding. *Child Development, 73*(6), 1715–1726.

37. Ainsworth, M. S. (1979). Infant–mother attachment. *American Psychologist, 34*(10), 932–937.

38. Bellis, M. A., Hughes, K., Ford, K., et al. (2018). Adverse childhood experiences and sources of childhood resilience: A retrospective study of their combined relationships with child health and education attendance. *BMC Public Health, 18*, 792.

39. De Bellis, M. D., & Zisk, A. (2014). The biological effects of child trauma. *Child and Adolescent Psychiatric Clinics of North America, 23*(2), 185–222.

40. National Scientific Council on the Developing Child. (2005). Excessive stress disrupts the architecture of the developing brain. Working Paper No. 3. http://www.developingchild.net/pubs/wp/Stress_Disrupts_Architecture_Developing_Brain.pdf. http://developingchild.harvard.edu.

41. Masten, A. S., & Barnes, A. J. (2018). Resilience in children: Developmental perspectives. *Children 17*, 5 (7): 98. doi: 10.3390/children5070098.

42. Howard, L. M., Molyneaux, E., Dennis, C. L., Rochat, T., Stein, A., Milgrom, J. (2014). Non-Psychotic mental disorders in the perinatal period. *Lancet, 384*(9956): 1775–1788.

43. Paulson, J. F., & Bazemore, S. D. (2010). Prenatal and postnatal depression in fathers and its association with maternal depression: A meta-analysis. *Journal of the American Medical Association, 303*, 1961–1969.

44. Bergström, M. (2013). Depressive symptoms in new first-time fathers: Associations with age, sociodemographic characteristics, and antenatal psychological well-being. *Birth, 40*(1), 32–38.

45. Leach, L. S., Poyser, C., Cooklin, A. R., & Giallo, R. (2016). Prevelence and course of anxiety disorder (and symptom levels) in men across the perinatal period: A systematic review. *Journal of Affective Disorders, 190*, 675–686.

46. Gover, V., Reynolds, R., Axford, N., & Barlow, J. (2019). In A. Emond (Ed.), *Health for all children* (5th ed.). Oxford: Oxford University Press.

47. Stein, A., Pearson, S. M., Goodman, R. H., et al. (2014). Effects of perinatal disorders on the foetus and child. *The Lancet, 384*(9956), 1800–1819.

48. Hyde, R., O'Callaghan, M., Bor, W., Williams, G., & Najam, J. (2012). Long lasting outcomes of infant behavioural dysregulation. *Pediatrics, 130*(5), 1243–1251.

49. O'Conner, T. G., Heron, J., Golding, J., et al. (2002). Maternal anxiety and children's behavioural/emotional problems at 4 years. Report from the Avon Longitudinal Study of Parents and Children. *British Journal of Psychiatry, 180*, 502–508.

50. Hecht, P. M., Hudson, M., Connors, S. L., et al. (2016). Maternal serotonin transporter genotype affects risk for ASD with exposure to parental stress. *Journal for the International Society for Autism Research, 9*(11), 1151–1160.

51. van Santvoort, F., Hosman, C., Janssens, J., van Doesum, K., et al. (2015). The impact of various parental mental disorders on children's diagnoses: A systematic review. *Clinical Child and Family Psychology Review, 18*, 281–299.

52. World Health Organisation (2012) Understanding and addressing violence against women: Intermate Partner Violence. https://apps.who.int/iris/bitstream/handle/10665/77432/WHO_RHR_12.36_eng.pdf;jsessionid=11B3991BA9E3137DBF45AA2AD7967D7A?sequence=1.

53. Heise, L., Ellsberg, M., & Gottemoeller, M. (1999). *Ending violence against women*. Baltimore, MD: Johns Hopkins University School of Public Health, Center for Communications Programs.

54. Office of National Statistics. (2018). Domestic abuse in England and Wales: Year ending March 2018. https://www.ons.gov.uk/peoplepopulationandcommunity/crimeandjustice/bulletins/domesticabuseinenglandandwales/yearendingmarch2018.

55. Howard, L. M., Oram, S., Galley, H., Trevillion, K., & Feder, G. (2013). Domestic violence and perinatal mental disorders: A systematic review and meta-analysis. *PLoS Med, 10*(5), e1001452.

56. Finney, A. (2004). *Alcohol and intimate partner violence: key findings from the research.* London: Home Office.

57. MacDowell, K. (2013). The combined and independent impact of witnessed intermate partner violence and child maltreatment. *Partner Abuse, 3*, 358–378.

58. Kishor, S., & Johnson, K. (2004). *Profiling domestic violence – A multi-country study.* Calverton, MD: ORC Macro.

59. Abramsky, T., Watts, C. H., Garcia-Moreno, C., Devries, K., Kiss, L., Ellsberg, M., Jansen, H. A., Heise, L. (2011). What factors are associated with recent intimate partner violence? Findings from the WHO multi-country study on women's health and domestic violence. *BioMed Central Public Health*, 11: 109.

60. World Health Organisation. (2020). Substance abuse. https://www.who.int/topics/substance_abuse/en/.

61. Shonkoff, J. P., Levitt, P., Bunge, S., et al. (2014). National Scientific Council on the Developing Child. Excessive distress disrupts the architecture of the developing brain. Working Paper 3. Centre on the Developing Child. Harvard University. https://developingchild.harvard.edu/wp-content/uploads/2005/05/Stress_Disrupts_Architecture_Developing_Brain-1.pdf.

62. Cleaver, H., Unell, I., & Aldgate, J. (2011). *Children's needs: Parenting capacity: Child abuse: Parental mental illness, learning disability, substance misuse, and domestic violence (PDF).* London: The Stationery Office (TSO).

63. Axford, N., Sonthalia, S., Wigley, Z., et al. (2015). The best start at home: A report on what works to improve the quality of parent–child interactions from conception to age 5. Early intervention foundation. https://www.eif.org.uk/report/the-best-start-at-home.

64. Olds, D. L. (2002). Prenatal and infancy home visiting by nurses: From randomized trials to community replication. *Prevention Science: the Official Journal of the Society for Prevention Research, 3*(3), 153–172.

65. Scottish Government. (2019). *Family nurse partnership in Scotland: Revaluation report.*

66. Fonagy, P., Gergely, G., Jurist, E., & Target, M. (2002). *Affect regulation, mentalization and the development of the self.* New York: Other Press.

67. Sadler, L. S., Slade, A., Close, N., et al. (2013). Minding the baby: Enhancing reflectiveness to improve early health and relationship outcomes in an interdisciplinary home-visiting program. *Infant Mental Health Journal, 34*(5), 391–405.

68. Brazelton, T. B., & Nugent, J. K. (2011). *The Neonatal Behavioral Assessment Scale.* Cambridge: Mac Keith Press.

69. Best Beginnings. (2020). Baby Buddy app. https://www.bestbeginnings.org.uk/baby-buddy.

70. Daly, H., Baum, A., Richie, J., et al. (2016). G317|Baby buddy app – A public health opportunity for new parents; evaluation of the first 46,000 downloads. *British Association for Child and Adolescent Public Health and British Association of General Paediatrics, 101*, A184–A185.

71. Walker, P. (2011). *Baby massage.* London: Carroll and Brown Publishers Ltd.

72. Asmussen, K. (2015). Infant massage: Understanding the evidence base. https://www.eif.org.uk/blog/infant-massage-understanding-the-evidence-base.

73. Solihull Approach. (2019). https://solihullapproachparenting.com/.

74. Stefanopoulou, E., Coker, S., Greenshields, M., et al. (2011). Health visitors view on consultation using the Solihull Approach: A grounded theory study. *Community Practitioner, 84*, 7.

75. MacBeth, A. (2015) Mellow Parenting: Systematic review and meta-analysis of an intervention to promote sensitive parenting. Mellow all about relationships. https://www.mellowparenting.org/papers/. Accessed 21 December 2021.

76. Vaez, E., Indran, R., Abdollahi, A., Juhari, R., et al. (2015). How marital relations affect child behavior: review of recent research. *Vulnerable Children and Youth Studies, 10*(4), 321–336.

# 15

# COMMUNICATION AND LANGUAGE DEVELOPMENT

JOANNE GIBSON ▪ JEAN COWIE ▪ MICHELLE SCOTT

## CHAPTER CONTENTS

INTRODUCTION

HOW DO CHILDREN'S SLC SKILLS DEVELOP?

RISK OF SLC NEED

IDENTIFICATION OF SPEECH, LANGUAGE AND COMMUNICATION NEEDS

THE ROLE OF THE HEALTH VISITOR

EARLY INTERVENTION APPROACHES

HOME LEARNING ENVIRONMENTS

SUPPORTING CHILDREN WITH LANGUAGE DIFFICULTIES IN THE EARLY YEARS

WORKING IN PARTNERSHIP: HEALTH VISITING AND SPEECH AND LANGUAGE THERAPY

CONCLUSION

## LEARNING OUTCOMES

To:

- describe speech, language and communication development in young children

- identify and critically appraise speech, language and communication needs in young children

- discuss the role of the health visitor in leading/promoting early interventions strategies to promote speech, language and communication development in young children

## INTRODUCTION

Speech, language and communication (SLC) development is a critical component of early development that has a significant impact on well-being outcomes in later life. Poor SLC development in children is not only linked to social disadvantage but is intergenerational and recurring (All Parliamentary Group on SLC Difficulties, 2013[1]; RCSLT, 2017[33]). Many children start school with immature or poorly developed language skills (Hartshorn, 2006[44,45]), go on to struggle with learning and, according to Moss and Washbrook (2016),[44,45] achieve poor outcomes in maths and English at the age of 7 years and low literacy skills when they reach 11 years. These children then are more likely to leave school with little qualifications and very poor job prospects. The early years, therefore, is a critical time of very rapid development that with early intervention and the right nurturing has the potential to better shape and improve outcomes for children and young people.

Health visitors have a key role in assessing, profiling and promoting SLC development in children, yet evidence (Communication Trust, 2017)[45] indicates that a third of the children and young people's workforce lack confidence in supporting SLC needs in children. This chapter,

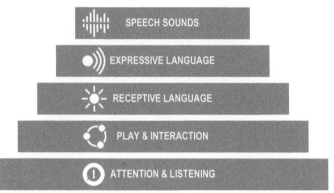

**Figure 15.1** ■ Language development pyramid. (Image from NHS Education for Scotland.)

therefore, will begin by exploring the components of SLC development relevant to the zero- to five-year age group, then go on to discuss factors influencing SLC development. Consideration will then be given to SLC needs and strategies to identify SLC needs in children. Finally, the role of the health visitor in leading early interventions and strategies to promote SLC development and minimise SLC need in young children will be discussed. Useful case studies and thinking spaces will be inter-dispersed throughout the chapter.

## HOW DO CHILDREN'S SLC SKILLS DEVELOP?

Children develop their SLC skills from birth and these skills develop through a child's early years and beyond. Indeed, many skills which contribute to the development of SLC are practised before the baby is born: for example, listening, absorbing language and recognising parental voices and rhythm. The early years is a critical time for the development of children's SLC skills as during this phase the brain is developing rapidly. This period of development is often referred to as a 'window of opportunity'.[2] During the first few years of life children will move through various stages of their communication development, developing skills in relation to talking, listening, interacting and socialising with others.

The pyramid above (Figure 15.1) is a popular visual illustration to represent the constituent parts of children's SLC skills.

The skills at the bottom of the pyramid act as a foundation for more complex skills to develop. Each of these areas is multifaceted and multi-layered. However, all these elements are important for children to communicate effectively and children require to develop skills in each of these areas in order to communicate successfully.

- Attention & Listening: Joint attention is one of the main building blocks for early interaction and communication. Joint attention develops within the first year of life and is the basis of the development of effective communication skills.
- Play: Play and interaction experiences teach children the value of communicating and interacting with others. Children learn the non-verbal rules of communication such as listening, looking and taking turns which form the basis of developing successful language skills.
- Receptive language refers to understanding. A child's receptive language skills develop in advance of their expressive language skills.
- Expressive Language refers to a child's ability to express their needs and wants. It includes their use of vocabulary, grammar and syn-

tax. It also refers to non verbal behaviours such as gestures.

▪ Speech refers to the sounds children use to make words and their ability to speak fluently with appropriate tone, volume and intonation.

It should be noted that children learn to develop their language skills at different rates and can vary considerably regarding the rate at which they reach the various 'milestones'. There are several reasons for this. Some children naturally acquire skills quicker than others; however, there may also be differences in the levels of stimulation they experience in the home language learning environment.[82] These differences in the way that children acquire language can make identification of needs challenging (Bates et al 1988).[46] However, there is a recognised pattern of progression for mastering these skills. The information in Table 15.1 may be helpful in ascertaining if children's language development is following a

| TABLE 15.1 |
| :--: |
| **Key milestones to ascertain if children is following the typical pattern of development and progress.** |

| Age (Years) | Expression | Comprehension | Speech |
| --- | --- | --- | --- |
| 1–2 | ▪ Will use babble which includes speech sounds.<br>▪ Begins to use single words – simple words initially like mama, dada.<br>▪ Begins to use 10–20 single words.<br>▪ By 2 can begin to combine words. | ▪ Understands simple naming words, e.g. body parts<br>▪ Recognises, brings you and points to familiar objects<br>▪ Responds to their name | ▪ Limited number of sounds in their words – often these are *p, b, d, m, n*<br>▪ Speech may not be clear<br>▪ May miss the ends off words<br>▪ Substitutes sounds for those that are easier to say, e.g. *car* becomes *tar*, *sun* becomes *tun* |
| 2–3 | ▪ Uses at least 50 words, including verbs, e.g. *run, jump*<br>▪ Uses 2–3 words together, e.g. '*daddy car*'<br>▪ Uses language skills for a variety of purposes | ▪ Understands verbs, e.g. *cry, jump, want*<br>▪ Can follow short instructions i.e. *brush dolly's hair*<br>▪ Understands simple questions i.e. '*where's mummy's car?*'<br>▪ Understands between 200 and 500 words | ▪ A range of new sounds are emerging – *f, k, g, t, w*<br>▪ May shorten longer words, such as saying '*nana*' instead of '*banana*'<br>▪ Sound substitutions are still evident especially with sounds such as *sh, ch, j, l, r, th* |
| 3–4 | ▪ Beginning to speak fluently<br>▪ Uses three to four-word sentences.<br>▪ Uses 'small' words like '*the*' and '*is*' and able to mark tenses. | ▪ Understands longer instructions<br>▪ Understands '*who*' '*where*' '*what*' questions<br>▪ Understands concepts such as colour, number and time related words | ▪ Speech is becoming clearer and mostly intelligible<br>▪ Most sounds are in use, new sounds emerging are *ch, j, sh, v, l, z*<br>▪ May shorten longer words, such as saying '*nana*' instead of '*banana*'<br>▪ Some sound substitutions are still evident especially with sounds such as *th* and *r*.<br>▪ May also have difficulty where lots of sounds happen together in a word, e.g. they may say '*pider*' instead of '*spider*' |
| 4–5 | ▪ Can hold a simple conversation using four- to six-word sentences<br>▪ Using 4000–5000 words.<br>▪ Uses longer, well-formed sentences and links sentences together with '*and*' and '*because*'<br>▪ Describes events that have happened<br>▪ Able to retell short stories | ▪ Understands conversations<br>▪ Understands '*why*' questions<br>▪ Understands more complicated language and abstract words, i.e. *behind, above, first, last* | ▪ Uses most sounds effectively<br>▪ Speech is intelligible<br>▪ Complicated words may still be difficult to produce<br>▪ May find *r* and *th* difficult to produce until around 6 years old |

typical pattern and if they are making the progress that is predicted for their stage of development. By understanding the stage their child is at in their language development, parents can start to implement helpful strategies which will support their children's next stage of language development.

## Zero to one year

Babies are born ready to interact and communicate with their caregivers. In the early days and weeks of their lives they will show a preference for their parent/caregiver's voice, will look at faces and may even try to copy facial expressions. Although infants under 1 year are not yet using words, they are learning important skills of communication such as back and forth interactions, attention skills and social play. They learn these skills by interacting with adults and taking part in early interactions. Initially, their primary means of communication will be crying; however, in the coming months they begin to learn about language use from the responsive interactions with their parents/caregivers. They learn that communication and interaction is rewarding, and their crying will start to change according to their needs. Young infants will be able to recognise and respond to familiar voices and will be soothed by these. They will begin to engage in more vocal play; for example, they may 'coo' in response to familiar voices and start to make vowel-like sounds such as 'oo' and 'a'. Babies will begin to smile and laugh, and these shared experiences will reinforce and reward positive communication and attachment. By six months they will be experimenting more with sounds and be able to use simple babble involving syllables. Between 6 and 12 months this babble is likely to be in the form of repeated syllables (da-da-da).[3]

Something important happens around the age of one, when children make an important connection about intentional communication. They start to realise that they can communicate purposefully with those around them and that this can be rewarding. One of the first signs of intentional communication is the use of gestures and pointing. Children often start to point at objects out of their reach.[4] They will use their point to gain someone's attention and send a purposeful message. Pointing has been linked positively to language development. Lüke et al (2017)[47] found that the more children point early in their development, the better their language abilities are when they are older. This may be due to parents responding to children's pointing by repeating the words, thus children are hearing models of the vocabulary that they need.

## One to two years

Children reach an important milestone in their language development around one year of age when they begin to use their first words. Evidence[5–7] from the literature indicates variance in the age of first word acquisition, ranging from as early as 9 months up to 18 months. Words may appear slowly initially and then begin to develop over time. Early words tend to be nouns: for example, names of foods, animals, family, toys etc. These tend to be simple words such as 'mama', 'dada', 'teddy'. Children may use one word to represent a larger chunk of information; i.e., say 'up' to mean 'lift me up'. Children may also over-generalise some words, such as calling all animals 'doggy'. Although it can be helpful to record the number of words a child uses at this age, Law and Roy[8] advise caution when asking parents how many words their child uses. This is because of the variation in development at this stage, and also the difficulty for parents to keep a track of all the new words that their child is saying. Nevertheless, children's use of babble at this stage becomes more sophisticated and will sound more like their native language. Their attempts at words may not be clear but may sound something like the words they are trying to say. They may miss some sounds at the end of words or substitute some harder sounds for easier ones.

As well as being able to express some words, children will recognise more common objects/words and be able to respond to simple requests and instructions from their caregivers. Their levels of understanding will be in advance of what they can express. Evidence[9] suggests that children may be able to understand five times more than they can express at this stage. For example, they will know their own name and that of close family members and familiar objects in their environment.

## Two to three years

In the second year of a child's life (24–36 months), children will begin to combine words together into short two-word phrases, eventually building short sentences. Their vocabulary will be developing rapidly at this stage. Children can often experience a 'burst' in their vocabulary development around this time, where they can be acquiring new words on a frequent basis, some studies estimating up to nine new words a day.[10] At this stage there can be variations between children's language development, even within siblings in families. Following this vocabulary spurt, children will begin to combine two words together and will begin to master early grammar such as adjectives and verbs. Interestingly, a study found that the more verbs a child had at 2 years of age, the more advanced their language skills were 6 months later.[11] According to Sim et al,[12] a child's vocabulary development at 24 months is correlated to their later language acquisition, with children presenting with a vocabulary of less than 50 or not yet joining words, being at greater risk of longer-term difficulties. Although children will be talking more at this stage, it is still common for their speech not to be clear. Usually parents/caregivers can tune into their child's speech, but unfamiliar adults may still not always understand what the child is trying to say. It is estimated that

50% to 70% of a child's speech should be intelligible to others at this stage.

As well as expressive language development, a child's receptive language development and what they can understand is equally important at this age. Children will be able to understand instructions and simple questions. They are typically able to understand around 400 to 500 words even though they might not be able to use all these words yet.[13] It can be challenging gaining an accurate reflection of what children can understand in their home environment. Wilson and Law[14] highlight that caution must be used to avoid potential parental bias in reporting of children's receptive language abilities. For example, a child may be so used to the routines in the home that they do not need to rely as much on the oral language used in instructions. It may therefore appear a child is understanding language, but in fact they are simply responding to cues in their environment and the predictability of their routine.

## Three to five years

Between 3 and 5 years, children will combine words into increasingly lengthy sentences and develop their use of grammar and vocabulary. They will be able to talk about their experiences and use their language skills to communicate, form friendships and learn more about the world around them. Their speech will become increasingly clearer and by the time they go to school, they can have effective conversations, have a large vocabulary and be largely intelligible apart from the sounds such as 'r' and 'th'.

Table 15.1 outlines the key milestones which children pass through. This can be helpful in ascertaining if children are following a typical pattern of development and if progress is being seen.

It is important to remember that children develop their SLC skills gradually through interacting with others and the environment around them. The home learning environment, the experiences children take part in and the interactions they have with others are all crucial to their language development. Therefore, parents and caregivers play a vital role in the development of children's SLC skills. Caregivers' responsiveness to their child's attempts at communication will help to draw the child's attention to the meaning of words and reinforce their efforts. Both the way in which parents speak with their child (often referred to as parentese) and the number of turns they take with their child in an interaction has been shown to accelerate children's language development.[50] Furthermore, children who are exposed to a lot of language that includes a variety of words and sentences tend to have stronger language skills.[15] Therefore, both the quality and quantity of parent/caregiver language stimulation use can influence a child's language development and the rate at which this develops.

## RISK OF SLC NEED

Speech, language and communication needs (SLCN) is an umbrella term used to describe difficulties children may experience in any area of their SLC development. Children may experience difficulty in one or all areas of their communication development. For example, they may have difficulty with their speech intelligibility or forming words and expressing them fluently. They may have expressive language difficulties such as a reduced vocabulary or have difficulty recalling words and expressing their ideas. Children may also present with difficulties in their receptive language and understanding information which is conveyed orally. Furthermore, they may struggle to use their language appropriately in social situations and when interacting with others. Lindsay et al. highlight that the term SLCN encompasses a wide range of needs and that the types of needs and their severity can change over time as children develop.[49]

## Subgroups of speech, language and communication needs

SLCN can be viewed in three broad sub-groups[49]:

(i) **Primary SLCN:** Primary SLCN is where language difficulties occur in the absence of any identified neurodevelopmental or social cause; for example, specific language difficulties or specific speech disorder. These difficulties are described as being specific and persistent in their nature.

(ii) **Secondary SLCN:** Children with cognitive, sensory or physical impairment as their primary need may have language difficulties as a secondary need; e.g., SLCN secondary to autistic spectrum disorder, a hearing impairment or learning difficulty.

(iii) **Lack of stimulation:** Children may also present with SLCN associated with limited experiences and lack of stimulation.

(Lindsay et al., 2010)

It is estimated that 10% of all children will have long term SLCN.[51] This is often referred to as the 'most common childhood disability' with as many as approximately two children in every class of 30 pupils experiencing language difficulties severe enough to hinder academic progress.[16]

There may be a variety of reasons why children experience difficulty in developing SLC skills. In some occasions there is no clear cause or explanation. SLCN may be caused by neurological conditions, a hearing impairment or a recognised health condition. It can also be caused by learning difficulties, or emotional and behavioural difficulties.[17] A literature review by Dockrell et al[18,53] identified several risk factors that exist for children in the development of their SLC skills. Furthermore, Dockrell et al[18] found evidence of a strong social gradient with speech and language development that is consistent with the findings from the Millennium Cohort Study,[40] and highlight that pupils entitled to free school meals and living in areas of social disadvantage are 2.3 times more likely to be identified as having SLCN. This has been explained in the literature[19] by the difference in the quality and quantity of parent interaction. Hart and Risley[20] found that children in higher socio-economic backgrounds heard a greater amount, and a more varied vocabulary which positively influenced their language development. High language ability parents have also been found to have more frequent turns with their children in interactions.[21]

The Growing up in Scotland longitudinal population study[22] (Growing up in Scotland studies) has continued to show on a yearly basis, the stark variation in language development at age 3 and 5 years between different socio-economic groups in Scotland. Bromley et al[37] found that at age 3 children from less advantaged families were outperformed by their more affluent peers, with Naven et al. finding that by age 5 a 13-month vocabulary exists between children from the most and least affluent families.[56] As part of this longitudinal study Bromley et al also examined home learning activities such as reading and found that these were performed more regularly in more affluent households.[57]

However, the links between social disadvantage and language development are complex, as SLCN can often co-occur with other disorders and disabilities.[23] It can be difficult in practice to distinguish between SLCN caused by environmental factors and SLCN caused by neurodevelopmental problems. Family history (genetics) also play a significant role and family history has been shown to increase the likelihood of SLCN (Newbury and Monaco, 2010).[52] This relationship is recognised to be a complex interplay of factors with social factors likely to be compounding genetic ones. Law et al[24] concur that it is likely social disadvantage exacerbates rather than causes SLCN.

The Royal College of Speech and Language Therapists[33] illustrate the intergenerational and recurrent nature of SLCN and highlight the longer-term impacts of SLCN (Figure 15.2.) The profound impact of SLCN extends well into adulthood in terms of quality of life, attainment and outcomes in general.[25] For example, vocabulary difficulties at age 5 are associated with poor literacy, mental health and employment outcomes at age 34.[54]

Studies have shown the positive benefits of engaging parents in learning strategies to support their child's language development. For example, Colmar found that when parents from socio-economic areas were trained in easily learned strategies to support their child's language development, then significant improvement in the children's language development were made.[55] Indeed, it is acknowledged that parents of young children with language difficulties who have received support and information early about how they can modify their interactions are likely to see improvements in their child's language skills, irrespective of their socio-economic status.

Although social disadvantage is a powerful risk factor, it does not inevitably lead to SLCN. Early intervention is key to mitigating risks, particularly intervention that focuses on the parent-child interaction. Health visitors, therefore, must be aware of the risk to SLC development in young children and offer appropriate early interventions and support to parents to help them provide the best home learning environment they can for children.

### THINKING SPACE

Consider what other risk factors exist for SLCN. For example, gender, socio-economic background, learning English as an additional language. Which risk factors are prevalent in the families you work with? How can these risks be mitigated?

What tools are available for you to use to assess a child's SLC skills?

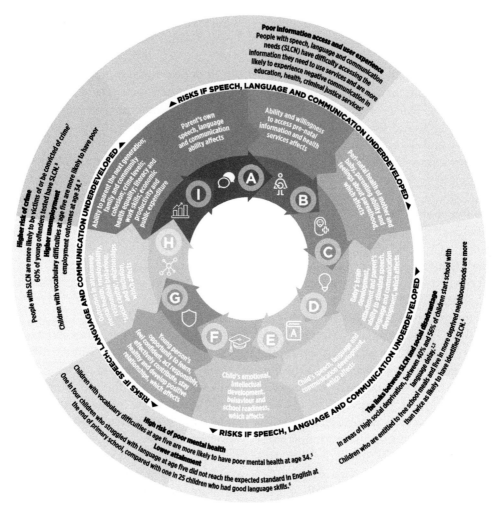

Figure 15.2 ■ The intergenerational cycle of speech, language and communication outcomes and risks. (Image from Royal College of Speech and Language Therapists).

## IDENTIFICATION OF SPEECH, LANGUAGE AND COMMUNICATION NEEDS

Health visitors have an important role in identifying developmental needs early. This early identification and detection can help ensure that children get access to the right support when they need it. However, identification of SLCN can be challenging in young children. This is due to the differences in the way in which some children acquire language, and in the accuracy and predictive

validity of the screening instruments which are available. Consequently, it can sometimes be difficult to ascertain the reason underpinning a child's language difficulties and whether indeed they require additional support and intervention.

Some children in the early years present with difficulties in their language development. Where this difficulty is due to environmental causes, it is recognised that their difficulties may be 'transient'. Sometimes referred to as 'late talkers' these children often present with a small vocabulary but are typically developing otherwise. Research[26] tells us that between 70% and 80% of these late talkers will catch up with their peers by the time they go to school. However, evidence suggests that even if these children do 'catch up' in respect of their language skills, some may continue to present with difficulties in relation to other areas such as behaviour, social skills and literacy.[27] According to Hawa and Spanoudis,[28] 20% to 30% of children described as late talkers will have ongoing language difficulties and need support and intervention to help them to progress.

'Developmental language disorder' is a term used to describe more specific and long-term language difficulties in children. A recent study by Norbury et al.[16] indicated a prevalence rate of 7.58% for developmental language disorder in the general population. For this group of children their language difficulties are evident in the absence of any other neurodevelopmental condition such as autistic spectrum disorder. Children with a developmental language disorder present with difficulties in one or more areas of their language development, including their expressive use of language or receptive skills and understanding of language. For example, they can find it difficult to express their ideas, wants or feelings, and may have a small vocabulary for their age or have difficulty building up sentences or using correct grammar. These children may also struggle to understand and make sense of words that they hear, and to follow instructions and make sense of the language they hear around them. Their social skills may also be affected, and they may have difficulty interacting with others or with social communication skills. For example, they may struggle to use their language skills effectively to have conversations, and to play and interact socially with others. For these children, their language difficulties are likely to have a significant impact on their educational progress and everyday interactions.

Although it can be difficult to identify which children are more likely to experience persistent language difficulties, there is some consensus in the literature of risk factors.[58-59] These are noted as:

- Limited babbling or sound play as an infant
- Family history of communication delay in immediate family
- Recurrent ear infections
- Limited consonant repertoire
- Lack of sequenced pretend play
- Mild delay in receptive skills
- Little or no use of communicative gestures
- Lack of verbal imitation
- Vocabulary consisting of mostly nouns and few or no verbs
- Poor social skills (with peers)
- Limited change in child's expressive language over time.

There are a variety of screening methods available to ascertain if children are experiencing difficulties with their language development. These are described as being direct or indirect. Direct methods include the use of specific speech and language assessment tools (i.e. Denver Developmental Screening Test; Hackney Early Language Screening Test; Language Development Survey). Direct language assessment tools have the advantage that observable behaviours are evaluated. However, no single tool or screen has been found to accurately identify persistent language difficulties in a single assessment.

Alternatively, indirect methods involve the parent by engaging them in parental reporting and observations. The Ages and Stages Questionnaire (3rd edition, ASQ-3) is an example of an indirect screening tool, as it is completed by a health visitor through conversations with a parent. Sachse[29] highlights the benefits of seeking parents' concerns and observations as it is accepted that parents generally provide a reasonable source of information about a child's development. By using indirect screening methods, information can be obtained quickly and easily, and in some occasions remotely as during the Covid-19 pandemic, without direct contact with the child. Nevertheless, some concerns have been raised about the reliability and objectivity of parental reporting.[30] Although parental reporting can be an accurate way of assessing a child's language development, Dockrell and Marshall[31] highlight challenges in relying on parental reporting alone. They advise that indirect methods should be used in combination with direct observation, assessment and consideration of risk factors.

Research by Berkman et al[32] highlights that individual screening methods display varying levels of diagnostic accuracy. This is due to the difficulty of some screening tools to accurately identify those who have a SLCN and require additional support, without over-identifying those who do not. Currently there is no 'gold standard' to guide screening for language difficulties. According to Law et al.,[38] screening assessments that take place at a single point in time are often not adequate for predicting language difficulties in young children. Indeed, there is no identified 'optimal age' for undertaking screening for language difficulties. As a result, many countries in the world do not advocate screening for language difficulties in young children Law et al[39]. Rather, Law et al.,[38] highlights the importance of assessing children's language development at multiple points in their development as this is more likely to create a picture of how the child is developing their language skills over time. Most universal screening programmes, such as the Healthy Child Programme (https://www.gov.uk/government/publications/commissioning-of-public-health-services-for-children/health-visiting-and-school-nursing-service-delivery-model) and the Universal Health Visiting Pathway (https://www.gov.scot/publications/universal-health-visiting-pathway-scotland-pre-birth-pre-school/) require children's language development to be assessed at multiple points over time and do not rely on a single assessment at a single point in time.

Screening of speech, language and development in children has its advantages and disadvantages. For example, potential adverse effects of screening include increased parental anxiety, over-referral of children to specialist services or conversely, under-identification of the children who require support long term. Screening is generally accepted to be of limited value if it is not followed by timely advice and support. Benefits of screening are recognised by early access to advice and health promotion, better support for parents and caregivers, and increased satisfaction with the support received. Screening can also assist in reducing health inequalities and ensuring that there is equal access to services from all groups in society.

Health visitors have the necessary skills and access to tools, such as the Ages and Stages Questionnaires (ASQ-3), to support their assessment of children's language development. Observation, assessment, consideration of risk factors, and professional judgement as well as ongoing monitoring over the early years of a child's life is crucial for informing decisions made about a child's speech and language ability and in identifying SLCN. Furthermore, close collaboration and liaison with specialist services such as Speech and Language Therapy is invaluable in supporting health visitors in the early identification of speech and language needs in young children and ensuring appropriate support and access to services for those that require it.

## THE ROLE OF THE HEALTH VISITOR

The Standards of Proficiency for Specialist Community Public Health Nurses identify 10 key standards for specialist community public health nursing, grouped under the following four domains[63]:

■ search for health needs
■ stimulation of awareness of health needs
■ influence on policies affecting health
■ facilitation of health-enhancing activities.

These standards and domains are particularly relevant to health visitors and their role in identifying and promoting SLC development in children.

In searching for health needs, health visitors are in a key position to identify children with, or at risk of SLCN. Moreover, in developing therapeutic relationships with families, health visitors should have an awareness of the communication needs and preferences of parents on their caseload. As alluded to earlier in this chapter there is an intergenerational pattern to SLCN in children that is strongly influenced by the SLC ability of parents.[33] Children of parents with poor SLC ability are at greater risk of developing SLCN. Reflecting on the public health role of health visitors, Law and Levickis argue that early SLC development in children is a public health issue that health visitors can help address.[60] In Scotland, SLC is the developmental domain of greatest concern within the 27- to 30-month child health review. The data also highlight that children living in the most deprived areas in Scotland have a greater risk of having SLCN.[61] This reflects the findings of McKean et al. who, in the Millennium Cohort Study, identified a social gradient in language skills across 5-year-old children.[62] In searching for health needs, therefore, health visitors have an important role in accessing national and local data relevant to child development, as well as identifying risk factors, and SLCN of individual children and their families in their caseloads.

Stimulation of awareness of health needs involves health visitors raising awareness of health and social needs at an individual and population level. Regarding SLCN of young children, health visitors can act as advocates for children and families and empower families to access information and to utilise resources that promote SLC development. This will involve health visitors working collaboratively with families and other professionals and agencies such as speech and language therapists and other early years workers.

Influence on policies affecting health requires health visitors to contribute to, and influence, the development of policy taking cognisance of the impact of policy on health. In practice this domain encompasses a range of strategies. For example, in relation to SLC development, health visitors should keep abreast of current research and evidence and use this to improve outcomes for children. This may require knowledge or application of quality improvement strategies such as 'test of change' that is, Plan-Do-Study-Act within their team or locality.

Health visitors, therefore, have a key role in early intervention and prevention and in supporting parents to give their child the best possible start in life. Public Health England as part of the Best Start in Life research programme have developed a language identification measure (ELIM) for Health Visitors to supplement current assessment processes at the 2 year child health review. As well as this assessment tool, a model of early intervention has been developed specifically for Health Visitors. The intervention supports families with key target behaviours for language development such as responsive interactions, shared book reading and focussed stimulation.

## EARLY INTERVENTION APPROACHES

As discussed earlier, babies are born ready to communicate. The innate behaviours of crying, watching faces and quietening to sound is forming their understanding of language, and the way a parent/caregiver interacts with their infant within the early years strongly influences their child's language development and abilities. Awareness of the frequency and quality of this parent-child interaction can serve as an early indicator to health visitors of the need for support or minimise language delay. Health visitors develop therapeutic relationships with families and knowledge of community supports enables them, within universal services, to work in partnership with parents to promote their child's development. The contact points health visitors make to families across the birth to five years continuum (Public Health England, 2018; Scottish Government, 2015) provide a substantial intervention opportunity to support families to promote their child's speech and language development.

Providing primary prevention and health promotion in the early years of a child's life is likely to result in greater improvements in reducing health inequalities than at any other stage of life.[64] Regarding speech and language development, the early years offers a 'window of opportunity' for children to build the foundations of successful language and communication abilities. This is supported by Adams and Cowley, who highlight that primary prevention in early childhood not only helps to reduce risk factors and prevent needs from arising, but also provides an opportunity to promote strategies and resources that enhance resilience and the ability to self-manage.[65] Regarding a child's language development, early intervention approaches are those that develop a parent's ability to foster their child's early language development. Parents, therefore, are a key resource and can have a tremendous influence on the SLC development of their children. The importance of the parent-child interaction for language development is well established.[66] Many early intervention approaches seek to build awareness and skills of parents in the strategies they use, and in turn this enables parents to promote language development in their children. Such interventions focus on the quality of the parent-child interaction and the nature and frequency of conversations that parents have with their children.

Health visitors work closely with families and establish meaningful and trusting relationships with parents that allow them to discuss a child's development including any concerns that the parent, or the health visitor, may have concerning the SLC ability of the child. Having a good rapport with parents, facilitates health visitors to raise any concerns about their child's SLC development and to involve parents in the decisions made, as well as in early intervention strategies to manage the concern. Such early support can help parents to see themselves as enablers in their child's developmental progress and to understand the key role they have in supporting their child's early language development. Learning to communicate, therefore, can be viewed as a joint endeavour between the child and their parent/caregiver. Children need to hear words around them to learn to communicate effectively. Consequently, parents need to be encouraged to talk frequently to their child to support their language development. This may simply be telling the child what they are doing as they are doing it. For example, mummy is washing the teacups; mummy is brushing your hair etc. The importance of parents talking to their children is based on research[20] which demonstrates that children who hear more words in interactions with their caregivers will have better language outcomes. Hearing words alone, however, is not enough. Studies (cited in Refs. [71–74]) have also demonstrated that the quality of the parent-child interaction is just as important as the quantity of words that children hear. Children need to hear words as part of sensitive and responsive interactions with their caregivers. These (cited in Refs. [71–74]) demonstrated that the quality of the parent-child interaction was important in children's development of language and a key predictor of later language proficiency. The following three key areas of parent-child interaction were highlighted as being important promoting language development:

- **Balanced conversations with equal turns,** (both nonverbal and verbal turns) allowing the adult and child to connect with each other in enjoyable back and forth interactions. Not an interaction which is dominated by the parent or involves lots of direct or testing questions.

- **Shared routines with words, objects, gestures and symbols.** These routines can be associated with the time of day (bath time, bedtime) or a familiar game (peek-a-boo) which is played in the same way each time. These routines are repetitive and predictable which allow for words and actions to be repeated and easily learned by the child.
- **Joint engagement** in activities which involve the parent and the child both attending and sharing meaning with each other. These are led by the child's interest and follow the child's focus of attention. Fundamental to these interactions are a parent's responsiveness to their child's communication attempts. These interactions are rich in words, objects, gestures and symbols.

Furthermore, children who participated in more frequent back and forth turns in an interaction with their caregiver were found in their study to have higher vocabulary scores.[67-71]

Consequently, the first three years of a child's life are particularly important for language development. Health visitors, therefore, have a key role in supporting parents to engage in positive interactions with their child from the day he/she is born in order to mitigate the risks of language delay and to effectively build the foundations for successful acquisition of SLC skills in their child.

## THINKING SPACE

It has been found that people remember and understand less than half of the information that we discuss with them. Some parents may have communication support needs themselves that you may not know about.

Consider the best way to communicate messages to families about positive parent-child interaction. How can you check if they have understood? Remember: coaching, role-modelling, audio/visual methods.

## HOME LEARNING ENVIRONMENTS

Cowley et al. and the Scottish Government emphasise the importance of therapeutic relationship-building and home visiting in health visiting practice.[72-73] In providing a person-centred, 'salutogenic' and universal service to all families in the UK, health visitors have the privilege of visiting families with pre-school aged children in the familiarity of their home. The home environment, however, is an important learning environment for young children. By visiting families at home, health visitors are better able to observe and assess the health and social needs of the family. For example, some families living in deprived circumstances may not have age-appropriate books and toys for their child, some households may be chaotic with families living in over-crowded conditions, other families may be subject to constant noise from the television, computer, radio, music and so forth. Some parents may have SLC difficulties themselves and not know how to interact and play with their child. Some young children, therefore, may lack stimulation and the opportunity to develop their SLC skills within their home environment.

Regarding parents with SLCN, health visitors by developing trusting and meaningful relationships with parents and meeting with them in the security of their home environment should be able to raise the subject of SLC need and discuss the parent's own communication preferences. Understanding the parents own communication needs and communication preferences is vital if health visitors are to break the intergenerational cycle of SLC need (RCSLT, 2017) and effectively support parents to promote SLC development in their own children. Golinkoff et al (2019)[76] highlighted the importance of shared book reading and appropriate play in promoting early language development. They found that pre-school children who participated in high quality reading, play and conversations with their caregiver had improved school readiness skills (maths, reading, vocabulary, problem solving) when they reached 5 years old. Shared book reading which includes the use of open-ended questions and an opportunity for the child to respond is a particularly powerful way of enhancing a child's language development.[75,79] This may be a challenge for parents with a SLC need such as difficulty reading, therefore, health visitors need to discuss the importance of these parents describing pictures in books with their children and formulating stories from the pictures. Health visitors also need to raise awareness of local resources and groups such as the library and age appropriate story telling sessions.

Within the home environment, consideration also needs to be given to background noise and parental distractions such as mobile phones. According to Erikson and Newman (2010),[77] young infants find it hard to focus on their parent's voice in the presence of background noise such as from the television or radio. Health visitors should encourage parents to prioritise some quiet time without any distraction to speak, play and interact with their child. Kildare and Middlemiss (2017)[74] highlight that mobile phones/technology can also be a distraction for parents and reduces their responsiveness to their infant's needs. For example, parents using mobile phone/technology are often more focused on the virtual conversation/communication and may miss important cues from their child.

Although the primary source of interaction and stimulation for young children will be their parents and caregivers, it should be noted that interactions with siblings and peers has also been attributed to positive language outcomes. Sometimes siblings have been viewed as a barrier to a child developing their language skills with references to older children 'speaking for the younger child'. However, literature does not support this idea with siblings considered to have a positive influence on language development. Topping et al. (2015) highlight that siblings and peers are a source of interaction, negotiation and joint planning which can enhance language development.

### Case Study 1

*Concern was initially raised about Andrew's speech and language skills at age 2 years. Andrew had approximately 20 single words. He was communicating via pointing and occasional single words. He was not yet joining any words together. He could follow simple instructions like 'where's the ball?' 'Point to your nose'. He could bring his Mum objects when requested. He was responding to his name and short commands.*

***Observations:*** *The Health Visitor observed that Andrew was keen to interact with others. He showed joint attention and was bringing his Mum objects, smiling and making appropriate eye contact and gestures.*

*The home environment was busy and there were not many toys. Andrew had three older siblings. Andrew's Mum reported he really enjoyed watching TV and playing on the iPAD. They were new to the area and not yet attending any playgroups or activities.*

***Assessment:*** *There were no concerns reported about any other aspects of Andrew's development and he was reaching other developmental milestones. The Health Visitor undertook assessment using the ASQ. He scored in the grey monitoring zone for his communication skills. His parents reported that Andrew developed his first words around 15 months. Since then other words have been slow to appear but have been developing steadily.*

***Early Intervention:*** *The Health Visitor spent time discussing and Role Modelling with Andrew's parents some parent-child interaction strategies*

- *Repetition was discussed with Andrew's Mum – it is very important to the acquisition of language. Infants and young children need to hear words over and over again before they will attempt to use them. Andrew's Mum was encouraged to repeat new words in different contexts for Andrew.*
- *Labelling – Andrew's Mum was encouraged to name a variety of vocabulary. Emphasising and stressing new words for Andrew. Remembering to point and name anything that Andrew shows an interest in. Andrew's Mum was encouraged to put into words what Andrew is trying to say.*

■ *Expanding Andrew's use of language by adding and extending his utterances. Adding one or two words. If Andrew says 'car' – you could say 'red car'.*

■ *Commenting: It was discussed with Mum that it is helpful to use short, simple sentences. Talking about what Andrew is doing and what he is interested in.*

*Discussion with Andrew's mum took place to help her to identify opportunities for her to interact with Andrew and use these strategies. It was discussed that by reducing his screen time there may be further opportunities for Andrew and his Mum to engage and communicate with each other e.g. during*

■ *Reading*
■ *Singing rhymes and songs*
■ *Routines*
■ *Play and taking turns back and forth*

*During these opportunities the Health Visitor discussed and demonstrated the importance of positive interaction such as getting face to face, taking turns, using a slow pace and allowing time (waiting) for Andrew to respond. Also, the importance of responding positively to Andrew's attempts at communication.*

***Signposting***: *The Health Visitor offered the family some resources to help them and suggested they attend a local playgroup. The Health Visitor also gave details of the local Speech and Language Therapy Drop In Clinic and telephone advice line so they could access further information if they needed this.*

*Goals were developed with the family and the Health Visitor agreed to review Andrew in 12 weeks. At the review Andrew's vocabulary had increased significantly and he was linking words together into short 2 to 3-word phrases. His parents were pleased with his progress.*

## SUPPORTING CHILDREN WITH LANGUAGE DIFFICULTIES IN THE EARLY YEARS

Children with language difficulties may have more difficulty in picking up cues in their environment. Therefore, it is important for their parents to pay attention to the way in which they are interacting with their child. They may need to use usual techniques more often or with increased intensity to support their child to develop their language skills. Therefore, interventions that focus on a parent-child interaction is an approach that is commonly used to support children with language difficulties in the early years. Originating from Parent Child Interaction Therapy (PCI) developed in the 1970's by Sheila Eyberg to support a child's behaviour, these approaches often use evidence-based interaction strategies between a parent and a child.[34] Often parents are supported through coaching to increase their use of positive parent child interaction strategies which facilitate language development. Ramírez et al[35] have shown this kind of intervention can be successful in boosting a child's language development with longer term outcomes being apparent. Tempel et al (2009)[78] also suggest that this kind of parent training can be an effective preventative intervention for children who are at risk of developing language difficulties.

Techniques in parent child interventions focus on language promoting strategies which parents can use in everyday conversations and interactions with their child. They build on the essential foundations of a positive parent child interaction where a parent is responsive to the child and engaged in joint interactions which build on the child's focus of attention and interests. Furthermore, the interactions seek to be balanced with equal turns back and forth with an adult allowing time and waiting for the child to initiate interactions. This act of 'waiting' and allowing a time delay for children to respond may need to be more emphasised for children with a language delay, giving them time to initiate an interaction or show what they are interested in. This positive back and forth interaction provides a platform for children to be engaged in language learning with their caregiver. Below (Table 15.2) is a summary of some parent-child interaction strategies

| TABLE 15.2 | |
|---|---|
| **Parental use of gesture** | In a systematic review of the literature Topping et al. found that parental use of gesture in interactions was found to support young children's use of gesture which in turn influences their vocabulary development.[79] |
| **Labelling words in context** | Repetition of key words and labelling vocabulary frequently across different contexts in a child's environment has been found to support child language learning. Some studies show that parent's emphasising and highlighting words through their pitch and tone can further support learning of vocabulary. |
| **Recasting** | Recasting is an adult's repetition of a child's utterance. Children have been found to benefit from hearing their attempts at communication repeated and modelled back. It confirms that the child's message has been understood and allows the child to hear their attempts modelled back to them in a mature form, that is, with the correct grammar or articulation. That is, child says '*daddy tar*' – parent could repeat back – daddy's car. |
| **Reducing directives/questions** | Frequent use of directive questions or commands has been found to correlate with delays in children's language development.[20] Therefore, parents are encouraged to use commenting on what is happening around the child and using open questions in replace of directive/testing questions to facilitate their child's language development. |
| **Expansions** | Expansion refers to when an adult repeats the child's utterance but modifies the child's sentence by adding new words or ideas. This allows the child to hear a more sophisticated and expanded model of language. That is, child says *daddy's car* – parent may say *yes – daddy's driving his car* |
| **Environmental arrangement** | By modifying the child's environment, parents are encouraged to seek opportunities for the child to communicate. For example, by offering the child a choice of items or placing items out of the child's reach for them to ask for. |

commonly used to support parents/carers of children with a language difficulties.

### Case Study 2

*At Lucas's 27-month review a concern was raised from the assessment that he was not yet communicating using many words. His parents reported that he had less than five single words. His parents were concerned.*

   **Observation:** *The Health Visitor observed that Lucas did not always use words consistently and would take an adult's hand to lead them to what he wanted. He used some vocalisations and gestures to communicate his needs.*

   *Lucas did not respond consistently to instructions or commands from his parents. He could share attention with an adult for short periods in play activities. His parents were trying to engage Lucas in play activities they had chosen. They tended to ask Lucas lots of questions to encourage Lucas to communicate.*

   **Early Intervention:** *The Health Visitor offered the parent some time role modelling and discussing some parent-child interaction strategies such as:*

- *Following Luca's interests and letting him take the lead in interactions.*
- *Getting down to Luca's level when interacting*

- *Pausing and Waiting: Allowing Lucas time to respond.*
- *Offering Lucas choices, for example, banana or apple and pausing for a few seconds to allow time for Lucas to communicate.*
- *Pace: Using a slow pace to allow time for Lucas to respond.*
- *Taking turns when playing games and singing rhymes.*
- *Using natural gestures when communicating with Lucas.*
- *Responding positively to Lucas's attempts at communication.*
- *Trying to avoid asking too many testing/direct questions.*

*The Health Visitor discussed some opportunities for using these strategies such as when reading, and during play, routines and people games. The Health Visitor set some goals with the family and made a referral to the local Speech and Language Therapy Service as well as giving written advice.*

   *Over the next few visits the Health Visitor introduced the following strategies:*

- *Repetition – repeating words for Lucas in lots of different contexts*

- *Copying back sounds or words Lucas uses to show you have understood and are listening*
- *Interpreting Lucas's attempts at communication and putting into words what he is trying to say. Emphasising and stressing words.*
- *Pointing and labelling words that Lucas shows an interest in*
- *Commenting: Using short, simple sentences. Talking about what Lucas is doing and what he interested in.*

## WORKING IN PARTNERSHIP: HEALTH VISITING AND SPEECH AND LANGUAGE THERAPY

Bercow[36] highlights that 10% of children and young people in the UK have a speech, communication and language need and that many of these children and young people do not receive the help and support they need. According to Bercow[36] this is due to poor understanding of SLC need by professionals and insufficient resourcing to support speech and language therapy services. Bercow[36] also highlights that to promote SLC development in young children and give them their optimum start in life, early years workers, including health visitors and speech and language therapists, need to work collaboratively. According to the RCSLT (2017), interprofessional and partnership working is key to reducing inequalities and breaking the intergenerational cycle of SLCN.

Knowledge of the components of SLC development, highlighted in the SLC pyramid discussed earlier in this chapter can help health visitors understand the stages children go through in their language development, as well as raise awareness of potential risk factors and how these might be mitigated. Taking a holistic view of the family, the home learning environment as well as the parents SLC preferences, health visitors can work with families building on their strengths and facilitating them to utilise the resources available to them in their own home and within the local community to promote SLC development in their child. Furthermore, knowledge of how speech and language develop and understanding of the elements identified in the SLC pyramid can aid health visitors in their assessment of a child's SLC ability. It can also help them to identify and more clearly articulate areas of concern when seeking advice, or requesting assistance, from their local speech and language therapist, or if indicated making a formal referral.

Health visitors have a key role working with families with young children and can make a significant contribution by intervening early and promoting SLC development. However, close collaboration between health visiting and speech and language therapy services is vital in seeking to ensure that those children who are most in need of support get it and have a chance of reaching their optimum potential in life.

### THINKING SPACE

Speech and Language Therapy Services. Close collaboration between agencies is vitally important to provide the best support to children, young people and their families.

- Do you know how to contact your local Speech and Language Therapy Service?
- What services are provided by your local Speech and Language Therapy department?
- What are the risks of over or under referral to Speech and Language Therapy services?
- What other services exist in your community that could support a child's SLC development?

## CONCLUSION

Speech language and communication (SLC) is an important aspect of childhood development that has significant outcomes for the life course of children and young people. Health visitors have a key role in leading and facilitating early intervention strategies to promote SLC development, giving young children their best possible start in life. This chapter has provided an overview of SLC development in young children, as well as the intergenerational impact of SLC need. The importance of identifying risks and intervening early to allay these risks as well as promoting SLC skills in young children and minimising SLC need has been discussed. The important role of health visitors in assessing and profiling SLC ability of young children and leading early intervention strategies to improve outcomes for children and young people has been highlighted.

## KEY LEARNING POINTS

- SLC development is a critical part of the healthy development of children.
- Health visitors need to be able to assess/profile speech language and communication development and identify factors that may lead to an increased risk of speech language and communication need in children.
- Health visitors should have the knowledge and skills to lead or facilitate early intervention strategies to promote SLC development in children and know when to refer to, or request assistance from, a speech and language therapist.

## REFERENCES

1. All Party Parliamentary Group on Speech and Language Difficulties (2013). The Links between Speech, Language and Communication Needs and Social Disadvantage. London: Royal College of Speech and Language Therapists (RCSLT). Available at: https://www.rcslt.org/wp-content/uploads/media/Project/RCSLT/appg-report-feb-2013.pdf.
2. Nelson, C. A. (2000). In *From neurons to neighborhoods: The Science of early childhood development*. In, J. P. Shonkoff & D. A. Phillips (Eds.), P.188, Washington, D.C., National Academy Press.
3. Vihman, M. (1996). *Phonological development: The origins of language in the child*. Oxford: Basil Blackwell.
4. Colonnesi, C., Stams, G. J. J., Koster, I., & Noom, M. J. (2010). The relation between pointing and language

development: A meta-analysis. *Developmental Review*, 30(4), 352–366.
5. Nelson, K., Rescorla, L., Gruendel, J., & Benedict, H. (1978). Early lexicons: What do they mean? *Child Development*, 49, 960–968.
6. Benedict, H. (1979). Early lexical development: Comprehension and production. *Journal of Child Language*, 6, 183–200.
7. Bates, E., Marchman, V., Thal, D., Fenson, L., Dale, P., Reznick, J. S., Reilly, J., & Hartung, J. (1994). Developmental and stylistic variation in the composition of early vocabulary. *Journal of Child Language*, 21(1), 58–123.
8. Law, J., & Roy, P. (2008). Parental report of infant language skills –A review of the development and application of the Communicative Development Inventories. *Child and Adolescent Mental Health*, 13, 198–206.
9. Menyuk, P., Liebergott, J. W., Schultz, M. C. (1995). *Early language development in full-term and premature infants*. Hillsdale, New Jersey: Lawrence Erlbaum.
10. Woodward, A. L., Markman, E. M., & Fitzsimmons, C. M. (1994). Rapid word learning in 13- and 18-month-olds. *Developmental Psychology*, 30, 553–566.
11. Hadley, P. A., Rispoli, M., & Hsua, N. (2016). Toddlers' verb lexicon diversity and grammatical outcomes. *Language, Speech, and Hearing Services in Schools*, 47, 44–58.
12. Sim, F., Haig, C., & O'Dowd, J. (2015). Development of a triage tool for neurodevelopmental risk in children aged 30 months. *Research in Developmental Disabilities*, 45(46), 69–82.
13. Bates, E., Thal, D., & Janowsky, J. S. (1992). Early language development and its neural correlates. In S. J. Segalowitz, & I. Rapin, (Eds). *Handbook of Neuropsychology*, 7: 69–110.
14. Wilson, P., & Law, J. (2019). Developmental reviews and the identification of disorders. In A. Edmond (Ed.), *Health for all children* (5th ed.). Oxford: Oxford University Press.
15. Saffran, J. R. (2018). Statistical learning as a window into developmental disabilities. *Journal of Neurodevelopmental Disorders*, 10(35), 1–5.
16. Norbury, C., Gooch, D., Wray, C., Baird, G., Charman, T., Simonoff, E., et al. (2016). The impact of nonverbal ability on prevalence and clinical presentation of language disorder: Evidence from a population study. *The Journal of Child Psychology and Psychiatry*, 57, 1247–1257.
17. Bishop, D. V. M., Snowling, M. J., Thompson, P. A., Greenhalgh, T., CATALISE consortium, The PLoS ONE Staff. (2016). Correction: CATALISE: A multinational and multidisciplinary Delphi consensus study. identifying language impairments in children. *PLoS One*, 11(12): e0168066.

18. Dockrell, J., Ricketts, J., & Lindsay, G. (2012). *Understanding speech, language and communication needs: Profiles of need and provision*. London: Department for Education research report. https://assets.publishing.service.gov.uk/government/uploads/system/uploads/attachment_data/file/557156/DFE-RR247-BCRP4.pdf.

19. Hart, B., & Risley, T. R. (2003). "The early catastrophe: The 30 million word gap by age 3." *American Educator, 27*(1), 4–9. www.aft.org/pdfs/americaneducator/spring2003/TheEarlyCatastrophe.pdf.

20. Hart, B., & Risley, T. R. (1995). *Meaningful differences in the everyday experiences of young American children*. Baltimore, MD: Paul. H. Brookes.

21. Gilkerson, J., & Richards, J. A. (2009). *The power of talk. Impact of adult talk, conversational turns and TV during the critical 0–4 years of child development*. Boulder, CO: LENA Foundation.

22. Knudsen, L., Currie, E., Bradshaw, P., Law, J., & Wood, R. (2019). *Growing up in Scotland: Changes in language ability over the primary school years*. Edinburgh: Scottish Government. https://www.gov.scot/publications/growing-up-scotland-changes-language-ability-over-primary-school-years/.

23. Tambyraja, S. R., Schmitt, M. B., Farquharson, K., & Justice, L. M. (2015). Stability of language and literacy profiles of children with language impairment in the public schools. *Journal of Speech, Language and Hearing Research, 58*, 1167–1181.

24. Law, J., Mensah, F., Westrupp, E., & Reilly, S. (2015). *Social disadvantage and early language delay*. Centre of Research Excellence in Child Language, Policy Brief.

25. Roulestone, S., Law, J., Rush, R., Clegg, J., & Peters, T. (2011). *Investigating the role of language in children's early educational outcomes*. Department of Education Research Report 134.

26. Paul, R. (1991). Profiles of toddlers with slow expressive language development. *Topics in Language Disorders, 11*(4), 1–13.

27. Ellis, E. M., & Thal, D. J. (2008). Early language delay and risk for language impairment. *Perspectives on Language Learning and Education, 15*(3), 93–100.

28. Hawa, V. V., & Spanoudis, G. (2014). Toddlers with delayed expressive language: An overview of the characteristics, risk factors and language outcomes. *Researchers in Developmental Disabilities, 35*, 400–407.

29. Sachse, S. (2008). Early identification of language delay by direct language assessment or parent report? *Journal of Developmental and Behavioural Pediatrics, 29*(1), 34–41. https://www.researchgate.net/publication/5551168_Early_Identification_of_Language_Delay_by_Direct_Language_Assessment_or_Parent_Report https://journals.

lww.com/jrnldbp/Abstract/2008/02000/Early_Identification_of_Language_Delay_by_Direct.6.aspx.

30. Pan, B. A., Rowe, M. L., Spier, E., et al. (2004). Measuring productive vocabulary of toddlers in low-income families: Concurrent and predictive validity of three sources of data. *Journal of Children's Language, 31*, 587–608.

31. Dockrell, J., & Marshall, C. (2014). Measurement issues: Assessing language skills in young children. *Child and Adolescent Mental Health, 20*(2), 116–125.

32. Berkman, N. D., Wallace, I., Watson, L., et al. (2015). Screening for speech and language delays and disorders in children age 5 years or younger: A systematic review for the U.S. Preventive Services Task Force. Rockville (MD): Agency for Healthcare Research and Quality (US) Accessible online from: https://pubmed.ncbi.nlm.nih.gov/26225412/. https://www.uspreventiveservices-taskforce.org/uspstf/document/evidence-summary30/speech-and-language-delay-and-disorders-in-children-age-5-and-younger-screening.

33. Royal College of Speech and Language Therapists (RCSLT) (2016). *Speech, language and communication capacity: A national asset*. https://www.rcslt.org/-/media/Project/RCSLT/rcslt-communication-capacity-factsheet.pdf?la=en&hash=24A0C48F479519A484B92B04A5C074C515254FF2.

34. Ramírez, N. F., Lytle, S. R., & Kuhl, P. K. (2020). Parent coaching increases conversational turns and advances infant language development. *Proceedings of the National Academy of Sciences of the United States of America, 117*(7), 3484–3491. https://www.pnas.org/content/117/7/3484.

35. Ramírez, N. F., Lytle, S. R., Fish, M., & Kuhl, P. K. (2018). Parent coaching at 6 and 10 months improves language outcomes at 14 months: A randomized controlled trial. *Developmental Science, 22*(3), e12762. https://www.onlinelibrary.wiley.com/doi/epdf/10.1111/desc.12762.

36. Bercow, J. (2018). *Bercow: Ten years on. An independent review of provision for children and young people with speech, language and communication needs in England*. RCSLT/I-CAN. https://www.bercow10yearson.com/.

37. Bromley, C. & Burley, S. (2010). *Growing up in Scotland: Health inequalities in the early years*. Edinburgh: Scottish Government.

38. Law, J., Charlton, J., & Amussem, K. (2017). *Language as a child wellbeing indicator*. Early Intervention Foundation [online]. https://www.eif.org.uk/report/language-as-a-child-wellbeing-indicator/.

39. Law, J., Boyle, J., Harris, F., Harkness, A., & Nye, C. (1998). Screening for speech and language delay: A systematic review of the literature. *Health Technology Assessment 1998, 2*(9), 1–184. https://www.crd.york.ac.uk/CRDWeb/ShowRecord.asp?ID=11998009012&ID=11998009012.

40. *Millenium Cohort Study.* https://cls.ucl.ac.uk/cls-studies/millennium-cohort-study/.

41. All Party Parliamentary Group on Speech and Language Difficulties. 2013. https://www.rcslt.org/wp-content/uploads/media/Project/RCSLT/all-party-parliamentary-group-on-slcn-inquiry-report.pdf The links between speech, language and communication needs and social disadvantage. London: Royal College of Speech and Language Therapists.

42. Royal College of Speech and Language Therapists Scotland. Speech Language and Communication Capacity. A National Asset. Edinburgh: RCSLTS; 2016.

43. Hartshorne, M. (2006). The Cost to the Nation of Children's Poor Communication. I CAN Talk Series – Issue 2. https://ican.org.uk/media/1592/2_the_cost_to_the_nation_of_childrens_poor_communication.pdf

44. Moss, G., Washbrook, L., & Eagle, S. (2016). Understanding the Gender Gap in Literacy and Language Development. Bristol: University of Bristol. http://www.bristol.ac.uk/media-library/sites/education/documents/bristol-working-papers-in-education/Understanding%20the%20Gender%20Gap%20working%20paper.pdf

45. The Communication Trust. (2017). Professional development in speech, language and communication: Findings from a National Survey. https://www.rcslt.org/wp-content/uploads/media/Project/RCSLT/1tctworkforce-development-report-final-online.pdf

46. Bates, E., Dale, P. & Thal, D., (2019). Individual Differences and their Implications for Theories of Language Development. The Handbook of Child Language, 95–151.

47. Lüke, C., Grimminger, A., Rohlfing, K. J., Liszkowski, U., Ritterfeld, U. (2017). In Infants' Hands: Identification of Preverbal Infants at Risk for Primary Language Delay. *Child Development, 88*(2), 484–492.

48. Lindsay, G., Dockrell, J., Desforges, M., Law, J. & Peacey, N., (2010). Meeting the needs of children and young people with speech, language and communication difficulties. International Journal of Language & Communication Disorders, 45(4), 448–460.

49. Lindsay, G., Dockrell, J., Desforges, M., Law, J. & Peacey, N. (2010). Meeting the needs of children and young people with speech, language and communication difficulties. *International Journal of Language & Communication Disorders, 45*(4), 448–460.

50. Ramírez, N.F., Lytle, S.R., Kuhl, P.K. (2020). Parenting coaching increases conversational turns and advances infant language development. *Proceedings of the National Academy of Sciences of the United States of America. 2020. 117*(7), 3484–3491. https://www.pnas.org/content/117/7/3484.

51. Bercow, J., (2018). Bercow: Ten Years On. An independent review of provision for children and young people with speech, language and communication needs in England. RCSLT / I-CAN. https://www.bercow10yearson.com/

52. Newbury, D.F., Monaco, A.P. (2010). Genetic Advances in the Study of Speech and Language Disorders. Neuron, 68, 309–320.

53. Dockrell, J., Ricketts, J., Lindsay, G. (2012). Understanding speech, language and communication needs: Profiles of need and provision. London: Department for Education research report. https://www.gov.uk/government/collections/better-communication-research-programme https://assets.publishing.service.gov.uk/government/uploads/system/uploads/attachment_data/file/557156/DFE-RR247-BCRP4.pdf

54. Schoon, I., Parsons, S., Rush, R., & Law, J. (2010). Childhood language skills and adult literacy: a 29-year follow-up study. *Pediatrics, 125*(3), e459–e466.

55. Colmar (2014) A parent-based book-reading intervention for disadvantaged children with language difficulties *Child Language Teaching and Therapy. 31*(1), 79–90.

56. Naven, L., Egan, J., Sosu, E. M., & Spencer, S. (2019). The influence of poverty on children's school experiences: pupils' perspectives. *Journal of Poverty and Social Justice, 27*(3), 313–331.

57. Bromley, C. (2009). Growing Up in Scotland: Year 3 – The Impact of Children's Early Activities on Cognitive Development. Edinburgh: Scottish Government.

58. Olswang, L.B., Rodriguez, B., & Timler, G. (1998). Recommending intervention for toddlers with specific language learning difficulties: We may not have all the answers, but we know a lot. *American Journal of Speech-Language Pathology. 7*(91), 23–32.

59. Camarata S. (2014). Early identification and early intervention in autism spectrum disorders: Accurate and effective? International Journal of Speech-Language Pathology, 16:1, 1–10

60. Law, J., & Levickis P., (2018). Early language development must be a public health priority. *Journal of Health Visiting. 6*(12), 586–589.

61. Public Health Scotland. (2020). Early Child Development. https://publichealthscotland.scot/publications/early-child-development/early-child-development-scotland-201920/

62. McKean, C., Wraith, D., Eadie, P., Cook, F., Mensah, F. & Reilly, S. (2017). Subgroups in language trajectories from 4 to 11 years: The nature and predictors of stable, improving and decreasing language trajectory groups. *Journal of Child Psychology and Psychiatry, 58*(10), 1081–1091.

63. Nursing and Midwifery Council (NMC). (2004). Standards of proficiency for specialist community public health nurses. London: NMC

64. Marmot, M. (2010). Fair society, healthy lives : The Marmot Review : Strategic review of health inequalities in England post-2010. London: The Marmot Review.

65. Adams, C., & Cowley, J. (2019). Ch8: Primary Prevention and Health Promotion in Childhood. In Emond, A. (Ed) 2019. Health for All Children (5th edn). Oxford: Oxford University Press.

66. Topping, K. J., Dekhinet, R., & Zeedyk, S. (2011). Hindrances for parents in enhancing child language. *Educational Psychology Review*, 23, 413–455.

67. McGovern Institute. Beyond the 30 Million Word Gap.http://mcgovern.mit.edu/news/news/research-news/beyond-the-30-million-word-gap/

68. Massachusetts Institute of Technology. Back-and-forth exchanges boost children's brain response to language. https://news.mit.edu/2018/conversation-boost-childrens-brain-response-language-0214

69. Romeo, R. R., Leonard, J. A., Robinson, S. T., West, M. R., Mackey, A. P., Rowe, M. L., & Gabrieli, J. D. E. (2018). Beyond the 30-Million-Word Gap: Children's Conversational Exposure Is Associated With Language-Related Brain Function. Psychol Sci. 29(5):700-710. doi: 10.1177/0956797617742725. Epub 2018 Feb 14. PMID: 29442613; PMCID: PMC5945324.

70. Trafton. A. (2018). Back-and-forth exchanges boost children's brain response to language. USA: Masachusetts Institute of Technology. https://news.mit.edu/2018/conversation-boost-childrens-brain-response-language-0214

71. Pryor, J. (2018). Beyond the 30 Million Word Gap: Back-and-forth exchanges boost children's brain response to language. Retrieved on April 7, 2018 from: http://mcgovern.mit.edu/news/news/research-news/beyond-the-30-million-word-gap/

72. Cowley, S., Whittaker, K., Grigulis, A., Malone, M., Donetto, S., Wood, H., Morrow, E., & Maben, J. (2013). Why Health Visiting? A review of the literature about key health visitor interventions, processes and outcomes for children and families. London: Kings College.

73. (2015) Universal Health Visiting Pathway in Scotland. Pre-birth to Pre-school. www.gov.scot/Publications/2015/10/9697/downloads (accessed 10 May 2018) Scottish Government.

74. Kildare, C. A., & Middlemiss, W. (2017). Impact of parents mobile device use on parent-child interaction: A literature review. Computers in Human Behavior, 75, 579–593.

75. Zhang, Y., Xu, X., Jiang, F., Gilkerson, J., Xu, D., Richards, J. A., ... & Topping, K. J. (2015). Effects of quantitative linguistic feedback to caregivers of young children: A pilot study in China. *Communication Disorders Quarterly, 37*(1), 16–24.

76. Golinkoff, R. M., Hoff, E., Rowe, M. L., Tamis-LeMonda, C. S., & Hirsh-Pasek, K. (2019). Language matters: Denying the existence of the 30-million-word gap has serious consequences. *Child development, 90*(3), 985–992.

77. Erickson, L. C., & Newman, R. S. (2017). Influences of background noise on infants and children. *Current directions in psychological science, 26*(5), 451–457.

78. Tempel, A. B., Wagner, S. M., & McNeil, C. B. (2009). Parent-child interaction therapy and language facilitation: The role of parent-training on language development. *The Journal of Speech and Language Pathology–Applied Behavior Analysis, 3*(2–3), 216.

79. Topping, K., Dekhinet, R., & Zeedyk, S. (2013). Parent–infant interaction and children's language development. *Educational Psychology, 33*(4), 391–426.

80. NHS Education for Scotland. 2018. 'Speech, Language and Communication: Giving Children the Best Possible Start in Life. Digital Speech, language and communication resource for health visitors available from: https://slctoolforhv.nes.digital/index.html

81. Public Health England. (2020). 'The Best Start in Speech, Language and Communication (SLC)' Guidance to help improve SLC in the early years including an Early Language Identification Measure and Intervention tool for Health Visitors to use with children aged 2 to 2 and a half available from: https://www.gov.uk/government/publications/best-start-in-speech-language-and-communication.

82. Law, J., Levickis, P., McKean, C., Goldfeld, S., Snow, P., & Reilly, S. (2017). Child language in a public health context. Melbourne: Murdoch Children Research Institute.

# 16

# MANAGEMENT OF COMMON CHILDHOOD AILMENTS AND ACCIDENT PREVENTION

VAL THURTLE

## CHAPTER CONTENTS

INTRODUCTION

ACCIDENT PREVENTION

HEALTH VISITOR ACTION IN ACCIDENT PREVENTION

SEARCH FOR HEALTH NEEDS

STIMULATION OF AN AWARENESS OF HEALTH NEEDS

INFLUENCE ON POLICIES AFFECTING HEALTH

FACILITATION OF HEALTH-ENHANCING ACTIVITIES

MANAGEMENT OF COMMON CHILDHOOD AILMENTS

ROLE OF THE HEALTH VISITOR

CONSIDER THE PATIENT

CARING FOR THE BABY OR SICK CHILD

CONCLUSION

## LEARNING OUTCOMES

*To:*

- outline the five dominant causes of unintentional injuries and critically review ways the health visiting service can seek to work with parents to prevent them.

- reflect on what is a 'common' childhood ailment and discuss with parents/carers ways of assessing the child and managing certain conditions in the home setting.

## INTRODUCTION

The focus of health visiting is prevention and health promotion as clearly outlined in the Principles of Health Visiting[1] and the Nursing and Midwifery Specialist Community Public Health Nurse domains.[2] The health visiting service sets out to take a preventative 'upstream' approach to all children and families, providing anticipatory guidance to promote well-being. While health visitors work with all families with a new baby, there are more interventions with those with increased needs seeking to reduce health inequalities and address the requirements of those who do not experience easy access to services.

Taking a proactive preventative approach could include any aspect dependent on the needs of the area, community, child or family and will differ over time; the focus is currently on 15 high impact areas.

This book has referred to many of these areas with the emphasis on working with parents to develop their personal and community assets, so they are in a position to support their child's health and developmental needs, preventing illness by immunisation, promoting well-being by nutrition and supporting good relationships.

This chapter focusses on high impact areas six and seven, the management of minor ailments and the reduction of accidents or unintentional injuries

## ACCIDENT PREVENTION

If prevention is a major part of the work of the health visitor, primary prevention stopping disease or injury before it ever occurs should be key for those working with babies and young children. Accident prevention is crucial as injuries to children are a major public health and inequality issue, as well as a cause of distress to individual children and their families. Quite rightly there is a concern with children sustaining intentional injuries, but accidents or unintentional injuries are more frequent. The Early Years High Impact Areas[5] set out the key contribution of health visitors to reduce accidents as a means of improving outcomes for all children.

Unintentional injuries in and around the home are a leading cause of preventable death, the most common cause of death in children over the age of 1 year,[6] and a major cause of ill health and serious disability for children under five. Between 2012/13–2016/17 in England an average of 55 children aged less than 5 years old died each year due to an unintentional injury, 370,000 children attended accident and emergency (A&E), and 40,000 were admitted to hospital as an emergency.[7] Others would have been managed in primary care or in the home. In Scotland in 2017/18, the rate of emergency hospital admission for unintentional injury per 100,000 males aged under five was 1150 compared to 995 for females.[8] In all the child age groups and countries, males were more likely than females to be admitted to hospital for an unintentional injury. No one intends to injure the child but many such accidents are predictable and could be averted. 'Unintentional injury' and 'accident' are used here interchangeably.

Accidents in the under-fives are a major health inequality. They are a result of the wider determinants of health and are influenced by the socio-economic setting, the physical environment in the home, together with over-crowding and homelessness, the education, knowledge and behaviour of parents and carers, the development of the child, the availability of safety equipment and consumer products in the home. Emergency hospital admission rates for unintentional injuries among the under-fives was 38% higher for children from the most deprived areas in England compared with the least deprived parts of the country.[9] In all parts of the United Kingdom, attendance at

A&E settings for children 0 to 4 years old is high,[10] though these will not always be the result of accidents. Treatment in any A&E facility has costs, the rate per day for an admission in 2018 was approximately £700–£1000 and the average short-term healthcare cost of an individual injury (all types) was £2494.[9] This does not take into account the health care and social care costs for longer term follow-up. Parents and carers bear the financial cost of loss of work, travel, extra child care for siblings and the emotional concern, the worry of coping with uncertainly and having a hurt and frightened child. Many reasons for attendance at A&E are avoidable or preventable if parents and carers were in a position to reduce the accidents.

## THINKING POINT

Is an accident and an unintentional injury the same or different?

## THINKING POINT

Why are accidents frequently linked with socio-economic deprivation?

Five causes account for 90% of unintentional injury hospital admissions for the under-fives,[7,9] and are considered below:

**Choking, suffocation and strangulation:** While deaths in under-fives have been reducing, inhalation of food and vomit is one of the causes of mortality in the under-twos; other causes are strangulation, perhaps by blind cords and suffocation with pillows, duvets and cot bumpers, which they do not need in the first year of life, as well as plastic bags or nappy sacks.

**Falls:** This is the most common cause of an emergency admission and includes falls from furniture, including beds and chairs; on and off stairs and steps; from or out of buildings, including windows and balconies as well as from being carried. We will all remember being involved in a fall that did not

get to hospital; inevitably hospital statistics show only part of the picture.

**Poisoning:** The two main risks to under-fives are medicines, which make up about 70% of poisoning admissions and household chemicals (such as liquid detergent capsules), leading to approximately 20% of admissions.[9] Children of about 1 year old most commonly ingest household chemicals and those about aged two go for medicines. No medicine container is completely child proof; they only slow the child down.

**Burns and scalds:** Though burns and scalds lead to a high number of admissions deaths are rare; however the injuries are expensive to treat and serious burns and scalds are disfiguring and disabling for young children. The causes of such injuries are hot drinks and hot fluids generally, hot appliances such as hair straighteners and heating appliances – for example, radiators and pipes – and bath water. The peak age for hospital admissions is 1 year,[9] with hot drinks causing the most injuries.

**Drowning:** Drowning is frequently lethal. For babies and young children, the main risk is the bath, though fish ponds and open water should not be forgotten. Babies and toddlers can drown in as little as five centimetres of water; they may not struggle or make any noise, giving no warning of what is happening.

## HEALTH VISITOR ACTION IN ACCIDENT PREVENTION

Public Health England[11] identified three key action areas in terms of preventing injuries:

- Providing leadership and mobilising existing services
- Supporting and training the early years workforce to enable it to strengthen its central role in helping to reduce unintentional injuries
- Focusing on five kinds of injuries for the under-fives.

Health visitors are not the only service involved in accident prevention, but these action points can be combined with the Principles of Health Visiting. The headings explore what is and should be happening.

## SEARCH FOR HEALTH NEEDS

Looking for health needs is required at national, community and individual levels. The preceding section has demonstrated the use of national reports to identify key areas of concern. Providing leadership and mobilising existing services involves working with directors of public health, directors of children's services, local children's trust boards and children's partnership boards, clinical commissioning groups and health and well-being boards in England, health and social care boards in Northern Ireland, NHS boards in Scotland and health boards and community health councils in Wales in order to take a strategic approach to identifying the extent of the issues in a particular area and the services already present.

More locally, a review of statistics – for instance, records of attendance at A&E facilities – may show the trends in types of accidents and the areas where they are most common, thus facilitating targeting or progressive universalism of health promotion strategies.

At a family level the health visitor will work with parents to identify the particular needs of the family in terms of the environment and the developmental level of their children.

## STIMULATION OF AN AWARENESS OF HEALTH NEEDS

Encouraging health promotion on the reduction of accidents is evident in The Healthy Child Programme (HCP)[12] and Early Years High Impact Area 5.[5] Anyone who is part of the early years workforce – including health visiting teams, school nurses, local authority children's services, early years settings and voluntary organisations – needs to be trained and supported, and to work together to provide local delivery of accident prevention interventions.

## INFLUENCE ON POLICIES AFFECTING HEALTH

A significant contribution to accident prevention is a population approach with laws and regulation; for instance, child-resistant medication containers, mandatory use of child car seats, controls on products used with young children, engineering and property regulations on windows and heating devices. Within health care the NICE guidelines[13,14] set out what should be done, with a particular focus on those living in disadvantaged circumstances.

## FACILITATION OF HEALTH-ENHANCING ACTIVITIES

Different approaches have been taken to improving home safety though a strong evidence base on the impact of injury is not always available: changes can be demonstrated in relation to practice but not necessarily to the incidence of injuries.[6,15,16]

Home safety education is the most obvious intervention and a meta-analysis of 22 randomised controlled trials,[17] albeit from some years ago, found home safety education and provision of equipment helped make homes safer, particularly in relation to restraints in cars, smoke alarm ownership and safe hot tap water temperature. Interventions were most effective when they combined health education, discussion of the issues, demonstrations, the provision of subsidised safety devices and reinforcement. Home safety education is most commonly undertaken in a one-to-one, face-to-face setting. There is evidence that such home-based parenting interventions reduce injury rates[18] and improve home safety.[19] Health visitors need to be able to discuss baby and child safety equipment and suggest what is needed and where it can be acquired or borrowed locally.

Discussion of home safety needs to be closely linked with child development stages. The five mandated contacts in England,[12] nine in Northern Ireland[20] and Wales[21] and eleven in Scotland[22] (see Chapter 4 for the model of health visiting practice in all four nations), together with taking a 'Making every contact count approach'[23] can be used to facilitate behaviour change in relation to the changing demands of the child and the preventative action that needs to follow. Using a specific model or electronic record system is useful to give prompts, but the experienced health visitor or community nursery nurse will be knowledgeable about areas of risk related to home safety at the key ages.

Taking a secondary prevention approach to home accidents, which aims to reduce the impact of an injury that has already occurred and prevent reinjury or recurrence, most health visiting services follow up the A&E attendance of which they are notified. A phone call to the parent may generate a defensive response or a carer who is guilt ridden that the accident took place or one keen to make changes in differing areas. The phone call or visit needs to be handled sensitively, with empathetic communication and input closely linked with the child's development stage, together with what they are likely to be able to do in the near future.

### Case study 16.1

Freya is the first child of parents who both work as teachers. She was born by normal delivery, was breastfed until 11 months and eats well. She has met all her developmental milestones. She is up to date with immunisations. At just 2 years of age she is in the 90th percentile for height, weight and head circumference. She walks confidently, can kick a ball with her right foot and can walk upstairs. She uses crayons to colour and can do simple puzzles. She understands commands and can make simple conversations with two to three words, such as 'What Daddy doing?' She is not toilet-trained. She sleeps 10 hours most nights, rarely waking.

Her mother Stephanie is pregnant with her second child. The health visitor has made an appointment to do an antenatal contact and finds the family have moved into a brand-new house, just a week before.

Is Freya at risk of having a home accident?

What type?

Should the health visitor discuss accident prevention?

If so, what areas should be his/her focus?

### THINKING POINT

Reflect on the organisation of health visiting in your UK country, and the mandated minimal number of contacts and the age of the child at these visits.

Identify and role play the delivery of a relevant (appropriate to the development needs of the child) injury prevention topic.

### THINKING POINT

Is there a law or regulation related to accident prevention that is required and for which we should be campaigning?

## MANAGEMENT OF COMMON CHILDHOOD AILMENTS

To discuss support and treatment for minor ailments raises the question 'What are they?' Perhaps they are defined as 'common or self-limiting or uncomplicated conditions which may be diagnosed and managed without doctor interventions'.[24] Recent estimates, following a study in parts of England and Scotland, suggest that 5% and 13% of consultations in emergency departments and general practice, respectively, are for minor conditions that could be managed in community pharmacies.[25]

Young children have a variety of ailments and the view of what is minor will be influenced by the context and severity of the illness, the previous history of the child and the experience of the parent or carer. Some conditions will indeed be self-limiting and require family care; others will be taken to and require (which may not be the same thing) A&E. More people generally attend A&E than was the case in the past.[26] This may be influenced by the availability of services outside the hospital, both in terms of the acceptability to the parent/carer, geography and opening times. Deciding what is minor involves assessment by the health worker or the parent.

## Assessment

Assessment is the first stage in the planning of care; it is the process of gathering information to make decisions about appropriate interventions.[27] Assessment of any child is central to the role of health visitor, whether in terms of health and well-being, interaction with parents and siblings, development, nutrition or the environment in which the family lives.

Assessment of a child hinges on communication with the parent and sometimes the child, together with observation of the child. The health visitor needs to identify what the parent sees as the problem. Figure 16.1 outlines what should be discussed, but beware a tick list approach.

## Observation

Observation of the child should be key in any interaction and recent use of telephone and video contacts has made this more difficult. There are different guidelines in different employing organisations to whether health visitors should examine (or even touch) a child but Figure 16.2 indicates what should be observed and considered by parent or health worker.

## Listening to the parent and carer

The parent knows their child and is best placed to note changes. Listening to their concerns is likely to be more effective than using a checklist approach, though that may be useful for the novice practitioner. The parent is likely to voice their most pressing or current worry.

## Symptoms of concern

Whether it is the parent or a health worker making the assessment, there are signs and symptoms that are not minor. They need to be taken seriously and acted upon. These include:

- **Difficulty breathing or respiratory distress.** This may be as a result of a virus or bacteria. The most serious respiratory diseases occur in the first 3 years of life.

| Areas for discussion |
|---|
| History of the child and the ailment |
| Presenting issue and details related to this |
| Past history, birth history, previous illneses, injuries |
| Allergies |
| Medication, immunisations |
| Growth and development |
| Nutrition (what and how they eat) |
| Nutritional assessment malnourished/ overweight using centile chart |
| Family medical history |
| Family context, parental concern, composition, siblings, parents' cultural religious tradition |

Figure 16.1 ■ Areas for discussion.

| General appearance, behaviour |
| Interaction with parents, siblings and peers |
| Posture, types of movement<br>   Head and neck control in young child |
| Pattern of breathing |
| Fontanelle (flat, swollen, bulging or sinking) |
| Pyrexical |
| Hygiene, clothing |
| Skin: colour, texture, temperature, moisture, lesions, rashes, tone, colour temperature |
| Hair texture and elasticity |
| Hearing reported and observed<br>   Understanding of speech |

Figure 16.2 ■ Areas for observation to be amended for age and development stage of the child.

Prompt medical attention is needed if the child grunts with each breath or has dips in their abdomen or between ribs as they breathe. It is an emergency if the child stops breathing or goes blue.

■ **Fever.** This is a common presentation in children and viruses are the most common cause; serious bacterial infections are rare but need to be found. Parents are used to taking a temperature and a temperature of more than 39 °C is worrying and in a baby of 0 to 3 months old a fever of over 38°C is of concern. Children can easily spike a temperature so a persistent fever raises more apprehension. If the fever is accompanied by other symptoms outlined here medical attention is needed.

■ **Pale and lethargic child.** The parents will know what their child is usually like so will recognise if they are less active or more floppy than usual. A high-pitched cry in a baby or a weak cry is of concern. It is a medical emergency if the child is unresponsive, has glazed eyes, does not focus on anything or cannot be woken. An epileptic fit always needs medical attention even if the child has recovered without medical intervention.

■ **A rash that started as pin pricks** spreads quickly and becomes purple or red blotches that do not fade under pressure.

■ **Diarrhoea and vomiting.** This is not unusual in children and for most children the symptoms are mild and transient. It is of concern if any sickness includes bile and if it leads to reduced urine output.

■ **Changes in eating and drinking patterns.** This happens with many children, ill and well, but a baby that has not taken fluids over an 8-hour period will have reduced urine output demonstrated in dry nappies. This does need medical attention.

Combinations of these signs and symptoms are unlikely to be minor. Even with other symptoms if the baby/child remains unwell or seems to be deteriorating further medical assessment is needed.

## ROLE OF THE HEALTH VISITOR

The health visiting service is not generally an emergency or treatment service, yet if they come across a child with symptoms as above, they and the parent or carer will seek emergency or medical treatment. Their role is far more likely to be one of facilitation, preparing the parent to manage minor illness in the future or talking through what could be done at the current time. Many health visitors can prescribe from the *Nurse Prescribers' Formulary for Community Practitioners*[28] and this might be used in managing some minor illness and conditions. Whether prescribing is involved or not the prescribing pyramid[29] (Figure 16.3) is a useful framework to use.

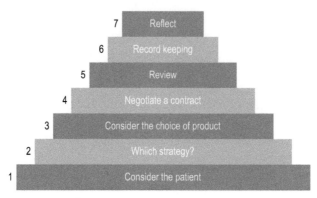

Figure 16.3 ■ The prescribing pyramid.[29]

## CONSIDER THE PATIENT

The issue of assessment, considered before, is part of this. The mnemonic WWHAM is useful, considering:

**W**ho has the health needs?
**W**hat are the symptoms?
**H**ow long have they been going on?
What **A**ction has already been taken?
Is any **M**edication in use?

### Which strategy?

Having identified the particular health need or minor ailment, it is the case of considering the options, including the giving of health information, pharmacological and non-pharmacological choices. For any approach both risks and benefits need to be considered and a plan identified with the parent/carer.

### Consider the choice of product

There may be cases when the health visitor wants to prescribe or they wish to help the parent/carer to decide on using over-the-counter preparations or those already in the home. In all cases the practitioner needs to consider how effective the product is and whether it is an appropriate treatment for the condition, age and history of the child. Prescriptions should be generic medicines, where practical, and safe; the practitioner should have an awareness of contraindications, interactions, cautions and unwanted effects.

### Negotiate a contract

Whatever is planned should be a shared decision, in partnership with carer/parent, so they have made an informed choice and are fully aware of what they need to do and what is likely to happen. A therapeutic relationship with the carer/parent is required that encourages two-way effective communication. Clear and accessible information needs to be provided by discussion, leaflets or reliable online sources. Honouring individual choices and beliefs is the hallmark of professional health care providers.[30] Being aware of the parent's values, accepting them and seeking clarification if necessary are essential if the person is to be respected. Taking this approach can also have a positive impact on concordance, both in terms of prescribing and whatever is agreed. In terms of medication, parents/carers need to be aware of what it is for, how to use it, the quantity involved, and how long it is to be used. There needs to be some 'safety netting', so they are aware of possible actions if the situation changes or deteriorates.

### Review

Follow-up of the child will establish that the situation proceeded as expected, will develop the relationship with the parent/carer and is a relevant learning experience for the practitioner.

## Record keeping

The Nursing and Midwifery Council Code[30] emphasises that nurses, midwives and nursing associates should keep clear and accurate records which are relevant to their practice. Whether paper or electronic records, they should be clearly written, dated and timed, without unnecessary abbreviations and jargon and should be contemporaneous and kept securely.

## Reflection

Reflection is how health and care professionals can assess their professional experiences. Reflection should be central to health visiting practice as it clarifies the issues and establishes the priorities for action, both in the episode under consideration and the planning for the future.

## CARING FOR THE BABY OR SICK CHILD

Minor illnesses, such as viral upper respiratory tract infections and others listed below, are commonplace with preschool children; it is estimated many have five such illnesses a year. Parents are not surprisingly anxious and need to be informed on how to manage minor illness and recognise the symptoms of concern for seeking medical attention discussed earlier. Ill babies and children become pale, listless, and do not want to eat; caring for the child involves ensuring they are given plenty of fluids and woken to be offered feeds if they are sleeping a lot. A temperature should be taken with a digital thermometer in the armpit and a reminder given that 37°C is normal. Babies and children generally, and certainly if they have a fever, should not be underdressed or over-wrapped. Pediatric liquid paracetamol can be given to address discomfort and keep the temperature down. The environment needs to be

quiet and peaceful and the child is likely to want increased care and attention.

It is important that the well-being of the child is monitored: how they look generally, their breathing, development of a rash, possible signs of dehydration by looking for a sunken fontanelle, dry mouth, sunken eyes alongside how much they are drinking and how much fluid they lose in vomit and wet nappies.

## Specific minor ailments

Inevitably this outline of conditions is not comprehensive. Further details are available from good textbooks[31] and reliable sites on the internet such as:

NHS Conditions. https://www.nhs.uk/conditions/

NHS Inform Ready Steady Baby. https://www.nhsinform.scot/ready-steady-baby

Ready Steady Toddler. http://www.readysteadytoddler.org.uk/

## Asthma

Asthma is a common lung disease, with intermittent narrowing of the bronchi, causing shortness of breath, noisy breathing, recurrent wheezing, a dry cough (particularly at night) and tightness in the chest.

Predisposing factors include a family history of atopy: that is, allergies, eczema, rhinitis, co-existence of atopic disease and bronchiolitis in infancy. Common triggers include allergies (to house dust mites, animal fur or pollen), smoking pollution and cold air, infections like colds or flu and exercise.

A doctor needs to make the diagnosis taking into account the baby's history, undertaking a clinical examination and reviewing bronchodilator responsiveness. There is currently no cure for asthma but treatment can control the symptoms. The aim of treatment and management is to help the child to lead as normal a life as possible, to minimise the need for relieving medication and to prevent severe attacks or exacerbations. Treatment is by a stepwise approach that includes short-acting inhaled bronchodilator therapy (relievers) (such as salbutamol) and prophylactic therapy (preventers) (such as inhaled steroids). As the severity and frequency of symptoms increases so does the addition of therapies until good control is reached, then treatment is stepped down. Advice on other measures is also given, such as parental smoking cessation and living with household pets. Regular reviews are needed by a nurse or doctor with additional asthma management training in primary care.

## Colic

Infantile colic is defined as paroxysmal uncontrollable crying in an otherwise healthy infant less than 3 months of age, with more than 3 hours of crying per day in more than 3 days a week and for more than 3 weeks.[32] The baby is hard to soothe or settle: they clench their fists and go red, perhaps giving the impression they have wind as they bring their knees up to their tummy or arch their back.

Colic is considered to be self-limiting and benign, but is a frustrating and frightening problem for parents and caregivers, who often consult a health worker. There is debate about the cause, querying abnormal gastrointestinal motility, different bacteria modifying motor function, behavioural issues such as family tensions or insufficient parent-infant interaction.

Parental concerns should be explored and the child assessed, looking for apnoeic episodes, cyanosis, respiratory distress, vomiting, or bloody stools as well as projectile vomiting and poor or decreasing weight gain. If the cause has not been identified, potential interventions are various, including diet modification for breastfeeding mothers or changes to formula milk, potentially excluding lactose. Simethicone (Infacol), which reduces intraluminal gas, is available over the counter but trials have not indicated that it is any more effective than a placebo[32]; currently there are no effective and safe pharmacological management options available over the counter or by prescription. Complementary treatments, including acupuncture, massage, herbal supplements, swaddling and chiropractic, are often suggested but there is insufficient evidence to recommend their use.

Instead, advice includes preventing and addressing wind by winding the baby after feeds, holding the baby upright during feeding to stop them swallowing air, holding and cuddling the baby when they are crying, gently rocking them in a crib or pushing them in a pram or giving them a warm bath. It is important to carry on feeding them as usual. Infantile colic, while self-limiting and benign, is distressing to parents, and therefore parental support is required.

## Crying baby

A crying child is upsetting to parents and the majority will have considered many of the following, but it is worth revisiting the options.

**Hunger or thirst:** The most common reason babies cry is because they are hungry. The simplest solution is to offer the breast, which provides comfort as well as nutrition; giving a bottle to the formula-fed child as well as a cuddle is part of responsive feeding.

**Nappy change:** A dirty nappy from urine or faeces is irritating to the skin. If not cleaned, it can cause pain and burning. A nappy, clothing that is too tight, or clothing that is rubbing will also lead to distress.

**Lack of stimulation or over-stimulation:** Babies do not like being ignored and can get bored; it is worth trying a toy, a song, or simply pick them up. Conversely, a busy day, with many visitors, may leave the infant over-stimulated. A move to a calm area or simple swaddling may help.

**Temperature of the environment:** It is appropriate to check the baby's hands and feet, forehead, and the nape of their neck to see if they are hot or cold, and remove or add clothes as needed.

**Teething:** see later.

## Constipation

Babies show substantial variation in bowel habit according to diet and if breastfed. Babies can look as if they are straining even when passing a liquid stool. Changing from breastfeeding to artificial and/or solids leads to changes in stool colour and consistency. This is not constipation; instead constipation is the painful passage of hard, infrequent stools.

Constipation is common in children, being prevalent in around 5% to 30% of the child population and affecting more boys than girls.[33] Preschool children may be viewed as constipated if they have not passed a stool at least three times in the previous week, the faeces are large and hard or conversely like little pellets. Children may strain or be in pain when they pass the stool and there could be some bleeding during or after passing the stool because it is large and hard. In children over a year of age soiled pants may indicate constipation, as diarrhoea leaks out around the hard, constipated stool.

In babies constipation may occur from hunger, over-strength feeds, and poor hydration; it is rare but possible for there to be a congenital abnormality, such as spinal cord lesions or Hirschsprung's disease. Constipation in children has many possible causes. These might include a limited diet, with little fruit and vegetables and minimal fibre, alongside an inadequate fluid intake. The amount of activity the child has may make a difference. Constipation can be associated with toilet training, with the child feeling pressured or being regularly interrupted while using the potty or perhaps resisting the training and withholding faeces. The child may be worried or anxious about, for instance, the arrival of a new baby, moving house or starting nursery. If a child becomes constipated they may find it painful to defaecate, which may mean they do not want to try to pass a stool, which creates a vicious circle; the more reluctant they are to defaecate the more constipated they become.

The management of short-lived or mild constipation and prevention of further constipation involves engaging the child and parents in promotion of a healthy diet, increased fluids and more exercise. If the child is afraid of the toilet it is a case of exploring ways to make toilet appealing; getting the child to sit comfortably on the toilet with feet supported (a footstool may help), avoiding punishments/reprimands and using simple rewards, such as a star chart or some sultanas. It is important to always respond to 'urge' and not to defer the need to defaecate.

Laxatives might be indicated, but few health visitor prescribers using the *Nurse Prescribers' Formulary for Community Practitioners*[28] would prescribe a laxative for a child and liaison with the general practitioners (GP) is needed.

## Fever in under fives

As noted before fevers in children are common. If the child does not have accompanying symptoms of concern and the temperature is not very high or persistent family care is needed. It is a case of keeping the child as comfortable as possible, probably giving paracetamol elixir. They need to be given small frequent drinks, particularly if the child is vomiting (as this is more likely to be retained). If the baby is breastfed this should be continued. Use of a fan or tepid sponging is no longer recommended. There is a need for observation of the child.

## Febrile convulsion

A febrile convulsion is a seizure in infancy or childhood, usually occurring between 3 months and 5 years of age, associated with fever but without evidence of intracranial infection or a defined cause. Febrile seizures are different from epilepsy, which is characterised by recurrent non-febrile seizures. Febrile convulsions present as tonic-clonic seizures, usually involving the whole body with widespread muscle contractions, muscular rigidity, intense jerking movements, and accumulation of saliva in the mouth. A febrile convulsion usually lasts for less than 5 minutes and the child may be sleepy for up to an hour afterwards.

Parents may not see a febrile convulsion as a minor ailment, but most children do not need hospital admission. Parents will need reassurance and education on how to safely manage a febrile convulsion, when to call for medical assistance, and appropriate follow-up. A child having a febrile seizure should be put in the recovery position. The adult with them should note how long the seizure lasts. Nothing should be put in the child's mouth during a seizure; there is the possibility they might bite their tongue. An ambulance needs to be called if it is the child's first seizure, if the seizure lasts longer than 5 minute or if the child is having difficulty breathing.

While febrile convulsions are not unusual, with approximately one in fifty children having a febrile convulsion by the time they are 5 years old, they should be reported to a GP. There is a need to say how long the seizure lasted, what happened to the child's body and if they recovered within an hour.

### Gastro-oesophageal reflux

Gastro-oesophageal reflux is when the stomach contents come back up into the oesophagus. For many babies this a normal event but for others it happens a lot and causes symptoms such as pain and weight loss or other problems, and is known as gastro-oesophageal reflux disease. Such reflux usually starts before a baby is 8 weeks old and gets better by the time the child is a year old. Babies with reflux tend to bring up milk or be sick during or shortly after feeding, cough or hiccup when feeding, be generally unsettled when feeding and swallow or gulp after burping or feeding.

Over-the-counter medication (e.g. Infant Gaviscon) aims to thicken stomach contents and help the stomach to empty faster. A Cochrane review[34] looked to see if medicines helped babies and children with reflux. They found little evidence to suggest that such medicines for babies younger than 1 year worked for functional reflux owing to small samples in the studies and the quality of the research; they found mixed evidence for infants with reflux disease.

Suggestions for management are likely to include advice on the baby's feeding position, holding the baby upright after feeding, possibly giving formula-fed babies smaller feeds more often and checking that the baby is sleeping flat on their back.

### Infections in children

**Otitis media:** This infection of the middle ear could be bacterial or viral. It is frequently experienced by children under four. It presents with pain, fever and the child pulling at or complaining about one or both ears. If examined with an auroscope there is a red bulging eardrum. Many cases will resolve without treatment and there is a move to manage the condition without antibiotics, giving paracetamol and fluids. If the child's temperature is very high and the ear infection remains unresolved after 3 days, medical intervention with antibiotics is needed. Recurrent ear infections can lead to chronic secretory otitis media (known as glue ear), linked with hearing loss. Medical attention is then required.

**Sore throat:** The most common cause of sore throats in children is a variety of viruses which are not treatable with antibiotics. These viruses can cause fever and a painful sore throat. Tonsillitis is linked with sore throats and inflamation of the tonsils. To help ease the symptoms the child needs to rest, drink cool fluids to soothe the throat and be given paracetamol or ibuprofen (do not give aspirin to children under 16). Sore throats and tonsillitis generally run their course but as with most childhood conditions a high temperaure and changing symptoms need referal to the the GP.

**Upper respiratory tract infections (URTI)** are extremely common and usually caused by viruses. They include the common cold. Most are mild and short-lasting, but can cause the child to feel unwell. Small children may have six to eight colds a year as they build up immunity to different viruses. The symptoms come on gradually and can include a blocked or runny nose, a sore throat, headaches, muscle aches, sneezing and a raised temperature. An URTI or cold usually resolves in a few days with paracetamol suspension and fluids. It may cause exacerbation of asthma and could lead to a febrile convulsion. Coughs often go with a cold, as mucus trickles down the back of the throat, but a cough that lasts longer than 3 weeks needs to be investigated by the GP.

A child with a very high temperature, or feeling hot and shivery, may have a chest infection, caused by bacteria rather than a virus, that needs review by a GP. Colds do not respond to antibiotics; they are best managed with rest and sleep, keeping warm and drinking plenty of fluids to avoid dehydration.

## Infectious diseases in childhood

**Chicken pox:** This is a viral illness that includes a rash of itchy spots which turn into fluid-filled blisters. They crust over to form scabs, and then drop off. Some children get many spots, whereas others only have a few. The spots are particularly likely to appear on the face, ears and scalp, under the arms, on the chest and tummy and on the arms and legs. Chickenpox is highly infectious during its early stages from the start until 5 days after the spots first appear. The incubation period of chickenpox is between 13 and 17 days after contact with the infected person. With no specific treatment for chickenpox, symptoms can be relieved with paracetamol (no aspirin to children under 16), to reduce the fever and calamine or cooling gels to ease itching, together with cool clothing and short nails to reduce the impact of scratching.

Pregnant women who contract chickenpox should make contact with the GP as there is a small risk of pneumonia, encephalitis and hepatitis for the mother. Between weeks 28 and 36 of pregnancy the virus can get into the body of the baby and become active in the early years of the baby's life, causing shingles. After 36 weeks of pregnancy the baby may be infected and could be born with chickenpox. The mother may be offered an antiviral medicine which is given within 24 hours of the appearance of the chicken pox rash.

**Measles:** This highly infectious illness most commonly affects young children. It was rare in the UK because of the effectiveness of the measles, mumps and rubella (MMR) vaccine. Concern about, and reluctance to have, all immunisation has led to its return and it is not usually seen as a minor illness.

**Scarlet fever:** This condition is a highly contagious bacterial infection spread by respiratory droplets. It causes a distinctive pink-red rash, usually starting on the chest and stomach before spreading to other areas of the body, which feels like sandpaper to touch and may be itchy. It generally starts with a sore throat, fever and headache, with the rash developing 2 to 5 days after infection.

Scarlet fever usually clears up after about a week but can be treated with antibiotics.

## Infestations

### Head lice

These wingless insects are most commonly found on children aged four to 16 but can infest anyone. They spread via head-to-head contact. Their eggs are known as 'nits' and are laid at the base of hair shafts and go on to hatch within 7 to 10 days. Lice pierce the scalp to feed on blood.

There is no known effective way of preventing the acquisition of head lice. The emphasis needs to be on early detection, by weekly combing wet, conditioner-covered hair with a light-coloured louse detection comb (fine-toothed) and early treatment to prevent spread to other adults and children. Once the child has head lice the scalp is itchy and the child scratches. Detection of a moving louse, not nits which may be empty shells, confirms the infestation. It is difficult to detect a moving louse on dry or damp hair unless there is a severe infestation.

Experts continue to debate the effectiveness of wet combing versus the use of insecticides. Wet combing is worth trying first and involves applying conditioner after washing and systematically combing all the hair with a fine-tooth, detector comb. The comb needs to be rinsed after each stroke to remove trapped lice and the process needs to be repeated on days 5, 9 and 13 to remove the immature headlice, known as nymphs. Infestation can be treated with insecticides, malathion, phenothrin, permethrin and carbaryl, which are available over the counter and by prescription. The preparations need to be applied in line with the instructions for a contact time of 12 hours and then repeated 7 days later. All close contacts of the person with the head lice should be examined and treated as necessary. Children do not need to be kept away from school or early years settings, but it is fair to let them know that head lice are about.

## Threadworm

Threadworm or pinworm is the commonest parasitic worm infestation in the UK and frequently occurs amongst children. The worm causes an anal itch as it leaves the bowel to lay eggs on the perineum. They are often seen as silvery thread-like worms in stools or at the anus. Scratching by the child transfers eggs to nails and hands, which are then ingested. Children over 2 years of age and other house members can be treated with mebendazole. Babies over 6 months of age can be given piperazine; both preparations are available over the counter or can be prescribed by a GP or by a health visitor prescribing from the *Nurse Prescribers Formulary for Community Practitioners*.[28] For children aged 6 months and under, rigorous hygiene measures, for 6 weeks but without medication, are recommended.

Prevention and reducing the possibility of reoccurrence includes promoting good hand washing with soap and warm water before meals, after going to the toilet, changing nappies and before handling food, as well as ensuring short and clean nails. Showering each morning, including the perianal area, to remove eggs from the skin is suggested as well as the changing of bed linen and nightwear daily for several days after treatment. Clothing and bedlinen should not be shaken as this may distribute eggs around the room. Thorough dusting and vacuuming of rooms are needed, together with damp-dusting surfaces in the bathroom. Washing and drying clothes and bedding on a hot cycle will kill pinworm eggs.

## Oral thrush

Oral thrush is a common fungal infection in the mouth, caused by candida albicans, and is marked out by white spots or patches on the baby's cheeks, gums, and palate. They look as if they should be easily wiped away but they are difficult to move and have a raw area underneath. Babies with oral thrush are often reluctant to feed and the breast-feeding mother may have thrush on her nipples, making them painful, red and cracked. Oral thrush is linked with persistent nappy rash, as the fungus moves through the gastrointestinal tract (see nappy rash below).

Oral thrush may need the prescription of an antifungal treatment. Both breastfeeding mother and baby need to be treated at the same time to ensure the fungal infection is not passed back and forth between mother and baby. The prescriber, health visitor or GP, may prescribe an antifungal treatment called nystatin oral suspension or potentially miconazole gel as well as an antifungal preparation for the mother. Negotiating the contract will include an outline on how to administer the preparation and a reminder about household hygiene related to sterilising bottles, dummies and other feeding equipment and separate towels for mother and baby, washing of hands before and after feeding, and before and after nappy changing.

## Skin conditions

**Cradle cap:** This is a harmless inflammatory skin condition that is common in babies at about 3 months of age and usually clears up of its own accord. However, it is not aesthetically pleasing, with yellow crusts on the scalp. It can appear on other parts of the body, such as the eyebrows, nose and nappy area. It does not irritate or cause the child pain. The cause is unknown and it is not caught from other babies. The strategy is to wash the baby's hair regularly with baby shampoo and gently loosen flakes or crusts with a soft brush. The crusts can be softened overnight with baby or olive oil and the baby's hair or scalp washed in the morning.

**Bites and stings:** In the UK common biting insects include wasps, bees, mosquitos, midges, ants, fleas, lice and bedbugs. There is little research evidence on the best way of managing such bites; most are self-limiting and managed at home.[35]

A puncture mark from the insect may be visible and the insect may have been seen and even identified. Reactions vary but may cause a red, swollen lump to develop on the skin. This may be painful or very itchy lasting a few hours or days. There may be a mild allergic reaction where a larger area around the sting or bite becomes swollen and painful; severe allergic reactions are unusual with insect bites and slightly more likely with bee and wasp stings. Such a severe allergic reaction, with breathing difficulties, dizziness and a swollen face or mouth, needs immediate medical treatment.

Home management of the majority of bites and stings will involve cold compresses and antihistamines. Information on prevention includes suggesting using clothing that covers limbs, especially in the early evening, the use of insect repellent, which can be used for infants over 2 months of age as well as pregnant and breastfeeding mothers.[35]

**Eczema:** Eczema is a long-term condition that causes the skin to become itchy, red, dry and cracked. The most common type is atopic eczema which mainly affects children but can continue into adulthood. Atopic eczema can affect any part of the body, but the most common areas to be affected are the cheeks, elbows outside or inside, knees backs or fronts, neck, hands and scalp.

Many children in the UK have eczema, with the majority developing the condition before the age of five, often before the child's first birthday. Children with atopic eczema have periods when the impact on the skin is less noticeable, and times when their symptoms are more severe. With some cases of eczema, it is possible to establish triggers that make the eczema worse, such as particular foods, fabrics, soaps or shampoos or washing powders.

While there is no cure for atopic eczema, treatments can ease the symptoms. There is a need to reduce the damage from scratching which can lead to more eczema and the risk of becoming infected or scarred. With babies with atopic eczema, anti-scratch mittens may stop them scratching their skin, and their nails need to be kept short and clean.

The main medications for atopic eczema are emollients (moisturisers) or topical corticosteroid ointments used to reduce swelling and redness during flare-ups. Emollients are moisturising treatments applied directly to the skin to reduce water loss and cover it with a protective film. They make the skin feel less dry and have a mild anti-inflammatory role. Emollients come in different forms: lotions, creams and ointments. The difference between them is the amount of oil they contain. Ointments containing the most oil can be quite greasy, but are most effective at keeping moisture in the skin. Children may need an ointment for very dry skin, a cream or lotion for less dry skin and an emollient to use instead of soap. Health visitors who have completed the V100 prescribing qualification and nurses with the V150 prescribing qualification can prescribe emollients. Corticosteroids may be required and are mainly used to reduce inflammation and suppress the immune system and are not a first choice of treatment.

**Impetigo:** Impetigo is a common and highly contagious skin infection that causes sores and blisters. It is common in young children 4 years old or under. It is caused by bacteria infecting the outer layers of skin. The bacteria can infect the skin through breaks in healthy skin, such as a cut, insect bite or other injury, and through skin damaged by other skin conditions, such as scabies or eczema. The infection is easily spread through close contact, such as physical contact or by sharing towels or flannels. The lesions are most commonly seen on the face, flexures and limbs. Blisters develop, which then burst to leave a small scabby patch of skin. The crusted lesions are often yellow in colour, itchy and spread in small clusters to surrounding skin.

Prevention and management are linked to good hygiene standards: ensuring clean hands when touching the child and cleanliness of toys, clothing and equipment. Each family member should have their own towels and facecloths. Impetigo usually gets better without treatment in 2 to 3 weeks, but treatment using an antibiotic oral or toppreparation will reduce the length of the illness and can reduce the chance of spreading the infection to others. Children should not be with those from outside the household until the lesions are healed or crusted, or 48 hours from starting the antibiotics.

**Prickly heat:** This condition, also known as heat rash or miliaria, is an itchy rash of small, raised red spots that cause a prickly sensation on the skin. Infants can get a prickly heat rash if they sweat more than usual, when it is hot and humid or if they're overdressed. The strategy is likely to be a reduction in the amount of clothing.

**Nappy rash:** Prevention of nappy rash is by far the preferable strategy. Skin in the nappy area needs protecting at every nappy change by washing (or use of a baby wipe) and by the application of a barrier cream. Nappy changing should happen at least after every feed and more frequently if needed. Skincare products should be non-perfumed to avoid irritation and dryness.

Nappy rash is marked out by redness, soreness, and broken with spots, pimples or blisters and possibly the skin feeling hot to the touch. Initial management involves more frequent nappy changing and cleaning, exposure of the nappy area to air by leaving the nappy off as long as possible and using a barrier cream. Persistent nappy rash is often associated with thrush, where the skin might look red or bright pink with small raised red spots. Here a prescribed, preparation from the GP or non-medical prescriber is needed, along with health promotion or a negotiated contract with carer on managing the nappy rash.

## Sticky eyes

Sticky eyes in new babies are common and are usually due to blocked tear ducts. They can be treated by regular swabbing with cooled boiled water.

## Teething

Signs of teething include: dribbling, wanting to chew or gnaw on anything, irritability, and red cheeks. Interventions might include giving the baby something hard on which to chew, such as a carrot or teething ring, and the use of over-the-counter teething gels. If the baby is in pain, paracetamol or ibuprofen can be given to relieve teething symptoms in babies and young children aged 3 months or older.

## Vomiting and diarrhoea

Most children experience vomiting in childhood. In most instances the symptoms are mild and transient. Different things are described as vomiting. Posseting or reflux describes the non-forceful return of milk, which usually resolves with the introduction of solid food (see gastro-oesophageal reflux earlier). Of concern to parents is the forceful ejection of gastric contents. This is likely to be from a particular cause – travel sickness, food poisoning or a symptom of a gastrointestinal infection, usually viral in origin. With such an infection the child may have diarrhoea, vomiting or a combination of the two. Projectile vomiting,

severe vomiting in which stomach contents can be forcefully propelled some distance away, is a symptom of pyloric stenosis, which usually develops in the first 3 to 6 weeks of life. Pyloric stenosis, which is not minor, is a thickening of the muscle where the stomach empties into the small intestine and blocks food from moving from the stomach to the duodenum of the small intestine. This requires paediatric assessment and, if diagnosed as such, surgery.

Breastfed babies have loose, often explosive 'mustard grain' stools and toddlers may have loose stools related to diet. Unusually loose or explosive stools, accompanied by vomiting, and/or an unwell child are likely to be an infection.

With diarrhoea and vomiting it is important to ensure the child has adequate fluids to prevent dehydration but to avoid giving fruit juice and carbonated drinks. Medication to stop diarrhoea is not advised and antibiotics are not usually given to treat diarrhoea and vomiting. Management of vomiting and diarrhoea at home involves carrying on with the baby's normal breast and bottle feeds, giving small feeds more often than usual if necessary. When a child is on solid foods it is a case of being guided by their appetite. The nappy area needs to be cleaned gently and thoroughly, after each episode of diarrhoea to avoid irritation to the skin and a barrier cream is even more important.

As with all minor ailments, medical attention should be sought if the condition deteriorates; for instance, green bile in vomit, presence of blood in the stool, or fails to improve.

Both in terms of preventing and managing vomiting and diarrhoea sound hygiene is required which involves regular washing of the carer's hands with soap and warm running water to prevent the spread of infection. This is required before handling food, including babies' bottles, before eating, after going to the toilet or changing the child's nappy, after cleaning up blood, faeces or vomit and after handling domestic rubbish. Surfaces need to be washed with detergent and with formula-fed babies, bottles need to be sterilised. Individuals in the same household should not share personal items, with each child having their own towels, toothbrushes, flannels or facecloths.

A child with diarrhoea and/or vomiting should not go to early years settings or mix with other children for 48 hours after their last episode of either.

### Case study 16.2

Idris was born at 41 weeks' gestation and is the second child of Stephanie and Edgar and younger brother of Freya. At 12 weeks he is completely breastfed and gaining weight well with a weight of 7.2 kg and length of 65 cm, putting him in the 95th centile for both. He is alert and smiling but reported to rarely sleep for more than 4 hours day or night. Stephanie brings Idris to the child health clinic with concern about the dry and red scaly areas in the creases of his elbows and knees.

What should the health visitor observe?
What should the health visitor ask?
What should the health visitor do?

## CONCLUSION

Prevention and health promotion are key to health visiting practice; managing minor illnesses and reducing unintentional injuries are high on the agenda throughout the United Kingdom and are currently high impact areas[5] within England.

This chapter has reviewed the extent of home accident injuries in hospital admissions for the under-fives and considered the five main causes: namely, choking, suffocation and strangulation, falls, poisoning, burns and scalds and drowning. Health visitors need to identify the needs of families, communities and population in terms of the reduction of accidents. The health visiting service will engage in health promotion on the reduction of accidents, working with others in the early years workforce. They need to be active in influencing policies that impact on accidents and use existing laws and regulations. Overall, they will be engaged in the facilitation of health enhancing activities related to home safety, whether it is home safety education and provision of equipment, discussion of home safety needs linked with child development stages and secondary prevention by the follow-up of earlier accidents and A&E attendance.

The concept of minor ailments together with many examples of such conditions was explored. The role of the health visitor in assessment and observation, and the facilitation of parents to do the same, was outlined. The prescribing pyramid was used as a framework for action, along with the mnemonic WWHAM and strategies for caring for the baby or sick child.

### KEY LEARNING POINTS

- Health visitors have a proactive role in supporting parents to prevent accidents in their children.
- Health visitors work collaboratively with parents supporting and signposting them to be able to access or borrow baby and child safety equipment.
- Health visitors have a role in supporting parents to assess and manage common childhood ailments in their children.

### FURTHER RESOURCES

**Websites**

**Accident prevention**

Child Accident Prevention Trust. (2020). Child accidents can be prevented. https://www.capt.org.uk/Pages/Category/safety-advice-injury-types. Accessed 19 June 2020.

*Be safe around dogs: Tips and advice for all family.* Drogs Trust. https://www.dogstrust.org.uk/help-advice/factsheets-downloads/bds%20parents%20leaflet.pdf. Accessed 19 June 2020.

Institute of Health Visiting, inpressInstitute of Health Visiting. Parent Tips – How to reduce unintentional injuries in children under 5 years (accident prevention). https://ihv.org.uk/wp-content/uploads/2015/10/PT-How-to-reduce-unintentional-injuries-in-children-under-5-FINAL-VERSION-3.6.19-1.pdf. Accessed 19 August 2020.

Making the link. 'Five for the under-fives': Preventing serious accidents for children under five. http://www.makingthelink.net/tools/five-under-fives-preventing-serious-accidents-children-under-five. Accessed 19 June 2020.

Safe Tea Keep hot drinks out of reach. https://safetea.org.uk/prevention/. Accessed 29 June 2020.

### Management of common childhood ailments

Asthma. UK Asthma and your child. https://www.asthma.org.uk/advice/child/. Accessed 20 August 2020.

Healthier together. https://what0-18.nhs.uk//. Accessed 20 August 2020.

Institute of Health Visiting. Parent tips. What can I do if my baby has oral thrush? https://ihv.org.uk/wp-content/uploads/2015/10/20-PT_Oral-Thrush_V4.pdf. Accessed 20.8.20.

Institute of Health Visiting. Good practice points for health visitors. Managing childhood illnesses. https://ihv.org.uk/wp-content/uploads/2020/04/GPP-Managing-childhood-illnesses-FINAL-VERSION-14.4.20.pdf. Accessed 2 September 2020.

Institute of Health Visiting. Parent tips. https://ihv.org.uk/wp-content/uploads/2020/04/PT-Coping-with-a-crying-baby-during-COVID19-FINAL-VERSION-14.4.20.pdf. Accessed 2 September 2020.

NHS Inform. Asthma. https://www.nhsinform.scot/illnesses-and-conditions/lungs-and-airways/asthma#treating-asthma. Accessed 2 September 2020.

NHS Inform Earache. https://www.nhsinform.scot/illnesses-and-conditions/ears-nose-and-throat/earache. Accessed 20 August 2020.

NHS. Fever in children. https://www.nhsinform.scot/illnesses-and-conditions/infections-and-poisoning/fever-in-children. Accessed 9 September 2020.

NHS Inform. Ready steady baby if your baby's ill. https://www.nhsinform.scot/ready-steady-baby/early-parenthood/caring-for-your-new-baby/if-your-babys-ill. Accessed 2 September 2020.

NHS Inform. Self-help guide. Fever in babies. https://www.nhsinform.scot/self-help-guides/self-help-guide-fever-in-babies. Accessed 2 September 2020.

NHS Inform. Skin rashes in children. https://www.nhsinform.scot/illnesses-and-conditions/injuries/skin-injuries/skin-rashes-in-children. Accessed 2 September 2020.

NICE National Institute for Health and Care Excellence. Head lice. https://cks.nice.org.uk/head-lice#!topicSummary. Accessed 2 September 2020.

NICE National Institute for Health and Care Excellence. Threadworms. https://cks.nice.org.uk/threadworm#!topicSummary. Accessed 2 September 2020.

SIGN. Asthma. https://www.sign.ac.uk/patient-and-public-involvement/patient-publications/asthma/. Accessed 2 September 2020.

### E-learning

IHV/ Child Accident Prevention Trust Child Accident Prevention e-learning – Module 1 and 2 https://ihv.org.uk/for-health-visitors/resources-for-members/resource/e-learning/child-accident-prevention-e-learning/.

RCPCH Spotting the sick child – online learning. https://www.rcpch.ac.uk/resources/spotting-sick-child-online-learning.

## REFERENCES

1. Council for the Education, Training of Health, Visitors. (1977). *Principles of health visiting.* CETHV.
2. Nursing, Midwifery Council. (2004). *Standards of proficiency for specialist-community public health nurses.* London: NMC.
3. Institute of Health Visiting. (2019). *Vision for health visiting health visiting in England: A vision for the future – full report.* iHV.
4. Emond, A. (Ed.). (2019). *Health for all children* (5th ed.). Oxford; New York, NY: Oxford University Press.
5. Department of Health and Social Care/Public Health England. (2018). Early years high impact area 5: Managing minor illnesses and reducing accidents (improving health literacy). Health Visitors Leading the Healthy Child Programme.
6. Kendrick (2017). Keeping Children Safe: A Multicentre Programme of Research to increase the evidence base for preventing unintentional injuries in the home in the under-fives.
7. Public Health England. (2018). Reducing Unintentional Injuries in and around the home among children under five years. Derby: Public Health England.
8. Information Services Division. (2019). Unintentional Injuries in Scotland Hospital Admissions: Year ending 31 March 2018. deaths: Year ending 31 December 2017. NHS National Services Scotland.
9. Public Health England. (2018). Reducing Unintentional Injuries among children and young people.
10. Public Health England. (2018). Public Health Profiles. A & E Attendances 0–5.
11. Public Health England. (undated). Reducing Unintentional Injuries in and around the home among children under five years. Report for Derby.
12. Department of Health (2009) The Health Child Programme: Pregnancy and the First Five Years of Life.

https://www.gov.uk/government/publications/healthy-child-programme-pregnancy-and-the-first-5-years-of-life.

13. National Institute for Health and Care Excellence. (2010). Public Health guideline [PH29]. Unintentional injuries: Prevention strategies for under-15s.

14. National Institute for Health and Care Excellence (NICE). (2010). Public Health Guideline PH30. Unintentional injuries in the home: Interventions for under-15s. NICE.

15. Kendrick, D., Smith, S., Sutton, A. J., Mulvaney, C., Watson, M., Coupland, C., & Mason-Jones, A. (2009). The effect of education and home safety equipment on childhood thermal injury prevention: Meta-analysis and meta-regression. *Injury Prevention. 15*(3), 197–204. https://doi.org/10.1136/ip.2008.020677.

16. Zou, K., Wynn, P. M., Miller, P., Hindmarch, P., Majsak-Newman, G., Young, B., et al(2015). Preventing childhood scalds within the home: Overview of systematic reviews and a systematic review of primary studies. *Burns, 41*(5), 907–924. https://doi.org/10.1016/j.burns.2014.11.002.

17. DiGuiseppi, C., Roberts, I. G. (2000). Individual-led injury prevention strategies in the clinical setting. *Future Child*, 10(1), 53–82.

18. Kendrick, D., Young, B., Simpson, J., Watson, M., Ilyas, N., Achana, F., et al. (2012). Home safety education and provision of safety equipment for injury prevention. *Cochrane Database of Systematic Reviews. 9.* https://doi.org/10.1002/14651858.CD005014.pub2.

19. Kendrick, D., Mulvaney, C. A., Ye, L., Stevens, T., Mytton, J. A., & Stewart-Brown, S. (2013). Parenting interventions for the prevention of unintentional injuries in childhood. *Cochrane Database of Systematic Reviews.* https://doi.org/10.1002/14651858.CD005014.pub2.

20. Department of Health Social Services and Public Safety. (2010). Healthy child healthy future. A framework for the Universal Child Health Promotion Programme. Department of Health Social Services and Public Safety.

21. Wales, N. H. S. (2016). *An overview of the Healthy Child Wales Programme.* Cardiff: NHS Wales.

22. The Scottish Government. (2015). Universal Health Visiting Pathway in Scotland: Pre-birth to pre-school.

23. Making Every Contact Count. http://makingeverycontactcount.co.uk/.

24. Jones, R., White, P., Armstrong, D., Ashworth, M., & Peters, M. (2010). *Managing acute illness.* King's Fund.

25. Watson, M. C., Holland, R., et al. (2014). *Community pharmacy management of minor illness (the MINA Study).* UK: Pharm. Res.

26. Baker, C. (2017). House of Commons Library Briefing Paper 6964: Accident and Emergency Statistics: Demand, Performance and Pressure.

27. Ballantyne, H., & Ballantyne, H. (2015). Developing nursing care plans. *Nursing Standard, 30*(26), 51–57.

28. National Institute for Health and Care Excellence (NICE). (2020). *Nurse Prescribers' Formulary for community practitioners.* NICE.

29. National Prescribing Centre. (1999). *Signposts for prescribing nurses – general principles of good prescribing.* NHS.

30. Nursing and Midwifery Council. (2018). *The Code. Professional standards of practice and behaviour for nurses, midwives and nursing associates.* NMC.

31. Brook, J., McGraw, C., & Thurtle, V. (2021). *Oxford handbook of primary care and community nursing* (3rd ed.). Oxford University Press.

32. Drug and Therapeutics Bulletin. (2013). Management of infantile colic. *BMJ, 10*(347), f4102. doi:10.1136/bmj.f4102.

33. NICE. (2017). Constipation in children and young people: Diagnosis and management [CG 99].

34. Tighe, M., Afzal, N., Bevan, A., Hayen, A., Munro, A., & Beattie, R. (2014). Pharmacological treatment of children with gastro-oesophageal reflux. *Cochrane Database of Systematic Reviews. 11.* CD008550.

35. Wilcock, J., Etherington, C., Hawthorne, K., & Brown, G. (2020). Insect bites. *BMJ, 370*(m2856), 242–244.

# 17 TRANSITION TO SCHOOL

JAMES McTAGGART ■ RUTH ASTBURY

## CHAPTER CONTENTS

INTRODUCTION

TRANSITION TO SCHOOL – OPPORTUNITIES AND CHALLENGES

WHAT IS TRANSITION?

DEVELOPMENT AND RESILIENCE

TRANSITIONS AROUND THE UK

## LEARNING OUTCOMES

*To:*

■ Understand the key features and experiences of transition to school for children and families.

■ Know the different frameworks for understanding starting school and the limits of 'school readiness' as an approach.

■ Understand the health visitor's influence and role in ensuring a good start at school.

■ Realise the anticipatory concerns and issues for particular populations.

## INTRODUCTION

The transition to school is a superficially simple moment that is in fact a wide range of different transitions spread over a length of time.[1] On the face of it, starting school is an issue that might seem far from the core of health visiting practice. In institutional terms, education becomes a universal part of children's lives and health recedes more into the background.

There are several good reasons why school entry is a key part of health visiting service delivery, however, in the first place, it is a moment when parents and carers are likely to be highly engaged and thinking ahead about their child, as well as looking back. It forms a 'touch point'[2] where parents and carers may be receptive to advice and health information as it is within the frame of starting school and the many futures that open up for the family as a result. Secondly, and related to this, parents and carers may well have unspoken worries and concerns about school that they feel safe and able to raise with their trusted health visitor. Being able to provide basic information and signposting is a core service that can improve parental self-efficacy and confidence and support a smooth start to school for children. Finally, transition to school is a major change for both child and family – supporting this to go well, assisting problem-solving and the transfer of relationships from health visitor to school staff lays a major foundation for resilience in the many further transitions that lie ahead.

Reflecting on the changes involved in transition to school, and the capacities it requires of children, parents/carers and professionals, will show that it is far from simple. The complexities are, however, well understood and reducible to a relatively small set of key assessment questions and intervention tasks. The core of any transition is not assessment, protocols, planning documents, policies or adult concerns, but the experience of the child. This chapter opens with an account of school entry from the point of view of the child. Understanding this will help the health visitor to support the family, but it is also important to take into account how the adults themselves may experience the changes. There will therefore be a section on parents' experiences of their children preparing for and starting school. This will then be set into the context of the experiences of the reflective practitioner, since health visitors are by no means passive in the process, and it has emotional and professional resonances that they need to be aware of and use to assist families.

## TRANSITION TO SCHOOL – OPPORTUNITIES AND CHALLENGES

### For children

Many people can remember their first day at school well into adulthood. Over time, we get used to school though, and it can be difficult for adults to remember quite how strange schools are as places, processes and social spaces. Sheer size looms in the memory of one author (JM), who remembers clearly the scale of the building, the difficulty of finding one's way around, and the enormous (seeming) size of the other children, both individually and as a large and noisy crowd. As well as new places, with different scales and strange smells, there are new people. Here, we are told, is a group of adults who we are now to trust and obey. Even if we already know them, it is a step from parent or childminder – or even from a small key worker group in a nursery – to this more professional relationship. Still kind and loving, but more distant, and strangely diluted and shared among other children. And again, even if we are used to a large family, or a group of children at nursery or childcare, here are many more small human beings, each with different characters and styles, all of whom must learn quickly to get along and share both resources and attention.

The rules are all different too, and not all of them are obvious. There are times when we play freely, like we used to, but at others we must sit *right here* and *like this*, while *doing that*. Then we are let out again to play, then brought into a large room with many others, where we must sit and stand or sing or clap. Used to simply asking an adult for help when the need presents, we must now wait a turn, or know somehow when is the right time and place, or use a new ritual like raising a hand.

Nor does a young child have to be a Marxist to realise, at least implicitly, that a new stage has begun where we must do things, or not do things, because that is what we must. Choices are becoming restricted for years (perhaps decades). School is something we must go to, whether or not we wish to or see why. It may be something we love, enjoy and find rich fulfilment in, but we are now part of the big world of work and obligation and don't know where it will lead us.

Finally, children may well see school as an exciting step, the beginning of being really 'grown up' and starting their learning in earnest. Many will be motivated by the thought of learning to do all those mysterious and difficult things that adults do every day – be it reading or writing or counting past ten. But it can turn out to be harder than it looks, and children need to be prepared for learning being a series of ups and downs, especially if through developmental or other needs they are likely to find it more of a challenge than others.

## THINKING SPACE

Either by yourself or as a group, discuss what you remember about starting school or changing schools later:

- What were you excited about?
- What were you worried about?
- Who helped you, and what did they do?

Now imagine you are a small child going to school for the first time:

- What might it look, sound, smell and feel like?
- What would a really good first few days look like?
- What could the adults do that might help? What might they say?
- What might they do that would make it harder? What might they say?

Now, as a group or on your own, can you come up with five key messages for parents about starting school?

It is worth dwelling on what transition to school feels like (looks like, sounds like, smells like) to young children because it is this experience that we need to address. Adult preoccupations with developmental levels, or reasonable adjustments, or how many letters a child needs to know, or whether they can write their name, must be set into this context rather than being the primary issues.[3] Children, even at a young age, are active makers of meaning. Early decisions as to whether school feels safe, nurturing, welcoming, a place where they feel at home and a challenge that they can both cope with and enjoy – these have ramifications not just for attainment and behaviour but for a lifetime of trust or otherwise in institutions, professions and sources of help.[4]

Even this very superficial pen portrait of a child's-eye view of transition to school makes clear that this is not something that can happen in an instant. The more unfamiliar and bewildering it is at first, the longer the process might take.

The more preparation of both child and school for their encounter with each other, the smoother the changes will be. Later sections will cover the kinds of assessment and approaches that can support this. But a key part of a child's preparation for transition is the narrative that parents place around it, including how they tolerate and answer the child's questions and concerns, as well as how effectively they can prepare their child cognitively, socially and physically to make the most of starting school. Understanding the parent experience of transition is therefore essential to supporting that of their children.

### Case study 17.1

Maisie has called you about her daughter, Amy, who is due to start school next autumn. Maisie is worried that Amy is 'young for her age', and Amy's aunt, who is a teacher, says that more time in nursery is needed.

- How can you find out what the law and local educational practice is on this issue where you work?
- What are the disadvantages of delaying school entry, thinking ahead over the next 10 years?
- How would you work with Maisie and the school to support her transition, or to help make deferral decisions if that is what educational assessment suggests is best?
- What are the issues that might make this harder for you? Where might you find help?

### For parents and carers

Starting school is a major change for parents and carers too,[1] even if the child in question is not their first. It is likely to be a mixture of looking forward and looking backwards. Many parents experience key developmental milestones as having elements of change and loss. For example, when a baby starts to crawl, they are becoming more independent and much as this is a joy, it also means they are starting to move away from their parents. Once a child starts school, babyhood is firmly in the past and while the future holds much promise, facing that future requires processing and letting go of any ambivalence.

Mixed feelings on the part of parents and carers may well become expressed either as anxieties or as avoiding facing up to the issues that transition presents. Parents and carers may focus on particular aspects of the transition where they feel higher levels of control or of helplessness, and health visitors can be helpful in setting those issues in context and signposting to information that can assist. The issues may be complicated by parents' and carer's own experiences of school, and memories of how they managed the transition. Many parents and carers may remember a school experience that was more directive and less inclusive than is the case today, including unhappy memories of discipline or of feeling that they were not learning or well supported. Others may have blissful memories and may need guidance to realise that for their child's particular temperament, history or developmental situation, challenges may lie ahead that need to be acknowledged and anticipated.

It is of paramount importance that parents are realistic about transition to school, and plan for any foreseeable issues, while presenting to the child faces of confidence and coping. They need to be able to contain their child's anxieties, or cope with their excitement, and tolerate sometimes repeated questions. Once again, health visitors who have built up relationships of trust over time, or who are skilled at establishing such relationships quickly with new clients, can be invaluable providers of containment and reassurance.

## WHAT IS TRANSITION?

### Multiple transitions and health visiting practice

The very term transition implies that in some way the child changes to accommodate what is required of them. However, if we revisit some of the theoretical frameworks which health visitors bring to their understanding of child development, in a social and cultural environment, this view can be questioned. All of the assessment tools used by health visitors across the UK, to gain insight and an understanding of children's worlds, use ecological frameworks such as the one designed by Bronfenbrenner.[5] This framework puts the child in the centre with various networks of support around them; networks which will change and expand over time as the child grows and develops. During times of transition the child remains at the centre but their relationships with the networks and environments change as they move from one micro-system to another. If we continue to take an ecological perspective the most important contributions to a child's well-being are the links which take place between each of the micro-systems and the meso systems. The stronger the links the better the outcomes for the child.[6]

By encouraging meaningful relationships between parents/carers and teachers, as they share their understanding around what the child needs to continue to learn and develop, health visitors will be strengthening these links which will, in turn, promote the child's well-being. Exploring with parents what their own experience of school was like? Perhaps finding out the nature of their relationships with their teachers? Did they have a favourite teacher? What was it that they valued about this teacher? This approach could lead to a positive discussion about current roles and responsibilities of teaching staff, including the focus on children's well-being which they share with parents.

So, whilst acknowledging that starting school is undoubtedly a time of change, and on the basis that children are required to accommodate this change (rather than needing to change themselves) is there anything else which health visitors can do to support parents at this time? If the child has an established ability to accommodate change this is going to be an advantage; however, it may be that parents don't appreciate the numerous small changes which have taken place in their child's life already and, in general, their child's remarkable capacity to cope. It can be helpful to distinguish between internal, vertical and horizontal transitions,[7] where internal transitions are the changes which take place within a setting, such as changing to a different nursery room at the age of three. Vertical transitions represent the major adjustments which take place within life, such as starting school, but there are horizontal changes taking place on a daily basis too. It is not unusual, in a pre-school year, for a child to be playing at home with a sibling and parent, to then be taken to a childminder's home where there are other children, and to nursery to interact with different children in a different setting. Each of these daily changes in activity can be viewed as horizontal transitions; and whilst perhaps not being perceived to have the same impact as vertical transitions each change still requires a degree of adjustment for the child, is preparation for major events, and creates opportunities to develop resilience.

Supporting parents to create opportunities for their child to be cared for in different environments by other responsible adults will help to develop their child's ability to understand new routines, build new relationships, and experience different social environments. This is all on the basis that the child has already developed secure attachments with their primary carers though, has an 'internal working model', which associates caring adults with a 'secure base' which they return to, and where all their primary needs are being met, so that they have capacity to explore and learn. Attachment theory (see Chapter 14) is another area where health visitors can bring known theory to practice, and with knowledge about the family will be able to listen and support in a realistic and therapeutic way. Where children are known to have experienced trauma, insecurity, or parents with unpredictable behaviour, this time, as with all times of change, may pose

challenges requiring additional support from other agencies.

## The reflective health visitor

Being a reflective practitioner is a Nursing & Midwifery Council (NMC)[8] requirement for a health visitor, and reflection is an important skill to be able to apply at this time of transition. Reflective practice is based on using a structured approach and in this context the health visitor will not only take account of their existing knowledge about each family but will also be encouraged to challenge their assumptions around how each family will manage at this time. As judgements inform decision-making a strong evidence base, through reflective practice, will support decisions around what to do next. This process, in turn, will support evidence-based practice, which is also an NMC requirement for health visitors.

Within all four nations of the UK there is an expectation that health visitors, as a minimum, review each child's records before transferring their responsibilities to others or closing down the record if all is well. By using the child's records as a reference point and reflecting on themes which have become evident over time, this will support any judgements which are being made. There are differences across the four nations around whether a direct contact takes place with all parents and carers at 4 to 5 years, and the nature of this direct contact if it does; however, the need to provide a person-centred approach is consistent, as is ensuring that the well-being of the child is supported and any needs are met. Consequently, if there is a strong evidence base to undertake a home visit, or to make contact by phone at this time, a reflective approach can support this justification.

For children who have been in receipt of an enhanced service during their pre-school years, for whatever reason, there may already be a pathway of further assessments, planning meetings with education colleagues and others, and direct referrals to a school nurse. Health visitors contributing to multi-agency discussions can provide a valuable perspective due to the opportunities they have had of getting to know families and their children over a significant period of time. For children and families where there has been a complex history, and particularly where the enhanced service from other agencies has been intermittent, clinical supervision may be required to enable health visitors to reflect with a colleague and tease out an optimum pathway of support during this transition period.

By its very nature a pandemic creates uncertainty for everyone, and this is particularly true of children and parents who have already experienced a level of uncertainty and disruption in their lives, and who may also have low levels of resilience. With these families, additional health visitor contacts may be indicated at this time in order to create the opportunity for parents and carers to talk over any concerns and to ensure that they have the contact details of people who can offer support in the future. These contacts should ideally be known personally to the health visitor as this will enhance a belief in the parents and carers that these support networks will be welcoming and effective.

Health visitors will be aware if their contact with families will be continuing as this is dependent on whether there are younger babies or children in the household. If a relationship with parents and carers is to continue after the child starts school the health visitor can continue to be a point of contact for the family; however, if this is the youngest or only child, there may also be a sense of loss for the health visitor when the relationship with the family naturally comes to an end. A sense of loss may be compounded by deep concerns around how the child and family will fair once their service's support has come to an end. These concerns are frequently relayed to school nurse colleagues. In addition to reflective practice creating an opportunity for health

visitors to question the root of their personal feelings can also support the development of a clear rationale around the nature of any concerns which exist. The analysis process, which justifies their concerns, will be recorded in the child's record, and can be used to articulate clearly the specific services which are deemed to be required in each case. Different areas of the UK have different structures for supporting vulnerable or troubled families and where a 0 to 19 team exists within the local area the health visitor may continue to be a point of reference for the school nurses. Where this structure does not exist, however, an effective professional relationship between health visitors and the local school nurse team will enable ongoing support to exist for families.

## DEVELOPMENT AND RESILIENCE

### Understandings of 'school readiness'

A key concern, whether of parents, policy makers or even, in their own terms, of children themselves is that they are 'ready' for school. Different countries have different ways of approaching this, although contrasts are not always so sharp in practice. In England, 'school readiness' is a widely accepted concept used in official documents and defined as a 'good level of development',[9] while in Scotland, the final nursery year and first school year are covered by a single curricular stage (Early Level) with an emphasis on continuity rather than change.[10]

There is a complex research literature on 'school readiness' and the factors that affect it,[3] and health visitors need to be critical consumers of these findings in order to help families. Over time, there has been a trend from quite narrow developmentally defined concepts of readiness – defined, for example, by score levels on developmental assessments – to understanding school readiness as a constructed concept with many levels of meaning. The latter kind of approaches understand any definition of 'ready' as more or less arbitrary and chosen due to particular concerns and emphases in wider society or the immediate professional context. Attitudes to school readiness as a construct also depend on underlying theories of development and learning. A more biological developmentalist view would emphasise factors within the child, such as vocabulary, self-care ability and dispositions. By contrast, more social views of learning would emphasise the interaction between the child's capabilities and the context, and the balance between being ready to learn and doing so in a context that adapts to and supports each child. To give one practical example, some would consider that children should have a given level of vocabulary and phonological awareness on starting school so that they are 'ready' for more formal reading instruction from day one. Others would point out that children naturally vary in these capacities into middle childhood quite apart from differences in experiences and stimulation due to social and family factors. The task is therefore for schools to provide instruction – formal or otherwise – at the appropriate level for each child while also working to fill developmental gaps. On this view the emphasis would be on schools being ready for children rather than children ready for school.[10]

However defined, the practical issue is to ensure that every child has a positive experience of starting school and that they are in a position to benefit from the opportunities it can bring. Readiness, understood pragmatically, therefore has three inter-related aspects – the readiness of the child, of the family, and of the school. Health visitors are in a position to influence all three, even if their main focus (and probably also that of parents and carers) will be on the child and their development and health. Given the conceptual and evidential complexities, the following sections provide a very brief orientation as to what matters for starting school according to each aspect.

## What matters for starting school?

Health visitors have a key role in dispelling myths about what children and families need to go to get ready for school, and also in promoting factors that do make a difference long term. Parents can be under considerable pressure to 'bring on' their children in certain aspects, and those who do not may encounter stigmatisation in communities or in the school system. For example, every summer, supermarkets push bright and colourful 'phonics' kits that will purportedly enable children to have a head start at school through knowing more sound-letter links. In fact, children would benefit far more from being read to and encouraged to scribble and draw than drilling meaningless graphemes during the summer holidays.

The following suggestions are therefore based less on what a child *should* be able to do, and more on the processes that will enable children to make the most out of starting school. If parents and carers can do these, they will also be ensuring that the family as a whole is ready for transition to school, since they will be actively involved in the child's learning, and confident in how to support them.

## Preparing children for transition

The section above, on the child's experience of starting school, will show some of the areas where advance preparation can make the change both smoother and more fruitful for both adults and children. This will also assist in future changes as it sets a pattern of resilience and adaptation that children and families can draw upon.[11] Some children need detailed and enhanced transition planning, and their issues are addressed below. But it is important that all children have a chance to see where they are going, to meet those who will be teaching and caring for them, and have their questions enabled and answered. Children may express concerns using very concrete and apparently trivial issues. For example, a question about whether the canteen serves the favourite brand of ketchup may be at root about worries about the food, the length of the day, being away from home or something quite different. Sensitive explanation and encouragement to talk and explore will reveal the underlying concerns if any. In addition, children often need to ask the same thing over and over, or about little aspects of detail. It is important that adults stay patient and respond to the needs.

For many children, going to school is a step up and a step ahead. They will be excited and pleased to be grown up, to wear their uniforms and walk to school. Others may cope with the changes well in advance by showing some regression in behaviour or self-regulation. This is not a sign of things going wrong or being done wrong. Parents will always be right to respond to the need as it presents itself – if children temporarily need more help with sleep, night worries, or need to move around more to let off steam, that is fine.

## Supporting parents' anticipatory concerns

Parents know their children best, and if they have concerns about school readiness, these are always to be taken seriously and acted upon sensitively. Reflex reassurance without reflecting with parents on the basis for their concerns and how they can be more fully assessed and addressed is unlikely to be helpful. Health visitors will bear in mind that parents' own experiences of education may not have been positive, and that they may well see aspects of their child that professionals do not. The reverse problem is also sometimes the case, that health visitors may be part of a professional group trying to encourage parents, who may be holding onto hopes that all will be well or their child will 'grow out' of difficulties, that their child needs assessment and support.

In order to assist, it is important that health visitors understand the local context of services, policies and eligibility. This chapter cannot cover these in detail as they vary from place to place and over time. Simply referring to another service, say speech and language therapy, without knowledge

of availability, accessibility or suitability merely results in delay, so-called 'did not attends' or a passing round of referrals between services and consequent stress to parents.

In addition, health visitors need to be up to date and confident in their knowledge of educational processes in their work area, especially with regard to special needs or additional support. Many schools offer open days, often as part of registration procedures, and many will be open to additional visits and conversations with parents and their children. If health visitors can confidently signpost to what is there, and advocate for the establishment of what is not, then they will be providing a service to parents whose value goes far beyond the information that is conveyed.

## THINKING SPACE

Imagine you have been working with a family, building a relationship with them, as their child grows from babyhood to starting school.

What will it be like saying goodbye …
■ For the parents?
■ For the child?
■ For you?

What would your messages for family and child be? How would you like them to remember you?

Are there cases where it would be harder to let go? Or easier? And how would you handle this?

## Particular concerns

*Children born preterm or with low birth weight, or who had traumatic deliveries or experienced intra-uterine growth retardation.*

With advances in healthcare over the last few decades, many more children born preterm, with low birth weight, or who needed high levels of care in special baby units, are now surviving and thriving into adulthood. Many such children do very well and require little additional support beyond the intensive early interventions. Others have levels of difficulty or disability that are clearly visible and well understood – for example, cerebral palsy or visual difficulties. There is also a sub-population of children, often born only moderately preterm, who have more subtle developmental issues that only come to light with the increasing demands on them following transition into school.[11,12] This section cannot provide a complete account of school transition for children born preterm or with low birth weight. However, health visitors should bear in mind that children who have had a complex birth or gestational history may need additional assessment and that their families may have understandable anxieties about starting school.

Health visitors need to be aware of local systems for supporting and identifying children born preterm or low birth weight, especially where there are gaps in transmission of knowledge or information. For example, most children receive high levels of continuing care from special care teams throughout their early years, but these may recede or withdraw as school age approaches. In addition, schools may not always be aware of a child's early history and much opportunity for prevention and adaptation can be lost while they become aware of issues without knowing the context. For example, expectations need to be relative to children's due date rather than actual birthday, and issues with behaviour may be misinterpreted as non-compliance or poor socialisation (or parenting), rather than linked back to visual or cognitive processing demands beyond what the child can cope with. Parents retain rights over information transfer, but health visitors should discuss with them carefully the pros and cons of making educators aware of children's early experiences and the impacts this may have on their education.

In general there is a linear relation with how preterm children are born and the levels and likelihoods of difficulty experienced in later life. There is also evidence for a partial 'cliff' with more significant issues for births earlier than 32 weeks. Each case will be individual with its own complexities, but the following domains are well-known areas of difficulty that may need anticipatory planning as well as adjustment and intervention during the early school years.

## Children and families who have experienced trauma and adversity

Chapter 11 provides an in-depth discussion of issues related to trauma and adversity. Health visitors will be aware that starting school may be both a time of great hope for families who have experienced adversity, but also a significant additional stressor.

It is important to take strengths-based approaches that also avoid making assumptions about children or families. There are some well-known associations of deprivation, for example, with delays in language development – but these will not necessarily hold for any given family. For example, families living in deprivation or difficult circumstances will have similar aspirations for their children's education and futures as other families, and will be equally prepared to support it.

Schools gather information about their catchment areas and the kinds of adaptations that may be needed to ensure that all children get a good start. These range from programmes to enrich language environments to providing opportunities for nurture experiences. Depending on local circumstances these will be either whole school approaches or targeted at smaller groups.

Health visitors can help the transition into school for all children by ensuring timely transmission of information and being part of reflective multi-agency teams that learn from both successful and less successful transitions for the future.

Some children will have experienced significant developmental trauma and have resulting gaps and difficulties in development. Health visitors will need to follow appropriate safeguarding processes (see Chapter 12) to ensure all children have the safety, positive relationships and stimulation they need to grow and flourish.

However, many families will be doing their best for their children in difficult circumstances, so it's important not to add further pressure by over-emphasising ideas such as 'readiness' for school. While this is a motivator for some, it may be more productive to emphasise the value of joyful playing and talking together using some of the ideas presented in Table 17.1.

## TRANSITIONS AROUND THE UK

Although there are some differences between the health visitor pathways and child health programmes across the four nations in the UK there are fundamental similarities; in each country the well-being of children is valued, and early intervention is implemented if required. In

| TABLE 17.1 | |
|---|---|
| **Promoting children's development through play and talking.** | |
| **Developmental area** | **Supporting processes** |
| Literacy | Reading with children, talking about content, telling stories with picture books<br>Telling stories (e.g. what did we do today?)<br>Modelling use of print and writing (shopping lists, etc)<br>Using and pointing out environmental print (e.g. road signs, shop labels)<br>Enjoying singing and rhyming<br>Opportunities to draw and scribble, especially on big surfaces or outside |
| Maths | Involving children in everyday activities involving quantities – laying tables, measuring ingredients, etc<br>Playing with jigsaws and shapes<br>Using language like 'more', 'up', 'bigger', etc<br>Playing matching games, and counting games<br>Songs and rhymes with numbers |
| Language and interaction | Lots of two-way conversations in quiet places<br>Giving children time to answer and building on their response<br>Reducing questions and making more comments and observations<br>Doing interesting things together that you can talk about later<br>Games with natural turn-taking, such as catch or ball passing; also, board or card games |
| Managing emotions | Understanding behaviour as expressing a difficult feeling and responding to that<br>Helping children calm themselves down; showing them what to do<br>Making sure children are not over-challenged<br>Modelling how to deal with difficulties and mistakes<br>Making time to listen to children and what they feel<br>Asking children for ideas how to make things better |
| Attention and memory | Games with natural turn-taking<br>Giving time before stopping one thing and starting another<br>Encouraging activities that the child most easily focuses on<br>Making sure the environment is not too stimulating or noisy<br>Many two-way conversations<br>Going over lists and what we need to take when going out<br>Repeated telling or reading of familiar stories to establish patterns<br>Telling back the story of the day<br>Physical activity that needs thinking as well – stop/start games, tag, etc |
| Social skills | If children unused to playing with lots of others, gradually introducing other children<br>Supporting turn-taking and sharing<br>Practise a new skill with your child before they try it with other children<br>Mistakes are natural – don't punish but explain and show what to do |

each area health visitors are encouraged to support all stages of transition, whether it is transition to parenthood, transferring into a new area, or starting school. All programmes are underpinned by the rich knowledge health visitors have around safeguarding and the negative impact adverse childhood experiences can have on an adult's life.

The *Healthy Child Wales Programme*[13] is delivered to families with children 0 to 7 years old, but still incorporates transfer to the school nurse at school entry. As in other areas the level of contact between professionals, and the parents or carers at this time, is proportionate to the child's or family's needs although there is the additional option of Flying Start health visitor teams supporting families in need. This proportionate approach is evident within other nations too – and although the *NHS Healthy Child Programme*[14] in England refers to the concept of progressive universalism the principles of strengths-based encounters, where relationship building is paramount, is also consistent across all countries. Despite the final universal assessment in England being at 2½ years using the Ages & Stages Questionnaire 3 (ASQ3)[15] there is still scope for further assessments if required, and a handover to a school nurse if appropriate at school entry.

In Scotland the *Universal Health Visitor Pathway*[16] builds on *Getting It Right for Every Child*[17] and includes a 4- to 5-year home visit to all families, which is an ideal time to identify concerns from the parents and carers' perspectives. If there is an established multi-disciplinary team working in partnership to support the child and their family, this home visit is in addition to the planning which will continue in partnership with the family and the team. Northern Ireland's *Healthy Child Healthy Futures Programme*[18] identifies a range of public health issues which need to be addressed at this stage; and they again reflect many of the same public health issues which are priorities across all four nations, including

a focus on immunisations, obesity, oral health, speech, language and communication, behaviour, and safeguarding.

The Covid-19 pandemic has had a significant impact on how health visitors are able to deliver all of their services across the whole of the UK, with virtual contacts being implemented where possible to keep families and professionals safe from spreading the virus. Reaching out to all parents of 4- to 5-year-olds to identify their specific concerns around their child starting school, and collating this information for local intelligence, is consistent with the health visitor's role in supporting population health.

Within all four countries School Nursing Services are currently under review, with health visitors giving voice to the requirements of children and families as they leave their care. This is again consistent with the expectations of a Specialist Community Public Health Nurse (SCPHN)[8] to not only search for health needs but to identify and promote solutions, which will meet their population's needs.

### Case study 17.2

Jack is a 5 year old in your caseload who is just about to start school after the summer holidays. You are in the summer term and made aware, by Jack's GP, that his mother has asked for a referral to another doctor as she was finding Jack's behaviour too difficult to handle. You email Jack's nursery teacher, to find out about his behaviour in nursery, and discover that he has frequently been absent during the previous term.

Jack is the youngest of three children in a home where single-mum Jane, has been prone to depression for the whole time that you have known the family. Jack has two older sisters: Sophie, who is going to High School after the summer, and Stacey, who is already in High School. You decide to undertake a home visit during school hours before you 'close' Jack's record.

On arrival it is Stacey who answers the door and welcomes you in. Jack, scantily clothed, is jumping up and down on the couch, and Jane is sitting on an armchair watching the television. You know Jane well and currently she appears in a low mood.

- What are your priorities?
- What are the strengths in this situation?
- What are you going to do now?

## KEY LEARNING POINTS

Transition into school is a big moment for children, families and health visitors. The superficially simple process of assembling lunchbox and uniform conceals a complex set of issues that play out over time differently for each child and family. Health visitors are well placed at this significant touchpoint to support children, families and educators to meet the presenting needs and anticipate future ones. While some children are particularly in need of advice and support at this juncture, for all children it is an opportunity for resilience building.

In this chapter we have explored:

- what transition is and what is meant by 'school readiness', as well as alternative frames
- what transition can mean for children, parents/carers and health visitors
- the opportunities and challenges which exist around this time
- ideas of activities which health visitors can suggest to promote a smooth school start for children and their parents/carers
- identification of child experiences which may 'get in the way' of a straightforward school start
- internal and external resources that health visitors have to support their practice.

## REFERENCES

1. Jindal-Snape, D. (Ed.). (2009). *Educational transitions: Moving stories from around the World.* Routledge.
2. Brazelton, T. B. (1992). In *Touchpoints: Your child's emotional and behavioral development.* Reading: Addison-Wesley.
3. Carlton, MP, Winsler, A. (1999). School readiness: The need for a paradigm shift. *School Psychology Review, 28*(3), 338–352.
4. European Commission. (2011). Communication from the Commission: Early childhood education and care: providing all our children with the best start for the world of tomorrow. Brussel, COM 66. European Commission.
5. Bronfenbrenner, U. (2005). *Making human beings human: Bioecological perspectives on human development.* Sage, Thousand Oaks, CA.
6. Brooker, L. (2002). *Starting school: Young children learning cultures.* OUP Press, Buckingham, UK.
7. O'Connor, A. (2017). *Understanding transitions in the early years: Supporting change through attachment and resilience.* Routledge. London
8. Nursing and Midwifery Council (Great Britain). (2015). *The Code: Professional standards of practice and behaviour for nurses and midwives.* NMC.
9. Public Health England. (2015). *Improving school readiness: Creating a better start for London.* PHE.
10. Realising the Ambition – Being Me: National Practice Guidance for Early Years in Scotland. (2020). Education Scotland.
11. Pritchard, V. E., Bora, S., Austin, N. C., Levin, K. J., & Woodward, L. J. (2014). Identifying very preterm children at educational risk using a school readiness framework. *Pediatrics, 134*(3), e825–e832.
12. Quigley, M. A., Poulsen, G., Boyle, E., Wolke, D., Field, D., Alfirevic, Z., & Kurinczuk, J. J. (2012). Early term and late preterm birth are associated with poorer school performance at age 5 years: a cohort study. *Archives of Disease in Childhood – Fetal and Neonatal Edition, 97*(3), F167–F173.
13. Welsh Government. (2016). *Healthy Child Wales Programme.* https://gov.wales/healthy-child-wales-programme. Accessed 10 October 2020.
14. Department of Health. (2009). NHS healthy child programme. http://www.healthychildprogramme.com/national-context. Accessed 10 October 2020.
15. Brookes (2021). Ages and Stages Questionnaire: ASQ-3. Brookes Publishing Co. https://agesandstages.com/products-pricing/asq3/
16. Scottish Government (2015). Universal Health Visiting Pathway in Scotland: pre-birth to pre-school. Edinburgh: The Scottish Government. https://www.gov.scot/publications/. Universal Health Visiting Pathway in Scotland: pre-birth to pre-school - gov.scot (www.gov.scot.
17. Scottish Government. (2004). *Getting It Right for Every Child (GIRFEC).* https://www.gov.scot/policies/girfec/. Accessed October 10, 2020.
18. Department of Health, Social Services and Public Safety. (2010). *Healthy child healthy futures programme.* https://www.health-ni.gov.uk/sites/default/files/publications/dhssps/healthychildhealthyfuture.pdf.

# INDEX

Page numbers followed by *f* indicate figures, *t* indicate tables, and *b* indicate boxes.

## A

ABC of Behaviour Change Theory, 193
Accident and emergency (A&E)
    childhood accidents, 324, 327
    facilities, 326
Accidents, children. *See* Childhood
    accidents
Accredited Educational Institutions
    (AEIs), 24
Adverse childhood experiences (ACEs),
    143, 148, 212, 213, 287, 290
Adversity. *See* Childhood adversity, trauma
    and
'A Fairer Healthier Scotland: A strategic
    framework for action 2017–2022', 73
Ages and Stages Questionnaire (ASQ), 10,
    11, 113, 114, 118
Air traffic control system, 281
'All our Health', 13
Alma Ata declaration, 13
American Psychological Association, 191
Antenatal contact, 137*b*, 137, 224
Antenatal/Postnatal Promotional Guides, 115
Anxiety, 252
    antenatal period, 254, 259, 260
    assessment, 116
    maternal, 257, 262, 264
    paternal period, 262
    perinatal period, 255
    PHQ-9, 256
    risk factors for, 255
Anxiety disorders, 253*b*, 254
Appropriate supports, for caregiver and
    child, 297
Arnstein's ladder of participation, 205
ASQ. *See* Ages and Stages Questionnaire
    (ASQ)
Assessment, 111
    Ages and Stages Questionnaire, 118
    childhood ailments, 328

clinical decision-making, 112
family health needs assessment, 115
flexible approach during, 113
framework, 149, 150*f*
matching agendas, 121
partnership working with parents, 119
perinatal depression and anxiety, 116
promotional guides, 115
risk, 149, 150*f*
and screening tools, 114, 115
strength-based approach, 121
tools
    barriers to using, 114
    multi-agency working, 115
    use of, 113
triangle, 186
virtual, COVID-19 pandemic, 122, 124*b*
working with family, 120
Assessment Framework Triangle, 115
Asthma, 331
Attachment
    antenatal period, 260, 261
    maternal–fetal, 260, 261
    and parental sensitivity, 291
    supporting positive, 295
    trauma and adversity, 217
Attachment theory, 284, 285*t*, 347
Attunement, 218
Authenticity, in therapeutic relationships, 92
Autistic spectrum disorder, 10
Autocratic leaders, 5
Autonomy, 47
Avon Longitudinal Study of Parents and
    Children (ALSPAC), 252, 260,
    262, 263

## B

Babies in Lockdown survey, 264
Baby Buddy app, 176*b*, 293

Baby Express newsletter, 292
Baby massage, 293
BAME communities. *See* Black and
    minority ethnic (BAME)
    communities
Beattie's model, of health promotion, 13, 15*f*
Behaviour, 191
    development in children, 148, 294
    effectiveness of providing information
        to change, 193
    health-promoting. (*See* Health-promoting
        behaviour, facilitation of)
    leadership, 11, 13
    management, 294
Behavioural disorders, 281
Behavioural theories, leadership, 5
Behaviour-change techniques (BCTs), 198
Best Start in Life research programme, 12
Beveridge's 'five giant evils', implications, 10
Biomedical interpretation, of health, 4
Biomedical model, 192
Bipolar disorder, 254
Bites and stings, 337
Black and minority ethnic (BAME)
    communities, 58, 59, 103
Black Lives Matter movement, 59, 103
Blackpool Better Start, 122
Boer War, 10
Brain architecture, 281
    impact of neglect on, 283
Brain development, 28, 216
    infant, 280, 283*b*, 283, 297
    trauma and adversity, in human, 211, 212
        fundamentals, 224
        physical environment, 217
        significance, 224
        social relationships, 218
Brazelton's Newborn Behavioural
    Observation (NBO), 293
Breast-feeding, 336

Brief interventions, 202
Broader interpretations, of health conceptualise, 4
Building and Strengthening Leadership, 61
Building community capacity, 196, 197, 204
Burnout, signs and symptoms of, 51
Burns and scalds, 325

## C

Capacity, 197
Care assurance, 142
Caregivers
  appropriate support for, 297
  babies ready to interact and communicate with, 3, 4t
    zero to one year, 5
    one to two years, 5
    two to three years, 6
    three to five years, 6
  containment and, 295
  nurturing, 295
  reciprocity, 90
  serve and return interactions, 283
  trauma and adversity. (See Childhood adversity, trauma and)
CBT. See Cognitive behavioural therapy (CBT)
Chartered Institute of Professional Development (CIPD), 4
ChatHealth, 123, 124b
Chicken pox, 335
Child Health Nurse, 23
Child Health Promotion Programme, 81
Childhood accidents
  accident and emergency, 324, 327
  prevention of, 323, 324
    action in, 325
    health-enhancing activities, 326
    secondary prevention approach to, 327
    significant contribution to, 326
Childhood adversity, trauma and, 209, 211, 214
  attachment, 217
  brain development, 211, 212
    fundamentals, 224
    physical environment, 217
    significance, 224
    social relationships, 218
  ecological and holistic approaches, 222
  factors, 223t
  impacts on development, 216
  implications, 211
  issues related to school transition, 351
  physical environment, 216
  presenting issues, 221

reflective practice, 225
resources, 217
stimulation, 220
touchpoints, 221
working with parents and carers, 224
Childhood ailments, 323
  asthma, 331
  caring for, 331
  chicken pox, 335
  colic, 332
  constipation, 333
  crying baby reasons, 332
  febrile convulsion, 333
  fever, 333
  gastro-oesophageal reflux disease, 334
  head lice, 336
  health visiting service, role, 329
  infections, 334
  infectious diseases, 335
  management of, 327
    assessment, 328f, 328
    changes in eating and drinking patterns, 329
    diarrhoea and vomiting, 329
    difficulty breathing/respiratory distress, 328
    fever, 329
    listening to parent and carer, 328
    observation, 328, 329f
  measles, 335
  oral thrush, 336
  otitis media, 334
  scarlet fever, 335
  skin conditions, 337
    bites and stings, 337
    cradle cap, 337
    eczema, 337
    impetigo, 338
    nappy rash, 338
    prickly heat, 338
  sore throat, 334
  sticky eyes, 339
  teething, signs of, 339
  threadworm, 336
  upper respiratory tract infections, 335
  vomiting and diarrhoea, 339
Child in Need Plans, 235
Child protection
  medical assessments, 235
  safeguarding. (See Safeguarding)
  scenarios, 90
Child Protection Information Sharing Project, 176b, 177
Children
  accidents. (See Childhood accidents)
  development

as adaptation, 215
and appropriate expectations, 296
early intervention and, 147
physical environment, 216
resources, 217
stimulation, 220
emotional mental health, 280
  domestic violence and abuse on, 289
  parental mental health difficulties on, 288
  risk factors, 287
  substance abuse or misuse on, 290
illness/diseases. (See Childhood ailments)
safeguarding, 93
  building effective, 231
  Covid-19, 234
  dangerous dynamics, significance, 237, 240b
  dynamics between child, family and worker, 233
  influence of value base and culture on competency, 236
  Karpman drama triangle, 237, 238, 242
  mandatory child protection training, 232, 233
  and promoting welfare, 187f
  statutory guidance, 238
  supervision process, 244, 245
  Troubled Families guidance, 238
  unconscious competence, 241
school transition. (See School transition)
SLC in. (See Speech, language and communication (SLC))
SLCN. (See Speech, language and communication needs (SLCN))
trauma and adversity. (See Childhood adversity, trauma and)
Children and Young People (Scotland) Act 2014, 80, 81, 96
Choking, 325
Cholera, 8, 9
Climbié, Victoria, 83
Clinical decision-making, 112
Clinical supervision, 54, 55
Coalition government, 17, 72
Cochrane Reviews, 134, 266, 334
Cognitive behavioural therapy (CBT), 50, 266, 267
Cognitive Continuum Theory, 113
Cognitive development, children, 148
Colic, 332
Collaborative communication, 138
Collaborative conversations, 91
Collective leadership, 7, 8
Collectivism, 6
Colonisation, 103

Communicable disease, 5, 8
  mortality from, 7
Communications technology, 175
Communities of Practice, 14
Community development, 13
Community leadership, 201, 202f
Community Practitioner and Health
    Visitor Association (CPHVA), 27
Community working, 98
Compassionate leaders, 8
Complex trauma, 213
Conscious competence, 241
Constipation, 333
Containment, 294, 295
Contemporary health visiting practice, 196
Contemporary public health, 3
Continuing Professional Development
    (CPD), 3
Convention of Scottish Local Authorities
    (COSLA), 73
Convulsion, febrile, 333
Core communication skills, 242
Coronavirus-19 (COVID-19), 12, 13, 63,
    100, 179, 353
  assessment process. (See Assessment)
  changes in times of crisis, 18
  dynamic assessment challenges, 234
  impact on maternal/paternal mental
    health, 264
  inequality, 58
  paternalism, 6
  safeguarding skills. (See Safeguarding)
  Scotland, 72
  SLCN, 10
  technology. (See Technology)
  utilitarianism, 6
  virtual assessments and impact of,
    122, 124b
Corporate Plan 2017–2021, 74
Council for the Education and Training of
    Health Visitors in 1977, 96
Council for the Education of health
    visitors (CETHV), 25
COVID-19. See Coronavirus-19
    (COVID-19)
Cradle cap, 337
Crimea War, 24
Criticality, public health
  first wave, 9
  fourth wave, 12
  second wave, 10
  third wave, 11
Cross-cultural competence, 103
Crying baby, reasons for, 332
Cultural capital, 200
Cultural relativism, 240

D
Data Protection Act, 186
Decision-making
  clinical, 112
  health-related, 193
  shared, 136
Democratic leaders, 5
Department of Health (DH), 3, 27, 186,
    255
Department of Health and Social Care in
    England, 281
Depression, 256, 257
  antenatal period, 254, 260
  maternal, 255, 262
  paternal, 252, 255
    estimated healthcare costs, 263
    vs. father–infant interactions, 262, 263
    integrative review of, 257
    during postnatal period, 263
  perinatal period, 252, 253b, 254, 261
  post-adoption, 259
  postnatal period, 102, 255, 262, 263
  risk factors for, 255
Depression identification questions,
    114, 256
Determinants of health, 13, 14f
Developmental language disorder, 10
Developmental trauma, 213
Diarrhoea, 329, 339
Digitally enhanced health service, 176, 178
Digital Red Book pilot, 176b
Digital skills
  core level of, 181, 181t
  essential framework, 181, 182b
Disguised compliance, 239
District Paediatric Nurse, 23
Documentation, 183
Domestic violence, mental health, 289
Donabedian model, 140, 141b
Drowning, 325
Dual processing models, 195

E
Early intervention, 142
  and child development, 147
  human ecology theory, 146f, 146
  investment in early years, 144
  maternal mental health, 142b
Early Intervention Foundation (EIF), 179,
    291, 292
Early Years High Impact Areas, 324
Eating disorders, 253b
Ecological approaches, childhood adversity
    and trauma, 222
Ecological model

Bronfenbrenner's ecological model,
    186, 226
  of child development, 186
  of health, 7, 115
Ecological systems theory, 284
Ecological theory, Bronfenbrenner's, 146f,
    146, 147
Ecological transactional approach
    (ETA), 234
Eczema, 337
Edinburgh Postnatal Depression Scale
    (EPDS), 116, 117, 142b, 252, 256,
    258, 263
Education Act, 1907, 10
Educational training programmes, 90
Effective relationship, establishment of, 90
EIF. See Early Intervention Foundation
    (EIF)
Electronic record system, 327
Emotional development, 294
  attachment theory, 284, 285t
  children, 148, 280
    domestic violence and abuse on, 289
    parental mental health difficulties
      on, 288
    risk factors, 287
    substance abuse or misuse on, 290
  ecological systems theory, 284
Emotional well-being, 47
Emotion work, 50
Empathy, 90, 119, 240, 294
Employment, 47
Empowerment approach, 6, 195, 196
England
  health visiting services provision, 83
  proportionate universalism, 32f, 32
  public health, 74
Environmental perspectives, public health, 7
EPDS. See Edinburgh Postnatal Depression
    Scale (EPDS)
Epidemiology, 3
Epigenetics, 28
Epigenome, 36
Ethnocentrism, 240
'European Court of Human Rights' Guide
    on Article 8 of the European
    Convention on Human Rights, 96
European Early Promotion Project in 2000,
    115
Evaluation
  capacity-building activities, 204
  outcome, 202, 203
  process evaluation, 203
  types, 202
Evidence-based early intervention, 38
Evidence-based medicine, 133

Evidence-based practice, 131, 133, 136
  care assurance, 142
  contemporary history of, 133*b*
  detrimental impact, 139
  and policy, 75
  professional judgement, 136*b*
  quality and, 138
  quality improvement and, 138
  quality monitoring and review, 140
  shared decision-making, 136
Evidence-based video feedback technique, 292
Evidence, hierarchy of, 134
  limitations of, 135
  research and, 135
'Experience-dependent' brain, 282
'Exploring What Matters', 62
Expressive Language, 3

F
Fair Society, Healthy Lives (Marmot Review), 27, 31
Falls, 325
Family foundations programme (FFP), 291
Family health needs assessment, 115
Family Nurse Partnership (FNP) programme, 90, 94, 122, 145, 291
The Family Partnership Model, 90
Family Resilience Assessment Instrument (FRAI), 115
Family Resilience Assessment Instrument Tool (FRAIT), 34, 115
Family Resilience Assessment Tool (FRAT), 82, 115
FASD. See Foetal alcohol spectrum disorder (FASD)
Father–infant interactions, paternal depression *vs.*, 262, 263
Febrile convulsion, 333
'Felt need', 29, 98
Female genital mutilation (FGM), 237
Fever, 329, 333
'The first 1001 days,' brain development, 224
First 1000 days, child's development, 23, 28, 37, 38
Flying Start, 35, 36, 40, 82, 293
FNP programme. See Family Nurse Partnership (FNP) programme
Focus of intervention, 13
Foetal alcohol spectrum disorder (FASD), 281
Four 'I's of transformational leadership, 6, 7*b*
4-5-6 Model of Health Visiting Support, 17, 18*b*, 32*f*, 32, 33
FRAI. See Family Resilience Assessment Instrument (FRAI)

FRAIT. See Family Resilience Assessment Instrument Tool (FRAIT)
Framework for the Assessment of Children in Need and their Families, 115, 186, 187*f*, 234
Francis Report (Report of the Mid Staffordshire NHS Foundation Trust Public Inquiry), 141
FRAT. See Family Resilience Assessment Tool (FRAT)
Freedom of Information Act, 186

G
GAD-2. See Generalized Anxiety Disorder 2-item (GAD-2)
Gastro-oesophageal reflux disease, 334
General Data Protection Regulation (GDPR), 186
Generalized Anxiety Disorder 2-item (GAD-2), 116, 117, 142*b*, 256
General practitioners (GPs), 40, 99
Getting it right for every child (GIRFEC), 80, 81, 115, 132, 146, 149, 353
GIRFEC. See Getting it right for every child (GIRFEC)
GIRFEC National Practice Model, 234
Glue ear, 334
Greenleaf Organisation, 6
Green perspectives, 7
Group-based programmes, 291, 294
Growing up in Scotland (GUS), 8, 71

H
Harvard Center on the Developing Child, 224
Harvard University Center on the Developing Child, 36
HCHF Programme. See Healthy Child, Healthy Future (HCHF) Programme
HCP. See Healthy Child Programme (HCP)
Head lice, 336
Health and Care Women Leaders Network, 58
Health and Social Care Act, 17, 18
Health and Social Care Board (HSCB), 81
Health awareness, changes in, 204
Healthcare, 77, 78
Healthcare Leadership Model, 14, 16
Healthcare Quality Strategy for NHS Scotland, 142
Health consequences, public health, 7
  first wave, 8
  fourth wave, 11

second wave, 10
  third wave, 11
Health Education England (HEE), 3, 55, 56, 62
Health-enhancing activities
  conversations, 90
  facilitation of, 17, 326
'Health Field' concept, 13
Health for health Professionals Wales, 63
Health information literacy, 137
Health needs
  awareness, stimulation of, 12, 326
  family assessment, 115
  search for, 326
  speech, language and communication needs, 12
Health-promoting behaviour, facilitation of, 191
  building community capacity, 196, 197, 204
  capacity, 197
  challenges, 197
  community leadership, 201, 202*f*
  community level/empowerment approaches, 196
  cultural capital, 200
  developments, 192
  develop trusting, 198
  evaluation
    capacity-building activities, 204
    outcome, 202, 203
    process evaluation, 203
    types, 202
  frameworks to guide intervention design, 199
  health visitor interventions, impact of, 202
  human capital, 200
  individual approaches, 197
  influential behaviour change theories, 194*f*
  instrumental theories, 193
  intention-behaviour gap, 193, 194
  political capital, 200
  pre- and post-1950s, 192
  social capital, 201
  social isolation, 197
Health promotion, 3, 12
  Beattie's model, 13, 15*f*
  behaviour. (See Health-promoting behaviour, facilitation of)
Health-related decision-making, 193
Health visiting service
  changes in times of crisis, 18
  changes to delivery, 17
  childhood ailments, 329
  contemporary, 196

early intervention, 36
equality, diversity and inclusion in, 103
foundations, 1
global perspectives, 23
history, 23
integrated services, 40
leadership development for, 10
need for service, 28
principles of, 16, 64, 182b, 182
    facilitation of health-enhancing
        activities, 17
    influence on policies affecting health, 16
    search for health needs, 16
    simulation of an awareness of health
        needs, 16
proportionate universalism, 31
    in England, 32f, 32
    in Northern Ireland, 33, 34f
    in Scotland, 34, 35f
    in Wales, 34
provision organisation, 79
    in England, 83
    in Northern Ireland, 81
    in Scotland, 80
    in Wales, 81
vs. public health, 15
school transition and, 346
team, 57
technology and. (See Technology)
United Kingdom, 24, 26b, 26t, 30, 31t
Health visitor, 112b. See also Health visiting
    service
case study, 57
essential digital skills for, 181, 181t
establishing an effective relationship for
    practice, 90
identity, 12
leadership skills required by, 16, 16t
reflective practice, school transition, 347
speech, language and communication
    needs, 11
transition from student to, 48
Health Visitor (HV) Implementation Plan,
    17, 28, 196
Health visitor interventions
design, frameworks to guide, 199
evaluation
    capacity-building activities, 204
    outcome, 202, 203
    process evaluation, 203
    types, 202
impact of, 202
Health Visitor Observation and
    Assessment of Infant Tool, 114
Healthy Child, Healthy Future (HCHF)
    Programme, 132, 353

Healthy Child Programme (HCP), 2, 4, 17,
    30, 32f, 115, 118, 120, 121, 326
agenda-matching assessment tools, 121
in England, 83, 255
health-promoting behaviour, facilitation
    of, 197
in Wales, 34, 81, 82, 115, 132, 255, 353
Heat rash, 338
Heckman Curve, 144, 145f
Hierarchy of evidence, 134
    limitations, 135
    research and, 135
Higher education institutions (HEIs), 27
High impact areas (HIAs), 324b
Holistic approaches, trauma and adversity,
    222
Home learning environments, 14
Home safety education, 326
Home-visiting programmes, 291
    targeted, 145
    and therapeutic relationships, 87, 95b
        authenticity, 92
        community working, 98
        developing trust, 94
        inclusive practice, 101
        safeguarding, 93
        trauma-informed practice, 101
        universal services, 95
Human capital, 200
Human ecology theory, 146f, 146
Human ethology, 287
Hypothalamic pituitary adrenal (HPA)
    axis, 260
Hypothetic-Deductive Model, 113

I

Identity, leadership, 12
iHV Vision for Health Visiting (iHV), 8
Impaired cognitive development, 262
Impetigo, 338
Inclusive practice, therapeutic
    relationships, 101
Industrial revolution, 8
Inequality, 58
Infacol (simethicone), 332
Infantile colic, 332
Infant mental health (IMH), 280
    domestic violence and abuse on, 289
    parental mental health difficulties
        on, 288
    risk factors, 287
    substance abuse or misuse on, 290
Infants
    attachment, 262
    brain development, 280, 283b, 283, 297

parent–infant interaction, 283
    'serve and return interactions', 283
father–infant interactions, paternal
    depression vs., 262, 263
massage, 293
parent–infant interaction, 283, 294, 296
reasons for crying, 332
Infections, childhood ailments, 334
    otitis media, 334
    sore throat, 334
    upper respiratory tract infections, 335
Infectious diseases, 192, 335
    chicken pox, 335
    measles, 335
    scarlet fever, 335
Information technology, 174, 177
Institute of Health Visiting (iHV), 3, 10,
    27, 39, 56, 57, 83, 120, 123
Institute of Health Visiting's Vision for the
    Future, 55
Instrumental theories, 193
Integrated services, health visiting, 40
Intention-behaviour gap, 193, 194
Inter-cultural competency (IC), 236, 237
Intermate partner violence (IPV), 289
Interpersonal therapy (IPT), 266, 267
Interpretation, of public health, 4, 5b
Intuition, 112, 233, 238
Investment, 47

J

Jameson Report, 25
Joint attention, 3
'Just and Learning Culture', 53

K

Karpman drama triangle, 237, 238, 242
Key performance indicators (KPIs), 65, 94,
    141, 175
Kings Fund, 2, 7
'Knowledge of use', 112

L

Lack of stimulation, SLCN, 7
Ladies Sanitary Reform Association, 24
Laissez-faire leaders, 5
Lalonde Report, 13
Language development pyramid, 3f, 3
Late talkers, children, 9
Laxatives, 333
Leadership, 4
    behaviour, 11, 13
    case study, 9b

Leadership (*Continued*)
    collective, 7, 8
    community, 201, 202*f*
    context of, 11, 12
    developing capability, 14
    historical development of, 5
    identity, 12
    purpose of, 11, 13
    role model, 15
    skills required by health visitors, 16, 16*t*
    transactional, 6
    transformational, 6, 7*b*, 7, 11
Leadership development model, 5, 10*f*, 10
Learning, public health
    first wave, 9
    fourth wave, 12
    second wave, 10
    third wave, 11
Liberal-individualistic perspectives, 6
Light therapy, 268
Local authorities, 11, 12, 17, 18
Local Government or Health Boards, 175

**M**

Making Every Contact Count (MECC), 13,
    14, 327
Manic depression. *See* Bipolar disorder
Massage, baby, 293
Matching agenda approaches, 121
Maternal Child Nurses, 23
Maternal Early Childhood Sustained
    Home-visiting (MESCH), 122
Maternal–fetal attachment (MFA),
    260, 261
Maternal mental health, 142
    antenatal, impact of, 259
    COVID-19 impact on, 264
    early intervention and, 142*b*
    postnatal, impact of, 261
Maternal Mental Health Alliance, 50
Maternity and Child Welfare Act of 1918,
    25
Measles, 335
MECC. *See* Making Every Contact Count
    (MECC)
Media-based methods, 292
Mellow Parenting, 295
Member of Parliament (MP), 38
Mentalisation, 240
Mentoring, 55
MI. *See* Motivational interviewing (MI)
Miliaria, 338
Millennium Cohort Study, 7, 12
Mindful listening, 50
Mindfulness-based interventions, 268

Mindfulness practice, 52
Mind-mindedness, 217
Ministry of Health, 10, 24, 25
Minor illnesses, 331
Mode of intervention, 13
Motivational interviewing (MI), 90, 91,
    198, 242
    assumptions, 243
    principles, 243
MUMSNET, 180
'My World Triangle', 115, 149, 186

**N**

Nappy rash, 338
'National Framework for Child Protection
    Education and Development in
    Scotland 2012', 232
National Government bodies, 175
National Health Service (NHS), 11, 17,
    25, 48
    black and minority ethnic communities,
        58, 59
    in England, 61, 63, 83
    financial situations of, 78
    in Scotland, 61
    staff survey, 50
    technology provisions in, 176*b*
    well-being and. (*See* Well-being)
National Institute for Health and Care
    Excellence (NICE), 37, 134, 142,
        256, 268
    antenatal/postnatal mental health,
        assessment, 116, 117
National Practice Model, 239
National Preceptorship Framework for
    Health Visiting, 55
National Risk Assessment Framework,
    239
National Scientific Council on the
    Developing Child, 287
National Service Framework for Children,
    30
NETMUMS, 180
Newborn Behavioural Observation
    (NBO), 292, 293*b*, 293, 294
New Labour government of 1997, 17
NHS. *See* National Health Service (NHS)
NHS Apps Library, 176*b*, 293
NHS Community Trust, 174
NHS Digital Library, 176*b*, 180
NHS Eatwell Guide, 204*b*
NHS Education for Scotland, 54
NHS Healthy Child Programme, 353
NHS Highland, 80
NHS Leadership Academy (NHSLA), 3

NHS Leadership Academy's Systems
    Leadership Development
    Framework, 9
NHS Leadership Competency Framework,
    3
NHS Leadership Framework, 4
NHS Long-Term Plan, 4, 75, 124*b*
NHS People Plan 20/21, 59
NHS SPINE, 177
NHS Staff and Learners mental Well-being
    Commission, 62
Nightingale, Florence, 24, 133
NMC Code of Conduct, 3
NMC Code of Professional Standards,
    Practice and Behaviour, 182
Non-communicable disease, 29, 192
Northern Ireland
    health visiting services provision, 81
    proportionate universalism, health
        visiting, 33, 34*f*
    public health, 73
Northern Ireland Health and Social Care
    Public Health Agency, 63
Notification of Birth Acts of 1907 and
    1915, 25
Nuffield Bioethics Intervention Ladder, 14
Nurse Prescribers' Formulary for
    Community Practitioners, 329,
        333, 336
Nursing and Midwifery Council (NMC),
    55, 111, 134, 141, 175, 182, 331, 347
Nurturing caregiver, 295
Nymphs, 336
Nystatin oral suspension, 337

**O**

OARS (open questions, affirmations,
    reflections, summaries), 91, 198
Obsessive compulsive disorder (OCD),
    253*b*, 254
OCD. *See* Obsessive compulsive disorder
    (OCD)
Open ended questions, affirmation,
    reflection and summaries (OARS),
    91, 198
Oral thrush, 336
Organisation for Economic Co-operation
    and Development (OECD), 141
Organisations, well-being, 60
Otitis media, 334
Ottawa Charter, 13
'Our Strategic Plan 2019–2022', 74
Over-the-counter medication, 330
    gastro-oesophageal reflux disease, 334
    teething, 339

## P

Parental contingent responsiveness, 283
Parental mental health
  difficulties of, 288
  representations of, 286
Parent child interaction (PCI) therapy,
  12, 16
Parent club, 176*b*
Parent–infant interaction
  development, 294, 296
  infant brain development, 283
Parenting – give it time, 176*b*
Parenting Northern Ireland (NI), 176*b*
Paternal depression, 252, 255
  estimated healthcare costs, 263
  *vs.* father–infant interactions, 262, 263
  integrative review of, 257
  during postnatal period, 263
Paternalism, 6, 193
Paternal mental health
  anxiety. (*See* Anxiety)
  COVID-19 impact on, 264
  depression. (*See* Depression)
  and well-being, 102
Patient Health Questionnaire 9 (PHQ9),
  116, 142*b*, 256
Patient-practitioner relationship, 193
Perinatal mental health (PMH), 251
  disorders, 252, 253*b*
    depression, 116
    financial implication of, 263
    identification, 255
    impact of, 262
    risk factors, 255
  interventions to support women and
    their families, 265
Personal protective equipment (PPE), 235
Person-centred approach, 34, 134, 136,
  267, 347
'PHE Strategy 2020–2025', 74
Physical development, children, 147
Physical environment, 216
'Plan, Do, Study, Act' (PDSA) cycle, 139, 140*f*
Play and interaction experiences, 3
Plunket nurse, 23
PMH. *See* Perinatal mental health (PMH)
Poisoning admissions, 325
Political capital, 200
Post-adoption depression, 259
Post-industrial society, implications, 11
Post-modern society, implications, 12
Postnatal depression, 102, 255, 262, 263
Postnatal psychosis, 253*b*
Postpartum psychosis, 254
Post-traumatic stress disorder (PTSD),
  253*b*, 254, 264

Poverty, 77, 217
Practitioner well-being, 45
PRAMS mnemonic, 216, 221, 223, 223*t*
Preceptorship, 49, 55
Pregnancy, 115
  alcohol use during, 281
  chickenpox, 335
  depression during, 252
  generalised anxiety disorder, 254
  Healthy Child, Healthy Futures
    programme, 81
  hormonal changes, 259
  intermate partner violence, 289
  maternal–fetal attachment, 260
  parental representations and, 286
  perinatal mental health, 251, 263
  physical and mental health outcomes, 290
  and postnatal period, 256
  selective serotonin reuptake
    inhibitors, 265
  stress and depression in, 289
Prematurity, 289
Prescribing pyramid, 329, 330*f*
Prickly heat, 338
Primary SLCN, 7
Proctor's model, 55
Professional judgement, 136*b*
Professional mission, 47
Professional practice, 45
Professional resilience, domains of, 60*f*
Proportionate universalism, 31, 40, 95
  in England, 32*f*, 32
  in Northern Ireland, 33, 34*f*
  in Scotland, 34, 35*f*
  in Wales, 34
Psychological trauma, 212
Psychosis, 253*b*
  postpartum, 254
PTSD. *See* Post-traumatic stress disorder
  (PTSD)
Public health
  changes in times of crisis, 18
  contemporary, 3
  definitions, 4
  5th wave in, 196
  foundations, 1
  health visiting *vs.*, 15
  history, 7
  interpretation, 4, 5*b*
  overview, 3
  priorities, 38
  promotion, 12
  'regimes' of, 8
  underpinning philosophies and
    perspectives, 6
    collectivism, 6

    environmental and green perspectives, 7
    liberal-individualistic perspectives, 6
    paternalism, 6
    socialism, 6
    utilitarianism, 6
  United Kingdom, 72
    England, 74
    Northern Ireland, 73
    Scotland, 72
    Wales, 74
  waves of, 8
    Beveridge's 'five giant evils'
      implications, 10
    industrial revolution implications, 8
    post-industrial society implications, 11
    post-modern society implications, 12
    war implications, 9
Public health agency (PHA), 74
Public Health England (PHE), 2, 74, 196
  preventing injuries, 325
  speech, language and communication
    needs, 12
Public health leaders, 8
  first wave, 9
  fourth wave, 11
  second wave, 10
  third wave, 11
Public Health Skills and Knowledge
  framework, 17
Puerperal psychosis, 253*b*

## Q

Quality, 138
  improvement, 138
  monitoring and review, 140

## R

Ready, steady, baby, 176*b*
Ready, steady, toddler, 176*b*
Receptive language, 3
Reciprocity, 90, 294
  leadership development and, 15
Record-keeping, 183, 185, 331
Records Management: NHS Code of
  Practice, 186
Reflection, 331
  for difficult conversations, 242
  school transition, 347
Reflective functioning, 217, 218
Reflective practice, 225
Reflective supervision, 245
Refuge, 235
Relationship-based therapeutic
  programmes, 291

Report of the Mid Staffordshire NHS Foundation Trust Public Inquiry (Francis Report), 141
Research-based evidence, 103
Resilience, 62, 215
  professional, domains of, 60*f*
  school transition, 348, 352*t*
    advance preparation for, 349
    issues related to trauma and adversity, 351
    particular concerns, 350
    school readiness, 348
    supporting parents' anticipatory concerns, 350
Resilience Framework, 115
Resilience Matrix, 115, 239
Resources, trauma and adversity, 217
Restorative practice approach, 53
Restorative supervision, 54, 55
Right from the Start (RFTS), 291
'Righting reflex', 91
Risk, 148
  assessment, 149
  management, 149
  toxic risk combinations, 239
Rogers' theory, 29
Royal College of Paediatrics and Child Health (RCPCH), 141
Royal College of Speech and Language Therapists (RCSLT), 8, 9*f*, 18
Royal Society for Public Health, 24
The rule of optimism, 239

**S**

Safeguarding, children, 93
  building effective, 231
  Covid-19, 234
  dangerous dynamics, significance, 237, 240*b*
  dynamics between child, family and worker, 233
  influence of value base and culture on competency, 236
  Karpman drama triangle, 237, 238, 242
  mandatory child protection training, 232, 233
  statutory guidance, 238
  supervision process, 244, 245
  Troubled Families guidance, 238
  unconscious competence, 241
Salutogenesis, 28, 29, 46, 90, 132
Scarlet fever, 335
School Nursing Services, 353
School readiness, 348
School transition, 343
  around UK, 352
  development and resilience, 348, 352*t*

  advance preparation for, 349
  issues related to trauma and adversity, 351
  particular concerns, 350
  school readiness, 348
  supporting parents' anticipatory concerns, 350
  and health visiting practice, 346
  opportunities and challenges
    for children, 344
    for parents and carers, 345
  reflective practice, 347
Scotland
  health visiting services provision, 80
  proportionate universalism, health visiting, 34, 35*f*
  public health, 72
Scottish Government (SG), 63, 71, 72, 235
  speech, language and communication needs, 14
Scottish Intercollegiate Guidelines Network (SIGN), 134
SCPHNs. *See* Specialist Community Public Health Nurses (SCPHNs)
Screening
  for adversity and trauma, 221
  speech, language and communication needs, 10, 11
  tools, 258
    Ages and Stages Questionnaire, 10, 114
    assessment and, 114, 115
    depression, 117
    EPDS, 116, 117, 142*b*, 252, 256, 258, 263
    GAD-2, 116, 117, 142*b*, 256
Secondary SLCN, 7
Secondary stress, 225
Selective serotonin reuptake inhibitors (SSRIs), 265
Self-awareness, 12
Self-care, 225, 295
Self-compassion, 49, 58, 269
Self-control, 195
Self-limiting, 327, 328, 332, 337
Self-regulation, 195
Sensitive care, 218
Serious Case Reviews, 233, 240
'Serve and return interactions,' child development, 283
*7 Habits of Highly Effective People* (Covey), 6
Shared decision-making, 136
Significant Case Reviews (SCRs), 233
Signs of Safety, 90
Simethicone (Infacol), 332
Simple trauma, 213
Six Cs of nursing, 222
Skin conditions, childhood ailments, 337
  bites and stings, 337

  cradle cap, 337
  eczema, 337
  impetigo, 338
  nappy rash, 338
  prickly heat, 338
SLAC record, 188
SLC. *See* Speech, language and communication (SLC)
SLCN. *See* Speech, language and communication needs (SLCN)
SLIC record, 187, 188
Social Baby DVD, 292
Social capital, 201
Social defence systems, 61
Social determinants of health, 31
Social development, 148, 294
Socialism, 6
Social isolation, 197
Social justice, 6, 7
Social learning theory, 15, 16
Social policy, 75
Social workers, 25
Societal context, public health
  first wave, 8
  fourth wave, 11
  second wave, 9
  third wave, 10
Socio-economic status, 47
Solihull approach, 143, 294, 295
Sophisticated dance, 90
Sore throat, 334
Specialist Community Public Health Nurses (SCPHNs), 3, 14, 17, 24, 27, 56, 102, 103, 182, 353
Specific, Measurable, Achievable, Realistic, Timely (SMART) approach, 139
Speech, 4
Speech, language and communication (SLC), 2
  parent-child interaction, 12, 16
  skill development, 3, 4*t*
    zero to one year, 5
    one to two years, 5
    two to three years, 6
    three to five years, 6
  support parents/carers, 16
  working in partnership, 18
Speech, language and communication needs (SLCN)
  Ages and Stages Questionnaires, 10, 11
  challenge for parents with, 14
  health visitor, role of, 11
  home learning environments, 14
  identification of, 9
  intergenerational cycle, 8, 9*f*, 14
  policies affecting health, 12
  risk factors, 7, 8*b*, 9*f*

screening methods, variety of, 10, 11
social disadvantage, 8
subgroups of, 7
Sticky eyes, 339
'Still face paradigm', 284
Stimulation
    awareness of health needs, 12, 326
    lack of, SLCN, 7
    trauma and adversity, 220
Strange Situation, 217, 285
Strangulation, 325
Strength-based approach, 90, 351
    assessment, 121
Strengthening Families approach, 239
Strengths-based models of working, 50
Stress
    categories of, 288t
    moderate and resolved, 219
    in pregnancy, 289
    secondary, 225
Stress hormone, 219
Stress inoculation, 219
Substance abuse, mental health, 290
Succinct information, 187b, 188
Suffocation, 325
Summarising information, 187b
Supervision, 49, 54
    appropriate, 295
    safeguarding, 244, 245
Sustainable Development Goals (SDGs), 13
Systems leader, 8
SystmOne, 176b


T

Targeted home visiting, 145
'Tea and Empathy group', 57
Technology, 173
    communications, 175
    digitally enhanced health service,
        characteristics of, 176
    to facilitate virtual consultations, 179t
    good usage of, 174b, 185b
    implications, 178
    information, 174, 177
    policy context for, 175
    poor usage of, 174b, 184b
    record-keeping, 183, 185
    workforce strategy, 180
Teething, signs of, 339
The Children (Northern Ireland) Order
        1995, 81
Therapeutic relationships, home visiting
        and, 87, 95b
    authenticity, 92
    community working, 98
    developing trust, 94

inclusive practice, 101
    safeguarding, 93
    trauma-informed practice, 101
    universal services, 95
Threadworm, 336
'Thriving at work', 63
Time constraints, 114
Towards Commissioning for Compassion, 61
Trait theories, leadership, 5
Transactional leadership, 6
Transformational leadership, 6, 7b, 7, 11
Transition to school. (See School transition)
Trauma
    and adversity. (See Childhood adversity,
        trauma and)
    complex, 213
    developmental, 213
    psychological, 212
    secondary, 225
    simple, 213
Trauma-informed practice, 101
Traumatic memories, 212, 213
'Triad of interconnected core practice', 34
Trust, development, 94
Tuberculosis, 192


U

UK Assessment Framework, 149
UK Confidential Enquiry into Maternal
        Deaths (CEMD), 265
UK Governments, technology, 175, 176
Unconditional positive regard, 92
Unconscious competence, 241
UNCRC. See United Nations Convention on
        the Rights of the Child (UNCRC)
Understanding the Needs of Children in
        Northern Ireland (UNOCINI), 234
Unintentional injuries, 324, 325b, 325
United Kingdom (UK)
    early years policy and practice in, 132
    health visiting, 24, 26b, 26t, 30, 31t
    national approach to public health, 72
        in England, 74
        in Northern Ireland, 73
        in Scotland, 72
        in Wales, 74
    school transition, 352
United Nations Convention on the Rights
        of the Child (UNCRC), 144
Universal Child Health Promotion
        Programme in Northern Ireland, 255
Universal Health Visiting Pathway,
        Scotland, 34, 80, 255, 353
Universal home visiting services, 95
Upper respiratory tract infections (URTI),
        335

URTI. See Upper respiratory tract
        infections (URTI)
Utilitarianism, 6


V

Vicarious trauma, 51, 225
Virtual assessment, COVID-19 pandemics,
        122, 124b
'Vision for Health Visiting', 65
Vomiting, 329, 339


W

Wales
    health visiting services provision, 81
    proportionate universalism, health
        visiting, 34
    public health, 74
War implications, waves of public health, 9
Well-being, 4, 45, 46, 131, 323
    domestic violence and abuse on, 289
    parental mental health difficulties on, 288
    paternal mental health and, 102
    practitioner, 45
    risk factors, 287
    substance abuse or misuse on, 290
    and work, 46
        benefits, 47
        dealing with reality, challenges, 64, 66b
        organisation, 60
        supporting individuals, 53, 54t
Welsh health visiting service, 35
Whooley questions, 114, 116, 117, 256
'Window of opportunity', 3, 13
Workforce strategy, 180
Worklessness, 47
Workplace compassion, 64b
Works
    with parents and carers, 224
    well-being and, 46
        benefits, 47
        dealing with reality, challenges, 64, 66b
        organisation, 60
        supporting individuals, 53, 54t
    with whole family service, 120
World Health Organisation (WHO), 13,
        26, 138, 140, 141
    health, 4
    health promotion, 13, 204
    well-being, 46
WWHAM mnemonic, 330


Y

Younghusband Report, 25